Fixed Prosthodontics

Fixed Prosthodontics

KEITH E. THAYER, D.D.S., M.S.

Professor, Fixed Prosthodontics
University of Iowa College of Dentistry
Iowa City, Iowa

YEAR BOOK MEDICAL PUBLISHERS, INC.
CHICAGO

Library of Congress Cataloging in Publication Data

Thayer, Keith E.
Fixed prosthodontics.

Includes index.
1. Crowns (Dentistry) 2. Bridges (Dentistry)
I. Title. [DNLM: 1. Denture, Partial, Fixed.
2. Crowns. WU 515 F566]
RK666.T48 1984 617.6′92 83-14591
ISBN 0-8151-8782-3

Sponsoring editor: Diana L. McAninch
Editing supervisor: Frances M. Perveiler
Production project manager: Dorothy J. Mulligan
Proofroom supervisor: Shirley E. Taylor

Contributors

Robert J. Connor, D.D.S., M.S.
Associate Professor
Department of Fixed Prosthodontics
School of Dentistry
West Virginia University
Morgantown, West Virginia

Asterios Doukoudakis, D.D.S., M.S., F.I.C.D.
Associate Professor
Department of Fixed Prosthodontics
School of Dentistry
Case Western Reserve University
Cleveland, Ohio

Walter W. Fingar, D.D.S., M.S.
Professor of Operative Dentistry
Assistant Dean for Admissions and Student Affairs
College of Dental Medicine
Medical University of South Carolina
Charleston, South Carolina

Albert T. Goldberg, D.D.S., M.S.
Professor
Department of Fixed Prosthodontics
School of Dentistry
Louisiana State University
New Orleans, Louisiana

Daniel L. Hall, D.D.S., M.S.
Associate Professor
Head, Department of Family Dentistry
College of Dentistry
University of Iowa
Iowa City, Iowa

Hani H. Hermes, D.D.S., M.S.
Detroit, Michigan

Peter M. Jackin, D.D.S., M.S., M.A.
Professor and Head
Section, Fixed Prosthesis
University of Manitoba
Winnepeg, Manitoba
Canada

Satish C. Khera, D.D.S., M.S.
Associate Professor
Department of Operative Dentistry
College of Dentistry
University of Iowa
Iowa City, Iowa

Arthur N. Kracht, D.D.S., M.S.
Assistant Professor
Department of Fixed Prosthodontics
College of Dentistry—Retired
University of Iowa
Colonel D.C.U.S.A.—Retired
Iowa City, Iowa

Kavita Nakra, D.D.S., M.S.
Assistant Professor
Department of Fixed Prosthodontics
School of Dentistry
Loyola University
Maywood, Illinois

Arun Nayyar, D.M.D., M.S.
Associate Professor and Director
Fixed Prosthodontics
Department of Restorative Dentistry
School of Dentistry
Medical College of Georgia
Augusta, Georgia

Miguel A. Pastrana, D.M.D., M.S.
Professor
Department of Prosthodontics
School of Dentistry
University of Puerto Rico
San Juan, Puerto Rico

Ronald J. Peterson, D.D.S., M.S.
Phoenix, Arizona

Iraj Shafagh, D.D.S., M.S.
Associate Professor
Department of Fixed Prosthodontics
College of Dentistry
University of Florida
Gainesville, Florida

Robert S. Staffanou, D.D.S., M.S., F.A.C.P., F.A.C.D.
Professor and Chairman
Department of Fixed Prosthodontics
Baylor College of Dentistry
Dallas, Texas

Keith E. Thayer, D.D.S., M.S., F.I.C.D., F.A.C.D.
Professor
Department of Fixed Prosthodontics
College of Dentistry
University of Iowa
Iowa City, Iowa

Vincent D. Williams, D.D.S., M.S.
Assistant Professor
Department of Family Dentistry
College of Dentistry
University of Iowa
Iowa City, Iowa

Contents

Preface xi
Acknowledgment xiii

1. History of Fixed Prosthodontics *By Keith E. Thayer, D.D.S.* **1**
Early Dentistry 1
Nineteenth Century Crown and Bridge 1
Twentieth Century Fixed Prosthodontics 3

2. Anatomical Structures *By Walter W. Fingar, D.D.S* **5**
The Hard Tissues 6
The Soft Tissues 9
The Supporting Tissues 9

3. Diagnosis and Treatment Planning *By Keith E. Thayer, D.D.S.* **12**
Review 19

4. Crown Foundations *By Hani H. Hermes, D.D.S.* **21**
Indications for Crown Foundations 21
Tooth Restoration 21
Tooth Preparation 22
Pin Selection 24
Pin Channel Preparation and Threaded Pin Insertion 25
Cemented Pins 26
Pulp Protection 26
The Matrix 27
Restorative Materials 27
Filling of the Cavity 28

5. Preparations *By Keith E. Thayer, D.D.S.* **31**
Retention and Resistance Form 31
Gingival Margins 32
Principles of Tooth Reduction 36
Restoration Design Modifications 48

6. Porcelain Fused to Metal Restorations
By Robert J. Connor, D.D.S. **53**
Restoration Considerations 53
Framework Design 55
The Metal Framework 59

The Porcelain Application 64
Reasons for Failures 67

7. Pin Retained Restorations *By Peter M. Jackin, D.D.S.* **70**
Use of Pins 72
Lingual Pin Veneer 72
Pinledges and Pinlays 77
Indications, Contraindications, and Uses 78
Problem Solving with Pins 80

8. Gingival Retraction and Tissue Management
By Keith E. Thayer, D.D.S. **83**
Gingival Retraction Modes 84
Clinical Techniques 86

9. Impression Materials and Techniques *By Satish C. Khera, D.D.S.* **91**
Prerequisites for Good Impressions 91
Impression Materials for Fixed Prosthodontics 93
Manipulation of Impression Materials 99
Dispensing and Mixing the Impression Materials 103

10. The Provisional Restoration *By Daniel L. Hall, D.D.S.* **116**
Requirements for the Provisional Restoration 116
Types of Provisional Restorations 117
Provisional Fixed Partial Denture for Multiple Adjacent Units 124
Cementation of the Provisional Restoration 131
Removal of the Intermediate Restoration 132
Summary 132

11. Interocclusal Records and Cast Articulation
By Asterios Doukoudakis, D.D.S. **134**
Rigid Materials 135
Waxes 136
Silicone Putty Materials 137
Registration Pastes 138
Recording Devices 139
Recording Techniques 139
Interocclusal Record Material Selection 140
Centric Relation Records 141
Centric Occlusion Records 143

12. Face-bow Transfer and Hinge Axis Location
By Robert S. Staffanou, D.D.S. **146**
Conclusion 159

13. Pantography *By Robert S. Staffanou, D.D.S.* **164**
Technique 173

14. Articulators *By Robert S. Staffanou, D.D.S.* **178**
Summary 189

15. The Working Cast and Removable Dies
By Arun Nayyar, D.M.D. **190**
Criteria for a Working Cast With Removable Dies 190
Selection of Die Material 191
Removable Die Systems 195
Use of Die-Spacers and Hardening Films 206
Articulation of the Working Cast 210
Commercial Dowel Pin Placement Systems 211
Removable Dies From Preformed Tray Systems 212
Clinical and Laboratory Considerations 213
Summary 216

16. Pontics and Pontic Form *By Keith E. Thayer, D.D.S.* **218**
Materials 218
Design 219
Ridge Modifications 226
Summary 226

17. Finishing and Fitting of Cast Restorations
By Iraj Shafagh, D.D.S. **228**
Laboratory Procedures 228
Patient Procedures 230
Finishing 233
Polishing 234
Polishing After Cementation 234
Armamentarium 234

18. Cementation in Fixed Prosthodontics *By Keith E. Thayer, D.D.S.* **236**
Temporary Cementation 236
Permanent Cementation Materials 237
Cementation Techniques 240
Restoration Fabrication Techniques 241
Cement Selection 241
Cementation Procedures 242

19. Acid-Etch Resin Bonded Cast Restorations
By Vincent D. Williams, D.D.S. **246**
Description of Technique 247
Periodontal Splints 250
Acid-Etch Application in Occlusal Treatment 250
Laboratory Procedures 252
Case Reports 255

20. Problems and Mechanics of Shade Selection
By Arthur. N. Kracht, D.D.S. ... **264**

21. Restoration of Endodontically Treated Teeth
By Miguel A. Pastrana, D.M.D. ... **276**
Diagnosis ... 276
Preplanning Endodontic Therapy ... 278
Construction of a Cast Post and Core ... 279

22. Orthodontic Considerations in Fixed Prosthodontics
By Kavita Nakra, D.D.S. ... **286**
Crossbites ... 287
Minor Tooth Movement ... 288
Management of Minor Tooth Movement ... 293
Pulpal Considerations ... 293
Alternatives to Uprighting Molars ... 294

23. Periodontal Considerations in Fixed Prosthodontics
By Robert J. Connor, D.D.S., and Ronald J. Peterson, D.D.S. ... **296**
Historical Background ... 296
Basic Principles for Root Resection ... 297
Endodontic Considerations ... 298
Restoring Partially Resected Multi-Rooted Teeth ... 300
Case Reports ... 300
Summary ... 311

24. Problems in Fixed Prosthodontics
By Albert T. Goldberg, D.D.S. ... **313**
Diagnosis and Treatment Planning ... 313
Patient Management and Mouth Hygiene ... 316
Preliminary Mouth Procedures ... 316
Tooth Preparation and Case Fabrication ... 319
Dentist-Laboratory Interaction ... 325
Summary ... 326

25. Fixed Prosthodontic Repairs *By Keith E. Thayer, D.D.S.* ... **327**
Causes of Failure ... 327
Summary ... 340

Index ... **343**

Preface

THIS BOOK is directed to both the dental student and the dental practitioner. The goal of the author and contributors is to present a wide range of information on the art and science of fixed prosthodontics. In addition to basic principles, multiple approaches to problems and techniques directed at solving them are recognized and presented.

Over the years there have been many advances in dentistry. Development and refinement of materials and procedures make the profession an ever expanding and dynamic challenge. No longer is it possible to say of an individual, as was said of Leonardo da Vinci, that he knows all there is to know in his world. It is also no longer possible for an individual to master all of the knowledge of even one specialty of one profession. It is the intention of the author and contributors to share the information they have mastered and the experiences they have encountered that may be useful to students and colleagues alike.

Dentistry cannot succeed without consideration of and attention to fundamentals. But fundamentals are not cast in concrete and dentists who have never broken Ante's law probably have not always served their patients to the fullest. Students and practitioners alike are limited only by their imaginations so long as their imaginations retain some reasonable restraint. Each new situation presents a challenge in problem solving.

Fixed prosthodontics is a demanding but rewarding specialty of dentistry. Sometimes, the greater the demands of a challenge, the greater the rewards of a solved problem and an objective achieved. "Trifles make perfection but perfection is no trifle," is a quotation attributed to Michelangelo. It is applicable to dentistry where attention to detail is always important whether it is in the performance of patient treatment or in the writing of a text.

Therefore, it is the hope of the author and contributors that this text will in some measure help the student and the practitioner approach the goal of perfection in fixed prosthodontics.

KEITH E. THAYER

Acknowledgments

THIS TEXT would not have been written without the Development Assignment Award supported by Dr. James H. McLeran, Dean of the College of Dentistry and approved by President Willard E. Boyd of the University of Iowa. Thanks are also extended to Dean Emeritus Loutfi M. Aboul-Ela and Dean M.S. El-Hadary of the Faculty of Dentistry, Alexandria University, who made my appointment as visiting professor at Alexandria University, Egypt, possible. It was during this time that the foundations for this text were laid.

The cooperation and efforts of the contributors of chapters have made possible a much more comprehensive presentation of material. All contributors hold Master of Science degrees from the University of Iowa, College of Dentistry granted during the 20 years from 1959 to 1979 that I was head of the department of fixed prosthodontics. The contributors are: Drs. Robert J. Connor, Asterios Doukoudakis, Walter W. Fingar, Albert T. Goldberg, Daniel L. Hall, Hani H. Hermes, Peter M. Jackin, Satish C. Khera, Arthur N. Kracht, Kavita Nakra, Arun Nayyar, Miguel A. Pastrana, Ronald J. Peterson, Iraj Shafagh, Robert S. Staffanou, and Vincent D. Williams. Their combined and varied experiences add an otherwise unattainable dimension to this work.

Thanks are extended to our four sons, James, Gregory, Scott, and Bradley, all of whom have expressed interest and offered encouragement in this project. They have all contributed indirectly to it through their efforts. The continuing long hours of attention and support by my wife, Nancy, in encouraging, proofreading and editing are gratefully acknowledged. Without her this work could not possibly have been completed.

KEITH E. THAYER

CHAPTER 1

History of Fixed Prosthodontics

KEITH E. THAYER, D.D.S.

THE FIRST ATTEMPT at fixed prosthodontic treatment may have been as early as 2600 B.C. Two molars bound together with a gold wire date to this period and are attributed to the work of the Egyptian Imhotep, who is known as the patron saint of medicine in Egypt, as Aesculapius was in Greece.[1] This is evidence that there may have been a specialty of dentistry in Egypt at that early date: fixed prosthodontics. But it is speculated that these molars were joined with the gold wire post mortem.[2] Regardless, this appears to be the oldest attempt at fixed prosthodontic treatment.[3]

EARLY DENTISTRY

Further concrete evidence of teeth being replaced with gold wire ligatures and bands dates from 400 to 600 B.C. in Syria. There is also evidence that the Syrians used gold wire ligatures for periodontal treatment. The technique spread to the Phoenicians who were such good navigators that they in turn spread their skills throughout their known world of the Etruscans, Romans, and Israelites until the time of Christ. There seems to be little or no further evidence or reference to replacing missing teeth until the late middle ages. By the late 1300s, cattle bone teeth were used as replacements in France, and by the 17th century ivory was being used.[4]

Our patron saint of dentistry, Saint Apollonia, was born in Alexandria, Egypt around 249 A.D. and was reportedly tortured by having her teeth broken and extracted.[1] During this same period of history there is extensive evidence of tooth mutilations in the Mayan culture. Teeth were serrated, grooved, and pointed by filing in Mexico and Central and South America for an esthetic effect. Metallic inlays were used on anterior teeth in this culture. The fact that some inlays were placed on lingual surfaces of anterior teeth raises the question of whether the inlays were done for decoration or esthetic effect alone.[1] The practice of tooth filing still exists today in some of the south sea islands.[5]

Early dentistry continued to flourish and progress primarily in western Europe and later in America until the 19th century. Among the leaders in the profession during this time were Pierre Fauchard and Claude Mouton in France, and John Greenwood in America.

Fauchard is credited with being a pioneer because he shared knowledge and experience through writing whereas others were still keeping their skills to themselves. Fauchard described the use of human teeth, which he preferred, for the fabrication of fixed replacements in detail.[6] He also used ivory and bone extensively and contributed the use of springs in denture construction.[7]

Claude Mouton published the first specialized book on prosthodontics. He described the fabrication of a gold crown as we know it today in detail. Perhaps he was inspired to develop his technique as a result of a child exhibited at a fair in Italy in 1593 with a golden molar. This has become known as the first gold crown, but at the time it was the center of debate and controversy for more than 100 years. The golden molar was attributed to such things as gold in the local water, the work of the devil, and the sins of the mother. Finally, it was disclosed that the gold crown had been fashioned and placed by a clever goldsmith.[6]

The first 100 years of dentistry in America, approximately 1620 to 1730 were termed the barber-surgeon era.[8] During the colonial period and through the beginning of the 19th century practitioners were known as "tooth drawers," "surgeon-dentists," and finally "dentists." The most famous records we have of this period are of George Washington's dentures. Dr. John Greenwood is attributed with having made two or three sets for Washington from 1789 onward. The dentures were probably carved from hippopotamus tusk. Washington's earlier dentures, when he still had one mandibular premolar remaining, were fabricated with wooden bases.[8]

NINETEENTH CENTURY CROWN AND BRIDGE

The 19th century began with the first dental implant in France (1807) when a molar with a gold root was implanted.[9] The Iron Duke's dentures were fabricated in England using natural teeth for the anterior replacements and ivory blocks for the posteriors. The maxillary and mandibular dentures were connected with the conventional spring of the time. The base of the maxillary denture was fashioned with gold whereas the mandibular denture base was of ivory.[10]

It was early in the 19th century that Fonzi (Italy) first used individual procelain teeth fused around metal pins, which in turn were soldered to a denture base. From this beginning, Ash and S. S. White monopolized the world market in porcelain teeth for the rest of the century. The Goodyear Dental Vulcanite Rubber Company was founded in the 1860s and pioneered the use of vulcanized rubber for denture bases. By the 1880s the Richmond crown was developed by incorporating the techniques of using a metal post in the root canal for retention, the flowing of solder for a backing, and the fusing of porcelain for a facing in single tooth anterior restorations. At the end of the century, appliances were being fabricated both in Germany and the United States that were recognizable as modern day fixed restorations.[11] Zinc phosphate cement, which remains a standard today, had been developed and was being widely used.

Dr. Chapin A. Harris published his monumental text, Principles and Practice of Dental Surgery, in Philadelphia in the 1840s. It was the first definitive text on all phases of dental surgery to be published and remained the standard for the profession here and abroad until the turn of the century.[7] It was Harris who first applied the principles of atmospheric pressure and capillary attraction to make possible the elimination of troublesome connecting springs between maxillary and mandibular dentures.

TWENTIETH CENTURY FIXED PROSTHODONTICS

The century began with major advances in dental gold castings. These castings were made using a variety of techniques. One technique used gravity and steam pressure that was developed from a wet asbestos pad pressed over a casting ring. A pattern had been invested in the ring and gold was melted in the investment crucible formed in the ring. This was a common and effective method. Later air pressure, centrifugal force, and vacuum pressure were employed individually and in combination to make castings.[12]

Dr. William Taggart presented his casting machine invention to the profession in 1907. He demonstrated the equipment and technique at a professional meeting in New York but wanted a royalty for every casting made using it. This eventually led to a court case that Taggart lost, in part, because of the fact that an obscure Iowa dentist by the name of B. F. Philbrook had presented essentially the same technique to his local dental society in 1896.

Methyl methacrylate was first used as a replacement for vulcanite as a denture base material in the 1930s. Soon thereafter it was used as a tooth-colored veneer in crowns and bridges. In the next 30 years numerous chemical and physical modifications of this method occurred. The composite resins, first introduced in the 1960s, are descendants of the original resins.[13]

From an historical perspective the 1950s were a truly revolutionary period for the development of fixed prosthodontics. Reversible hydrocolloid had been available and in use before this time, but it was not until the elastomeric impression materials were introduced that the indirect technique, so necessary to fixed prosthodontics, was really developed and became routine with the general practitioner. Starting with the polysulfide polymer rubbers and continuing with silicones, polyethers, and vinyl polysiloxanes, accurate impressions of prepared teeth are now within easy reach of every practicing dentist.

Along with the elastomeric impression materials and the refining of the indirect technique came a second major breakthrough in material and technique—the porcelain-fused-to-metal process. This made personalizing of esthetic tooth repair and replacement possible to a degree never before available.

To complement the two material developments of the decade a mechanical invention was applied to dentistry in the form of the air rotor handpiece. It was now practical, from both patient and dentist standpoints, to prepare teeth for fixed restorations by using the newly developed materials and techniques. Since then dentistry has progressed to the point where millions of units of fixed prosthodontics are produced annually by American dentists alone!

REFERENCES

1. Weinberger B.W.: *The History of Dentistry,* Vol. 1. St. Louis, C.V. Mosby Co., 1948.
2. Hoffmann-Axthelm W.: Is the practice of dentistry in ancient Egypt an archaeological fact? *Bull. Hist. Dent.* 27:71, 1979.
3. Harris J.E., Iskander Z., Farid S.: Restorative dentistry in ancient Egypt: An archaeological fact. *J. Mich. Dent. Assoc.* 57:401, 1975.
4. Hoffmann-Axthelm W.: The history of tooth replacement. *Quint. Int.* 70:81, 1970.
5. Horton M.: Tooth filing in Bali. *Cal.* April 1982, pp. 23–25.
6. Hoffmann-Axthelm W.: The history of tooth replacement. *Quint. Int.* 70:69, 1970.
7. Harris C.A.: Classics in dental history: Of the atmospheric pressure and capillary attraction method of applying artificial teeth. *Bull. Hist. Dent.* 24:106, 1976.

8. Weinberger B.W.: *The History of Dentistry*, Vol. 2. St. Louis, C.V. Mosby Co., 1948.
9. Bobbio A.: The first endosseous alloplastic implant in the history of man. *Bull. Hist. Dent.* 20:1, 1972.
10. Henry C.B.: The Iron Duke's dentures. *Br. Dent. J.* 125:354, 1968.
11. Hoffmann-Axthelm W.: The history of tooth replacement. *Quint. Int.* 70:77, 1970.
12. Hagman H.C.: The evolution of metal castings for dentistry. *Bull. Hist. Dent.* 24:98, 1976.
13. Peyton F.A.: History of resins in dentistry. *Dent. Clin. North Am.* 19:211, 1975.

CHAPTER 2

Anatomical Structures

WALTER W. FINGAR, D.D.S.

THE STUDY OF any part of the human body must leave us amazed at its complexity and efficiency and the study of the teeth and their supporting structures is no exception (Fig 2–1). Indeed, no investigator can be anything but amazed at the efficient design of these structures and their ability to withstand the functional stresses and external trauma that they are subjected to. We must realize, however,

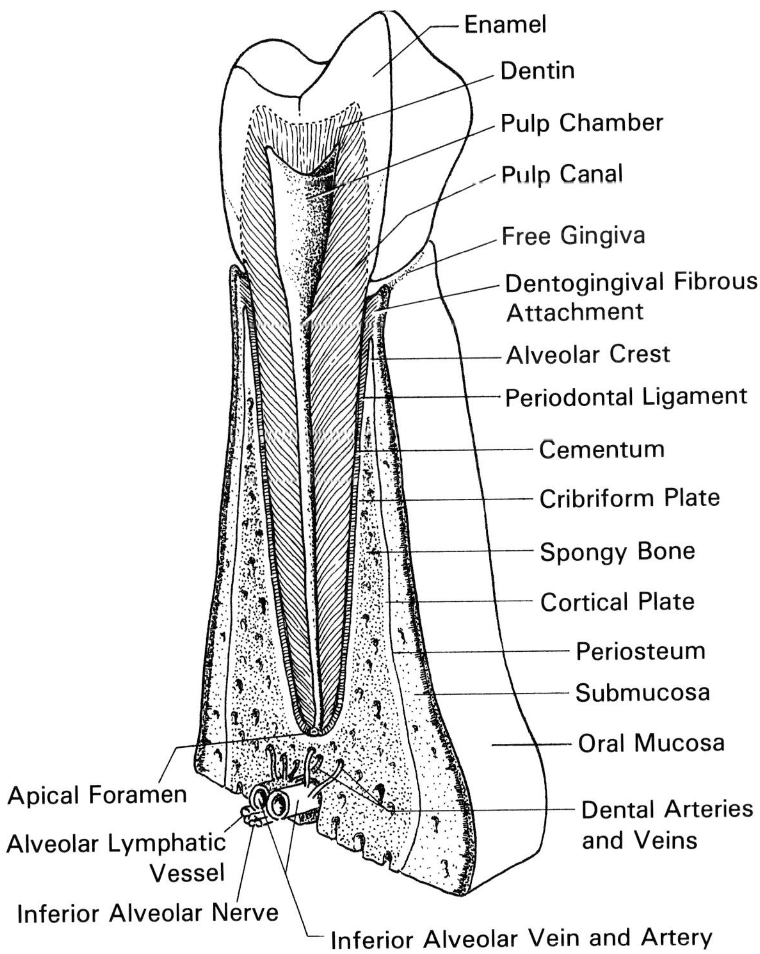

Fig 2–1.—Longitudinal cross section of a premolar.

that in spite of their near perfect design, the teeth and their supporting structures sometimes do succumb to the hazards and abuses of their environment. This is a sobering thought for any of us who would design replacements for these structures. The task is at times awesome and as we approach it two things are certain:

1. There will be failures no matter how capable and careful the operator is. We should be challenged, not discouraged, by these inevitable failures; and

2. Failures can be kept to a minimum only if there is a proper respect for the task at hand and if this respect is coupled with a thorough knowledge of the techniques and a dedication to extreme care in their employment.

Inherent in the proper use of the latest and best techniques is the need for a thorough knowledge of the nature of the structures involved. This chapter is intended to present the basic information necessary for such an understanding. It should be noted, however, that there is not enough space here for the presentation of all the information existing on this subject. This chapter can only be a start. Hopefully it will serve as a synopsis of the subject from which continuing, deeper study will evolve.

THE HARD TISSUES

The Enamel

THE DENTAL ENAMEL is the densest and hardest naturally occurring material in the body. In spite of this, it can be worn away and fractured in the mouth. This is a good indication of how severe the stresses on the teeth are and it should be reason enough to respect and give careful consideration to the forces that will be applied to any fixed restoration that is placed in the mouth. Materials that are placed in the mouth and that are expected to endure the stresses that enamel endures obviously must be hard and strong.

To better understand this remarkable material we should look at its composition. Enamel is 96% to 98% inorganic substance with 90% being hydroxyapatite, which is crystalline in nature. In addition, the enamel contains water, organic substances, minerals, and a wide variety of trace metals. Together these form this extremely hard and durable substance.

Structurally, the enamel is composed of millions of calcified rods or prisms that traverse the entire width of the enamel. Each rod is separated from its neighbor by a thin layer of organic material, the matrix. These rods are laid down by a specialized cell that is developed from the inner epithelium of the enamel organ, the ameloblast.

Whereas enamel must be hard so that it can function properly, it is prone to splitting and chipping. But it does have sufficient strength to withstand the normal pressures of mastication.

The enamel is semitranslucent and can sometimes assume the hues of the underlying dentin. It is subject to dissolution by acid solutions that are sometimes found in the mouth. The surface enamel is less susceptible than the inner enamel. The application of fluorides to the surface of the enamel further decrease the solubility of the surface.

The term "selectively permeable" is often applied to the enamel. We know that compared with other hard tissues of the body, the enamel is relatively impenetrable to outside solutions. However, it has been shown that dyes and certain radioactive substances do penetrate the enamel surface through flaws and cracks and perhaps by osmosis through the enamel substance itself.

In dealing with the enamel then, we should keep in mind that although the enamel substance is seemingly impenetrable, it is vulnerable by way of imperfections such as cracks and other flaws. Also, it is the "selectively permeable" nature of enamel that allows us to alter it with topical treatment substances such as fluoride.

The Dentin

Dentin constitutes the main portion of the tooth structure, and it runs almost the entire length of the tooth. It is covered by the enamel in the crown and by cementum in the root. The internal surface forms the walls of the pulp cavity. Dentin is not as hard as enamel but it is harder than bone or cementum.

To best understand the nature of dentin we must consider its formation. The odontoblast is the cell responsible for the formation of dentin and unlike the ameloblast, which loses its vitality once it has formed the enamel, the odontoblast retains its vitality after it has formed the initial bulk of the dentin (primary dentin) and lives on within the pulp cavity to form additional dentin.

Clinically, dentin is composed of approximately 75% inorganic matter, mainly calcium phosphate in the form of hydroxyapatite, and 25% organic matter, which is for the most part collagenous. The inorganic matter is laid down by the odontoblast in the form of tubules, each tubule being laid down by a single odontoblast. Contained within the lumen of each tubule are protoplasmic extensions called odontoblast processes. Because odontoblast processes exist in the dentin it is considered a living tissue that has the capacity to react to physiologic and pathologic stimuli. These stimuli may produce changes within the dentin such as the laying down of secondary dentin or sclerotic dentin.

Secondary Dentin

There are two types of secondary dentin: physiologic and reparative. Physiologic secondary dentin is easily seen histologically as a regular and somewhat uniform layer of dentin around the pulp cavity. It is believed to be formed without external stimulation by the odontoblasts after the bulk of the dentin (the primary dentin) is laid down. It can be distinguished from primary dentin only by the fact that the tubules in secondary dentin appear to take a different directional pattern than those in primary dentin. According to most investigators, this type of dentin has a slower rate of growth and accounts for the slowly decreasing size of the pulp cavity that occurs with age. The clinical significance of smaller pulp cavities in older persons and larger pulp cavities in younger persons is well known.

Reparative secondary dentin is formed in response to irritation. It appears as a localized deposit on the pulp cavity wall usually beneath an external source of irritation such as dental caries, erosion, or abrasion. This reparative layer of dentin serves to insulate the pulp from the irritation of external stimuli.

Sclerotic Dentin

Sclerotic dentin occurs within the primary dentin and is the result of a change in the structural composition of the early primary dentin. The tubules in sclerotic dentin are obliterated by the calcification of the tubular content. The resultant dentin is more highly mineralized than regular dentin and is therefore harder and less pervious to external irritants. As in the case of reparative secondary dentin, the appearance of sclerotic dentin is in response to external stimuli such as carious lesions, erosion, and abrasion. Consequently, it is assumed that this is also a defensive mechanism that affords the pulp a protection from external irritations.

The dynamic way in which the dentin gives protection to the pulp is remarkable and must be understood by the clinician as he or she is working against the processes that threaten the vitality of the pulp—caries, abrasion, and erosion. Moreover, the clinician introduces many irritations to the tooth in the form of high-speed cutting and chemical irritants. Therefore, there must be some understanding of the abilities of the tooth to adjust to the trauma that is inevitably inflicted.

The Cementum

The third hard tissue of the tooth is the cementum. This is the tissue that covers the root portion of the tooth. Cementum is the material of the tooth into which periodontal ligament fibers are incorporated, thereby providing an attachment of tooth to bone.

There are two types of cementum: acellular (primary) and cellular (secondary). Acellular cementum is found on the cervical portion of the root and contains no cells. This cementum contains a large number of fibers from the periodontal ligament (Sharpey's fibers) and plays an important part in the attachment of the tooth to bone. Cellular cementum covers the apical portion of the root and, as its name implies, contains cementocytes in individual spaces (lacunae) that communicate through a system of anastomosing cementum canaliculi. This type of cementum bears a close resemblance to bone. Cementocytes form both cellular and acellular cementum by apposition of layers (lamellae) one over the other.

Formation of cementum, like the formation of dentin, is a continuous process that lasts throughout life. It is a part of the process of continuous tooth eruption. The teeth erupt in an effort to keep pace with occlusal and incisal wear on the tooth structure. As the tooth erupts, there is less root length left in the socket. This shortening is compensated for by the laying down of cementum on the root and by the formation of bone at the crest of the alveolus. The net effect is that the tooth erupts to compensate for occlusal and incisal wear, but there is no loss of support because the root length is replaced in the alveolus by the laying down of new cementum on the root.

Cementum, in addition to showing continuous deposition, is subject to resorption that is brought on by trauma such as occlusal loading and orthodontic movement. The cervical area of the cementum is particularly susceptible to erosion and when this occurs troublesome problems are presented for the dentist who is attempting to restore the teeth.

Extreme thickening of the cementum (hypercementosis) is often seen in teeth and its cause varies. It can be caused by an excessive tension on the teeth that is caused by orthodontic appliances or by a total loss of function because of the loss of antagonist teeth. Hypercementosis is thought to be hereditary in some cases and may also occur with certain systemic diseases such as Paget's disease. Hypercementosis can often be seen in the area of periapical irritation arising from pulp disease and is thought to be a compensation for the loss of fibrous attachment resulting from the irritation.

In summary, it could be said that the deposition and resorption of cementum constitutes yet another of the body's mechanisms for adjusting to the extreme functional demands and sometimes traumatic forces to which the teeth are subjected.

THE SOFT TISSUES

The Dental Pulp

The dental pulp occupies the central portion (pulp cavity) of the tooth and is surrounded by dentin. Virtually all of the soft tissues of the tooth are housed within this cavity.

One of the primary functions of the pulp tissue is to maintain the odontoblastic layer and the odontoblast processes. The odontoblasts arise from the mesodermal tissue of the pulp. The blood and lymph of the pulp tissue provide nourishment for the cells that line the chamber walls (odontoblast layer). The blood is carried into the tooth by way of the dental arteries and there is usually one artery entering each foramen. Inside the pulp cavity the blood vessels branch into many arterioles and supply the abundant capillary beds, which are in turn drained by two or three veins. The overall vascular bed is enriched by a profuse lymphatic network that closely parallels the capillaries and services the same structures.

The pulp contains nerve fibers, many of which go directly to the odontoblast layer. Others have endings in the lining of the vessels and control the distribution of blood. Nerve fibers have been discovered passing from the pulp tissue into the odontoblastic processes, but the exact mechanism involved in the innervation of the dentin is a controversial subject.

Many different types of cells that serve many different purposes are found in the pulp. Reticuloendothelial cells, wandering cells, and fibroblasts can all be found in the pulp. This demonstrates the many complex functions going on within this tissue that is a support for all the functions within the other tooth tissues.

The integrity of the pulp is of vital importance to the proper function of the tooth. Indeed, we have already shown how many of the compensating mechanisms of other tooth tissues serve to protect the dental pulp and to maintain its integrity. Obviously, the dentist must always be conscious of the condition of the pulp in any tooth on which he or she operates. Indeed, the procedures must be gauged so as not to compromise the vitality of this important tooth structure.

THE SUPPORTING TISSUES

The Gingiva

The gingiva is that part of the oral mucous membrane that covers the alveolar processes of the jaws and surrounds the necks of the teeth. It is divided into the marginal, attached, and interdental areas.

The marginal gingiva surrounds the teeth in a collar-like fashion and is demarcated from the adjacent attached gingiva by a shallow linear depression, the free gingival groove. The attached gingiva is continuous with the marginal gingiva. It is firm, resilient, and lightly bound to the underlying cementum and alveolar bone. The interdental gingiva is that portion of the gingiva that occupies the space between the teeth apically from the contact area.

The gingiva covers the underlying tissues that serve to invest and attach the teeth to the jaws.

The Periodontal Ligament

The periodontal ligament is that structure that surrounds the root of the tooth and connects it with the bone. It is composed of connective tissue and is continuous with the connective tissue of the gingiva. This ligament has a fibrous connection with the marrow spaces of bone through the vascular channels of the bone.

The most important feature of the periodontal ligament is the way in which its principal fibers are arranged in groups at different angles to form a "hammock-like" suspension for the tooth. This suspension serves to absorb the impact of forces exerted on the tooth and also to attach the tooth securely to the supporting bony structures. There are five groups of principal fibers: the transseptal group, the alveolar crest group, the horizontal group, the oblique group, and the apical group.

The transseptal group of fibers extend interproximally over the alveolar crest and are embedded in the cementum of the adjacent teeth. These fibers can almost always be found clinically, even when periodontal disease has destroyed the alveolar bone.

The alveolar crest group of fibers extend obliquely from the cementum just beneath the epithelial attachment to the alveolar crest. These fibers serve to counterbalance the coronal thrust of the more apical fibers and to resist lateral tooth movement.

The horizontal group of fibers extend at right angles to the long axis of the tooth, from the cementum to the alveolar bone. They function in much the same way as the alveolar crest fibers.

The oblique group of fibers is the largest group in the periodontal ligament. They extend from the cementum of the tooth in a coronal direction to their attachment in the alveolar bone. These fibers bear the major share of the load exerted on the tooth by vertical masticatory stress.

The apical group of fibers radiate from the cementum of the tooth and attach to the base of the tooth socket.

In a remarkable way, the principal fiber groups of the periodontal ligament serve as "shock absorbers" for the tooth. They transfer the shock of occlusal forces to the bone and they attach the tooth firmly to the bone. Any alteration of these vital functions by way of destruction of the fibers and/or the bone drastically alters the capabilities of the teeth to survive and function. Periodontal disease causes both fibers and bone to be destroyed. Therefore, the periodontist and the fixed prosthodontist must work together continuously. The condition of the periodontal ligament is of extreme importance in the formation of any treatment plan and is never to be overlooked.

The Alveolar Process

The alveolar process is the bone that forms and supports the tooth sockets (alveoli). It consists of an inner socket wall that is called the alveolar bone proper (cribiform plate), the supporting alveolar bone, and the facial and lingual plates of compact bone.

The hard and rigid appearance of the alveolar bone makes it appear to be the most stable of the supporting structures. This is not true, however, as the alveolar bone is in a constant state of flux. There is a sensitive balance between bone formation and bone resorption that is regulated by local and systemic influences. Bone is resorbed in areas of pressure and formed in areas of tension.

The alveolar bone supports the teeth during mastication and its condition, must, therefore, be considered at all times. A knowledge of the ability of the alveolar bone to change in response to the various forces that are placed on the teeth is an absolute necessity for the operator who would in any way alter those forces.

REFERENCES

Ainamo J., Loe H.: Anatomical characteristics of gingiva. A clinical and microscopic study of the free and attached gingiva. *J. Periodontol.* 37:5, 1966.

Anderson D.J., Ronning G.A.: Dye diffusion in human dentin. *Arch. Oral. Biol.* 7:505, 1962.

Atkinson H.F., Saunsbury P.: An investigation into the hardness of human enamel. *Brit. Dent. J.* 94:82, 1953.

Benzer S.: The development and morphology of physiological secondary dentine. *J. Dent. Res.* 27:640, 1948.

Bergman G.: Microscopic demonstration of fluid flow through human dental enamel. *Arch. Oral. Biol.* 8:223, 1963.

Bhussey B.R., Bibby, B.G.: Surface changes in enamel. *J. Dent. Res.* 36:409, 1957.

Box H.K.: Evidence of lymphatics in the periodontium. *J. Canad. Dent. Assoc.* 15:8, 1949.

Brannstrom M.: Sensitivity of dentine. *Oral Surg.* 21:517, 1966.

Breitner C.: Tooth supporting apparatus under occlusal changes. *J. Periodontol.* 13:72, 1942.

Glickman I.: *Clinical Periodontology,* ed 4. Philadelphia, W.B. Saunders Co., 1972.

Goldman H.M., Cohen, D.W.: *Periodontics,* ed 4. St. Louis, C.V. Mosby Co., 1959.

Gottlieb B.: Histology consideration of the supporting tissues of the teeth. *J. Am. Dent. Assoc.* 30:1872, 1943.

Johansen E.: Microstructure of enamel and dentin. *J. Dent. Res.* 43:1007, 1964.

Kramer I.R.H.: Alveolar bone in health and disease. *Dent. Pract.* 12:327, 1962.

Kronfield R.: Biology of cementum. *J. Am. Dent. Assoc.* 25:1451, 1938.

Little M.F., Ceuto E.S.: Some chemical and physical properties of "altered" enamel. *J. Dent. Res.* 38:674, 1959.

Lungeland L.: Tissue changes in the dental pulp. An experimental histological study. *Odontol. Tidskr.* 65:239, 1957.

Lowater F., Murray M.M.: Chemical composition of teeth. V. Spectrographic analysis. *Biochem. J.* 31:837, 1937.

Nylen M.U., Scott D.B.: Electron microscopic studies of odontogenesis. *J. Ind. State Dent. Assoc.* 39:406, 1960.

Orban B.: *Oral Histology and Embryology,* ed 2. St. Louis, C.V. Mosby Co., 1949.

Orban B., Sicher, H.: The oral mucosa. *J. Dent. Educ.* 10:94, 1945.

Provenza D.U.: The blood supply of the pulp with emphasis on capillary circulation. *Circ. Res.* 6:213, 1958.

Schafer W.G., Hine M.K., Levy B.M.: *A Textbook of Oral Pathology,* ed 2. Philadelphia, W.B. Saunders Co., 1963.

Stack M.V., Fearnlead R.W.: Tooth Enamel: Its Composition, Properties and Fundamental Structure. Baltimore, William & Wilkins Co., 1965.

Wainwright W.W.: Penetration of teeth by radioactive materials. *J. Dent. Res.* 33:767, 34:28, 1954.

Yoon S.H., Brudevold F., Gardner D.E., et al. Distribution of fluorine in the teeth and fluorine level in water. *J. Dent. Res.* 39:845, 1960.

CHAPTER 3

Diagnosis and Treatment Planning

KEITH E. THAYER, D.D.S.

DIAGNOSIS IS THE art or act of recognizing a disease from its symptoms. Dental diagnosis is a result of an evaluation of the oral conditions of a patient. Treatment planning is the development, in greater or lesser detail as the case dictates, of the type and sequence of treatment necessary to address the disease or conditions that require attention.

To arrive at a reasonable, effective, and accurate diagnosis a variety of data must be collected.[1] A good medical and dental history is the foundation for data collection (Fig 3–1). There must be enough information included in the history to alert the dentist to ask additional specific questions if the history and clinical examination combined so indicate. The history form should not be so elaborate and inclusive that it becomes cumbersome and redundant. It should provide a good overview of the general health and dental concerns and attitudes of the patient.

The next step in the diagnosis is a thorough clinical examination of soft and hard oral tissues (Figs 3–2 and 3–3). These findings should be recorded on appropriate forms so that the information is easily and accurately accessible.

First, the conditions of the soft tissues are observed and recorded. General oral hygiene, tissue appearance, attached gingiva, and gingival sulcus depths are noted. The size and position of the tongue and the consistency and amount of saliva are valuable observations for data collection. The lip line should be recorded while the patients converses or laughs to identify what areas of what teeth, both maxillary and mandibular, are visible. This will help to determine esthetic requirements for any fixed restorations.

Location, size, and type of existing restorations are recorded. Any detectable carious lesions are noted on the record. Missing teeth and types of replacements, if any, are also recorded.

This is followed by an evaluation of the occlusion. An occlusion questionnaire (Fig 3–4) may be used routinely or if occlusal symptoms are present. At least, general occlusal relationships including the initial tooth contacts in the joint controlled mandibular position (centric relation) must be recorded (Fig 3–5). This is the retruded position or the uppermost, rearmost unstrained relation of the heads of the condyles in the glenoid fossae. Any vertical or horizontal change in the mandibular position from this relationship to maximum intercuspation should be recorded. This is the position from which the mouth can comfortably close and chew, and may be referred to as centric occlusion.[2] During treatment, if the teeth are

Update ________

HEALTH QUESTIONNAIRE

Reason for seeking treatment? ________

Patient ID

Date

PLEASE CIRCLE THE APPROPRIATE ANSWER

1. Are you in good health? . . . . YES NO
2. Has there been any change in your health within the past year? . . . . YES NO
3. Date of last physical exam ________
4. Are you now under medical care? . . . . YES NO
5. If so, for what? ________
6. Have you ever had a serious illness or operation? . . YES NO
7. If so, explain ________
8. Do you have or have you ever had any of the following diseases?
   a. Rheumatic fever or rheumatic heart disease . . . . YES NO
   b. Congenital heart disease . . . . YES NO
   c. Cardiovascular disease (heart trouble, heart attack, coronary insufficiency, coronary occlusion, high blood pressure, arteriosclerosis, stroke) . . . . YES NO
   d. Allergy . . . . YES NO
   e. Asthma or hay fever . . . . YES NO
   f. Hives or a skin rash . . . . YES NO
   g. Fainting spells or seizures . . . . YES NO
   h. Diabetes . . . . YES NO
   i. Hepatitis, jaundice or liver disease . . . . YES NO
   j. Inflammatory rheumatism (painful swollen joints) YES NO
   k. Arthritis . . . . YES NO
   l. Stomach ulcers . . . . YES NO
   m. Kidney trouble . . . . YES NO
   n. Tuberculosis . . . . YES NO
   o. Persistent cough or cough up blood . . . . YES NO
   p. Venereal disease . . . . YES NO
   q. Epilepsy . . . . YES NO
   r. Other ________
9. Do you have pain in chest upon exertion? . . . . . . YES NO
10. Are you ever short of breath after mild exercise? . . YES NO
11. Do your ankles swell? . . . . YES NO
12. Do you get short of breath when you lie down, or do you require extra pillows to sleep? . . . . YES NO
13. Do you have to urinate (pass water) more than six times a day? . . . . YES NO
14. Are you thirsty much of the time? . . . . YES NO
15. Have you had abnormal bleeding associated with previous surgery, extractions or accidents? . . . . YES NO
16. Do you bruise easily? . . . . YES NO
17. Have you ever required a blood transfusion? . . . . . . YES NO
18. Do you have any blood disorders such as anemia, etc.? . . . . YES NO
19. Have you ever had surgery or x-ray treatment for a tumor, growth, or other condition? . . . . YES NO
20. Are you taking any of the following?
   a. Antibiotics or sulfa drugs . . . . YES NO
   b. Anticoagulants (blood thinners) . . . . YES NO
   c. Medicine for high blood pressure . . . . YES NO
   d. Cortisone or steroids . . . . YES NO
   f. Aspirin . . . . YES NO
   g. Dilantin or other anticonvulsant . . . . YES NO
   h. Insulin, tolbutamide, Orinase or similar drug . . . . . YES NO
   i. Digitalis or drugs for heart trouble . . . . YES NO
   j. Nitroglycerin . . . . YES NO
   k. Birth Control "pill" . . . . YES NO
   l. Any other? ________
21. Are you allergic to or have you ever reacted adversely to any of the following?
   a. Local anesthetics . . . . YES NO
   b. Penicillin or other antibiotics . . . . YES NO
   c. Sulfa drugs . . . . YES NO
   d. Barbiturates, sedatives, or sleeping pills . . . . YES NO
   e. Aspirin . . . . YES NO
   f. Any other? ________
22. Have you had any serious trouble associated with any previous dental treatment? . . . . YES NO
   If so, please explain ________
23. Do you have any disease, condition, or problem not listed above? If so, please explain ________
24. Are you employed in any situation which could expose you to x-rays or other ionizing radiations? . . . . YES NO
25. Date of last dental exam ________
26. Have you ever had orthodontic treatment (worn braces)? . . . . YES NO
27. Have you ever been treated for any gum diseases (gingivitis, periodontitis, trenchmouth, pyorrhea)? . . YES NO
28. Do your gums bleed when you brush your teeth? . . . YES NO
29. Do you grind or clench your teeth? . . . . YES NO
30. Have you often had toothaches? . . . . YES NO
31. Have you had frequent sores in your mouth? . . . . . YES NO
32. Have you had any injuries to your mouth or jaws? . YES NO
   If so, please explain ________
33. Do you have any sores or swellings of your mouth or jaws? . . . . YES NO
34. Are you interested in keeping your teeth? . . . . YES NO
35. Have you been satisfied with your previous dental care? . . . . YES NO
   If not, please explain ________

WOMEN

36. Are you pregnant? . . . . YES NO
37. Do you have any problems associated with your menstrual period? . . . . YES NO

The undersigned agrees that the information above is accurate.

________ Signature ________ Date

Fig 3–1.—A good medical and dental health questionnaire is an important part of any diagnosis.

being restored to centric occlusion and the initial tooth contact in centric relation is not being restored, that contact should remain as the initial contact in centric relation. If any possible change in vertical relation is contemplated the interocclusal space should be observed and recorded.

Radiographs are a valuable aid in any diagnosis. Depending on the previously gathered data the dentist may require a panoramic radiograph, a full mouth survey of periapical and bite wing radiographs or selected individual radiographs. Periapical radiographs are necessary to diagnose the supporting mechanisms of individual

I. Pt. Info. a. I.D.	DIAGNOSIS AND TREATMENT PLAN	16) Gingiva (measure pockets)
	c. Date of Birth	17) bone loss
	d. Physician	
	e. Physician's Phone	18) mobility
b. Date of Exam	f. Dental Insurance Co.	
	g. Prior Approval	19) Non-Vital Teeth
h. Entrance Complaint		
II. Historical Information		20) Periapical Lesions
1) History of Entrance Comp.		
		21) Caries
2) Medical History		
		22) Impacted Teeth
3) Dental History		
		23) Fractured Teeth
III. Soft Tissue Exam		24) Extractions
4) Skin		
		V. Additional Considerations
5) Neck		25) Potential Cusp Fracture
6) Lips		26) Strategic Teeth
7) Mucosa		27) Occlusion
8) Tongue		28) Musculature
9) Floor of Mouth		29) Tempromandibular Joint
10) Salivary Glands		30) Study Casts
11) Palate		31) Shade and Mold
12) Oropharynx		32) Consultations Tests, Etc.
		33) Patient Attitude
IV. Dental Exam		
13) Deciduous Teeth		34) Case Presentation
14) Missing Teeth		35) Articulator Setting
15) Oral Hygiene		36) Prognosis

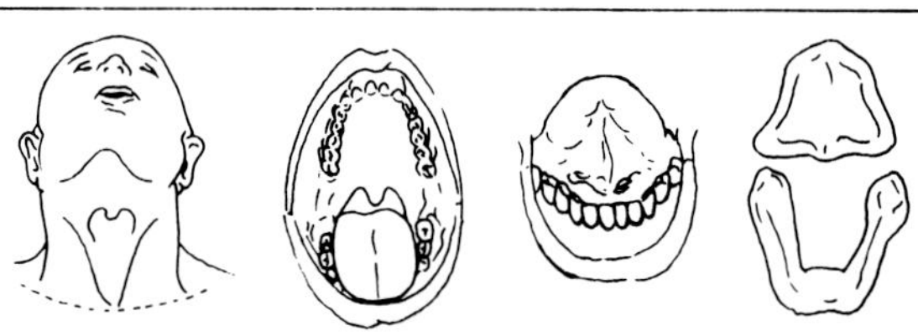

Fig 3–2.—A wide variety of factors involved in the diagnosis and treatment plan can be listed to check. Open space is allowed for comments and observations.

teeth and periapical conditions, whereas panoramic radiographs give an excellent overall view of bone and teeth relationships and any gross lesions. Teeth that may need crowns or that are being considered as fixed appliance abutment teeth should be tested for vitality at this time. Profile and full face photographs, as well as intraoral photographs may be helpful in treatment planning and case presentation. They also provide the patient with a before and after comparison.

Finally, alginate impressions should be made of both ärches to obtain casts to be used in diagnosis and treatment. Depending on the complexity of the case and the experience of the operator, the casts may serve only for fabricating custom impres-

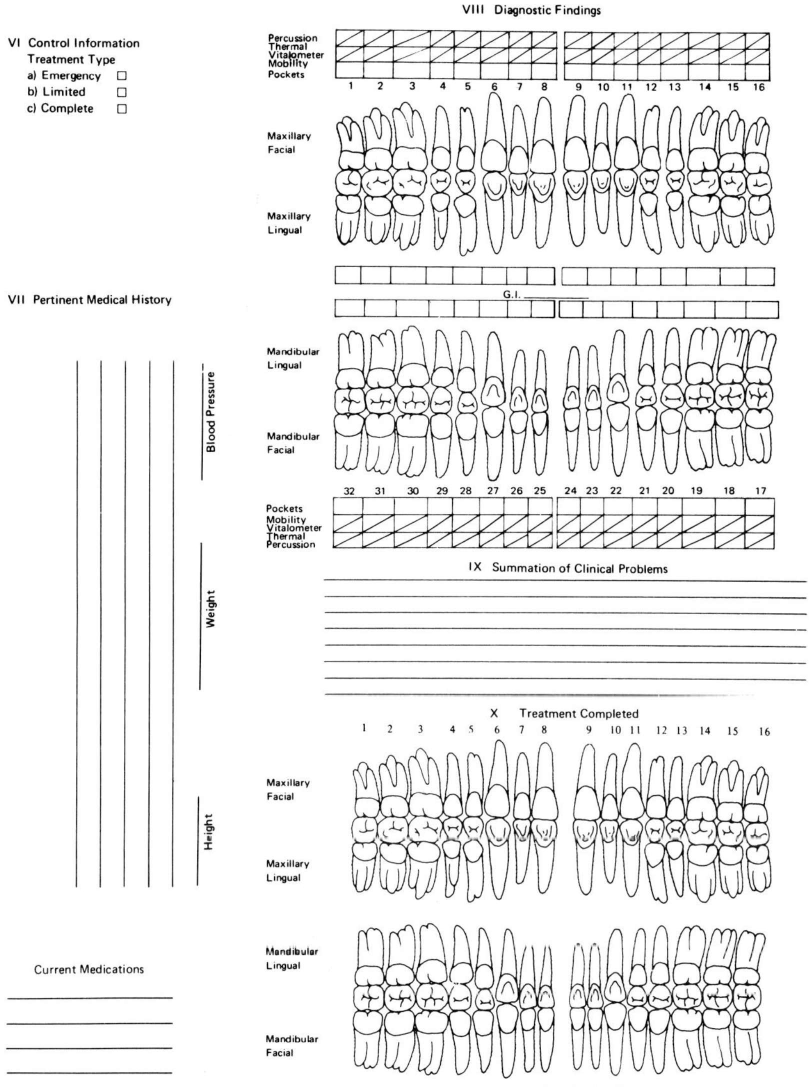

Fig 3–3.—A tooth chart is invaluable in recording caries and missing teeth as well as existing restorations and replacements. With color coding, radiographic findings may also be recorded.

sion trays or as an opposing cast in laboratory procedures. In any extensive case, the casts should be mounted as diagnostic casts. This should be done with the aid of a face-bow transfer and interocclusal centric and eccentric records on a semiadjustable articulator. More accurate diagnostic casts are obtained with the aid of pantographic tracings and the use of a fully adjustable articulator for mounting.

The diagnostic appointment is complete when all data that is necessary for treatment has been secured. Caries index tests, diet analysis, and blood and urine samples may be obtained as needed or the patient may be referred to a medical doctor. Any additional questions that are pertinent may be asked. Sometimes items such

OCCLUSION QUESTIONNAIRE

Patient ID

Date

PLEASE CIRCLE THE APPROPRIATE ANSWER

1. Have you been made aware of clenching or grinding your teeth at night? . . . . YES NO

2. Do you ever wake with tired jaw joints or muscles like you had been chewing gum all night? . . . . YES NO

3. Do you clench or grind your teeth during the day? . . . . YES NO

4. Do you ever have pain in your jaw joints, the side of your face or in or around your ears? . . . . YES NO

5. Do you have frequent head___, neck___, shoulder___, aches or pains? How many days per week?_____ . . . . YES NO

6. Do you have such an ache or pain now? . . . . YES NO

7. Does your jaw joint ever pop or click? . . . . YES NO

8. Do you ever have difficulty in opening your mouth widely or in closing? . . . . YES NO

9. Which side do you chew on? Right___ Left___ Both___

Signature Date

Fig 3–4.—An occlusion questionnaire is helpful in recording information about joints and muscles.

as the patient's occupation are helpful for treatment planning. If the patient has not had or taken an opportunity to express their dental concerns or desires during the appointment this should surely not be overlooked.

After the diagnostic appointment all of the gathered data are studied, reviewed, and correlated and a treatment plan is developed for a case presentation (Fig 3–6). For some patients there is only one reasonable and effective treatment plan. For others there may be two or more viable options that would vary in time and effort as well as in cost. The patient should be made aware of all reasonable options of treatment.

When extensive dental treatment that will have a marked effect on the size, shape, or position of teeth and that may result in changes in esthetics, phonetics,

OCCLUSAL ANALYSIS

PATIENT ______________________________

DATE ______________ ________, 19 _____

INITIAL TOOTH CONTACT	1	2	3	4	5	6	7	8	9	10	11	12	13	14	15	16
	32	31	30	29	28	27	26	25	24	23	22	21	20	19	18	17

MANDIBULAR DISPLACEMENT: Anterior _____mm. Vertical _____mm. Lateral: to the left _____mm. to the right _____mm.

GUIDANCE FROM CENTRIC RELATION:	1	2	3	4	5	6	7	8	9	10	11	12	13	14	15	16
	32	31	30	29	28	27	26	25	24	23	22	21	20	19	18	17

WORKING DEFLECTIVE CONTACTS:	1	2	3	4	5	6	7	8	9	10	11	12	12	14	15	16
	32	31	30	29	28	27	26	25	24	23	22	21	20	19	18	17

NON-WORKING DEFLECTIVE CONTACTS:	1	2	3	4	5	6	7	8	9	10	11	12	13	14	15	16
	32	31	30	29	28	27	26	25	24	23	22	21	20	19	18	17

PROTRUSIVE GUIDANCE CONTACTS:	1	2	3	4	5	6	7	8	9	10	11	12	13	14	15	16
	32	31	30	29	28	27	26	25	24	23	22	21	20	19	18	17

HORIZONTAL OVERLAP: _____mm. VERTICAL OVERLAP: _____mm.

ECCENTRIC BRUXISM FACETS:	1	2	3	4	5	6	7	8	9	10	11	12	13	14	15	16
	32	31	30	29	28	27	26	25	24	23	22	20	21	19	18	17

Fig 3–5.—The occlusal analysis is important whether the intent is to restore the patient to centric relation or centric occlusion. It is important that any new restoration does not provide a different initial tooth contact in centric relation if the teeth are being restored to centric occlusion.

and function is contemplated, a diagnostic wax-up should be made and diagnostic transitional restorations fabricated to verify the predicted esthetic, phonetic, and functional results.[3, 4]

A diagnostic wax-up is done best on articulated casts. Articulated casts also provide the optimum opportunity to observe and study the occlusion and to identify working and nonworking contacts that may or may not need to be reproduced in the restorations. Variations in the plane of occlusion that may need to be changed in the restorations, tipped teeth that may effect retainer choices, paths of insertion, and preparation modifications are all observed. All of these factors are important when a treatment plan is being devised.[4]

All of the factors identified from the diagnostic data should be considered when the treatment plan is being constructed. Specific examples include clinical crown length of teeth to be restored or used to retain fixed partial dentures. In the case of short crowns, crown lengthening procedures should be considered and can be done with the orthodontic or periodontic approach. Special attention should also be

PATIENT ID

PERIODONTAL CLASSIFICATION
I II III IV

CALCULUS
A B C D

XII. Treatment Priority

Priority	Treatment	Priority	Treatment
	Oral Pathology		Endodontics
	Radiology		Operative (major)
	Oral Diagnosis		Operative (minor)
	Dental Hygiene A B C D		Fixed Prosthodontics
	Oral Surgery		Removable Prosthodontics
	Periodontics		Orthodontics

XI. Treatment Plan

a) Tooth No.	b) Problem	c) Proposed Treatment	d) Code	e) Fee		

Fig 3–6.—Proposed treatment should be prioritized for sequence as well as need. If there are viable alternate treatment plans these may be listed separately, or coded, regarding sequence or fee.

given to teeth that are overerupted into longstanding edentulous spaces. Crowning such teeth for the purpose of improving the occlusal plane is frequently necessary. It is not unusual for patients who require tooth replacement to have had periodontal treatment previously. Such cases are always at greater risk because any fixed partial denture increases the need and the difficulty of maintaining good oral hygiene. Before fixed restorations are planned for such patients it should be determined that they are willing and able to maintain good oral hygiene.[5]

Biomechanic and physiologic design criteria must be considered and met when treatment is planned.[6] Biomechanically, the stress bearing capacity of the restoration must exceed its stress gathering capacity. Ante's law[7] is a good starting point for making this decision. It proposes that the periodontally supported root area of the abutment teeth should equal or exceed the average periodontally supported root area of the teeth to be replaced. Obviously, other parameters have an effect on stress bearing and gathering capacities. In addition, the quality of supporting bone is important. The elimination of all excurcive contacts in the occlusal scheme greatly reduces the lateral loads on posterior teeth and by reducing the size of the food table of the restoration the vertical loads of mastication may be reduced. If the fixed restoration is opposed by a removable denture the resultant load will be less. A reduced load also results when the patient is less muscular. Unless one or more of these factors are favorable, or can be accomplished in the design, Ante's law should be followed.

Physiologic design criteria include establishing contours that will provide a balance between protection and stimulation of the soft tissues. Ideally, margins should be placed in enamel where they can be more accurately finished. Supragingival margins should be used whenever possible. They are easier to prepare, make impressions of, fit and finish, and maintain and observe in the future. Frequently, however, esthetic and retentive demands and requirements indicate subgingival margin placement. Tooth defects from fracture, caries, or restorations may also require subgingival margin placement.[6]

Every missing tooth should be replaced as soon as the ridge is healed, whenever possible or practical. Complete ridge healing should be allowed with the patient wearing a temporary removable partial denture if there is an esthetic requirement. Immediate type fixed replacements are not recommended.

Frequently, removable replacements must be incorporated into the treatment plan depending on the number and location of missing teeth. In such combination cases clasp bearing teeth may be indicated for fixed restorations in preparation for the removable appliance. The design, shape, and choice of materials for these restorations are critical to the success or failure of the case.[8] Important considerations in the planning of such restorations include the plane of occlusion, path of insertion of removable partial denture, amount and location of retentive contours, rests and existing restorations, or caries and caries index. In some cases, the use of precision attachments may be indicated. Combination cases are links of a chain where if one link fails, the entire case fails or is impaired.[9]

REVIEW

A fixed partial denture is a means of replacing one or more missing teeth that uses one or more remaining teeth. It includes one or more replacement teeth (pontics) and one or more abutment teeth with their retainers to support and maintain the pontic.

There are basically three types of fixed partial dentures.[10] First, there are those in which the pontic or pontics are rigidly attached to all abutment retainers and may be referred to as fixed-fixed restorations. Second, broken-stress restorations in which the pontic is rigidly attached to one retainer and gains support and stability from the other retainer through a precision or semiprecision attachment using some type of dovetail slot and lug arrangement. Broken-stress restorations are also referred to as fixed-movable and are used primarily where all of the abutment teeth cannot be prepared with a common path of insertion or where pier abutments are involved. The cantilever fixed partial denture is the final type. This depends on one abutment tooth supporting and retaining the pontic, and it should be used with caution. The term extension pontic is sometimes applied to restorations where two or more abutment teeth, both of which are not adjacent to the edentulous space, are used. Whether these abutments are adjacent to each other or separated by yet another pontic, they significantly improve the physics of leverage and rotational loads that are such a problem with the customary cantilever restoration.

In addition to general diagnosis information, treatment planning of individual fixed restorations should include consideration of:

1. The number and location of missing teeth. Long span replacements may require multiple abutments for support and retention. Intermediate or pier abutments, with pontic spans on both sides, need special attention as they are more difficult in attaining good marginal fit and are subjected to greater loading because of the fulcruming effect;
2. Functioning stress and dietary habits of the individual patient;
3. Periodontal and periapical conditions of the abutments, including mobility and vitality;
4. Condition of the abutment teeth regarding caries, restorations, or fractures;
5. The occlusal relationships and any special forces that might effect the design;
6. The patient's oral hygiene, a prediction of its likelihood for change in the future, and its possible effect on caries index and periodonal disease; and
7. Esthetic considerations that may be of concern to the patient.

REFERENCES

1. Brehm T.W.: Diagnosis and treatment planning for fixed prosthodontics. *J. Prosthet. Dent.* 30:876, 1973.
2. Beyron H.: Point of significance in planning restorative procedures. *J. Prosthet. Dent.* 30:641, 1973.
3. Preston J.D.: A systematic approach to the control of esthetic form. *J. Prosthet. Dent.* 35:393, 1976.
4. Greeley J.H.: Planning for fixed prosthodontics. *J. Prosthet. Dent.* 20:412, 1968.
5. Bull A.W.: Diagnosis: A factor in the success of fixed partial dentures. *J. Prosthet. Dent.* 24:498, 1970.
6. Eissmann H.F., Radke R.A., Noble W.H.: Physiologic design criteria for fixed dental restorations. *Dent. Clin. North Am.* 15:543, 1971.
7. Ante I.H.: The fundamental principles of abutments. *Mich. State Dent. Soc. Bull.* 8:14, 1926.
8. Preston J.D.: Preventing ceramic failures when integrating fixed and removable prostheses. *Dent. Clin. North Am.* 23:37, 1979.
9. Lorey R.E.: Abutment considerations. *Dent. Clin. North Am.* 24:63, 1980.
10. Booth J.M., Storridge N.A., Alexander A.G.: Simple bridges replacing single missing teeth: Examination and treatment planning. *Apex.* 5:119, 1971.

CHAPTER 4

Crown Foundations

HANI H. HERMES, D.D.S.

A GREAT DEAL OF EFFORT is put into planning and designing a foundation for any type of structure because a structure without a proper foundation is not viable. The same applies to any prosthodontic procedure. We should not only be concerned with the esthetics and external aspects of a crown or fixed partial denture but should be equally concerned with its underlying support. The best restoration is only as good as its foundation.

The foundations of crowns or fixed partial dentures include the abutment tooth and its supporting periodontal tissues. The coronal portion of the tooth to be crowned or to be used as an abutment is critical to the success of the final restoration. Therefore, crown foundations or build-ups should be approached as an integral part of diagnosis and treatment planning.

The objective of a crown foundation is to enable the teeth to support and retain crowns or fixed partial dentures where such support and retention is otherwise deficient.

INDICATIONS FOR CROWN FOUNDATIONS

Serious consideration should be given to the replacement of existing restorations before abutments for crowns or fixed partial dentures are prepared. Unless there is clear evidence that such restorations are sound, they should be removed and replaced.

The following are definitive indications for crown foundations:

1. Untreated carious lesions;
2. Defective existing restorations;
3. Suspicious looking existing restorations;
4. Restorations that are projected to have minimal remaining retention after the completion of the crown preparation because of the gross removal of tooth structure; and
5. Restorations that are structurally weakened after completion of the crown preparation because of a gross reduction in bulk.

TOOTH RESTORATION

Before any clinical procedure, thorough clinical and radiographic examination of the tooth is mandatory. The examination should include pulpal and periodontal tissue health and occlusion. Careful exploration of the extent of tooth destruction, especially near the gingiva, is important. The gingival margin of the defective or restored tooth structure should be amenable to full coverage by the margin of the preparation. If not, measures should be taken to expose it surgically to allow complete restoration. This can be done easily with electrosurgery, if conditions permit. Pulpal health should be evaluated and, if in doubt, endodontic treatment should be performed before final crown foundation restorations.

Teeth that require cast restorations are usually so extensively destroyed that ideal or classic cavity preparations are not possible.[1] The design of modified cavity preparation requires complete comprehension and proficiency in the execution of the basic principles, ranging from outline form to finishing. Organization and planning rather than short cuts improve speed and efficiency. Adherence to these principles is the key to success.

There are five steps in the actual restoration:

1. Anesthesia (if necessary);
2. Tooth isolation;
3. Tooth preparation;
4. Pulp protection; and
5. Build-up of the tooth.

The sixth step, finishing and polishing the restoration, is needed if the final preparation for the casting is to be delayed for some time.

TOOTH PREPARATION

Rubber dam isolation is important to assure quality and to protect the patient from accidental aspiration of foreign objects such as pins. The merits of rubber dams are well known.[2, 3]

Tooth preparation should be done with conservation of tooth structure in mind. This principle becomes increasingly important when we are dealing with extensively damaged teeth. Conservation should be exercised pragmatically and not by compromise. Any suspect tooth structure should be completely removed. This includes structurally weakened, undermined, and carious tooth structure. Existing defective restorations should be completely removed.

After the removal of old restorations, bases, and defective tooth structure, a reappraisal of the remaining sound tooth structure is necessary. The projected crown preparation should be visualized to determine if the existing tooth structure will remain sound after preparation. The operator needs to have a clear idea of the amount of tooth structure to be removed for the crown preparation. Generally, the occlusal surface is reduced 1.5-2 mm for cast restorations and 2-2.5 mm for ceramometal restorations with porcelain occlusal surfaces.[1, 4] The external axial and proximal surfaces of the tooth are usually reduced by 1-1.5 mm during crown preparation (Fig 4–1). The remaining tooth structure should be sound after the tooth reduction; otherwise, it is removed and the area is included in the preparation.

All sloping surfaces should be converted to vertical and horizontal surfaces to be parallel or perpendicular to the anticipated occlusal forces (Fig 4–2).[1] The floor of the preparation and gingival seat should be made perpendicular to the occlusal forces. This may result in step form, without necessarily making it in one level (Fig 4–3). This improves retention and resistance and conserves tooth structure.[5]

The biggest problem in restoring extensively damaged teeth is retention of the restoration. To achieve any degree of retention, at least two opposing walls are

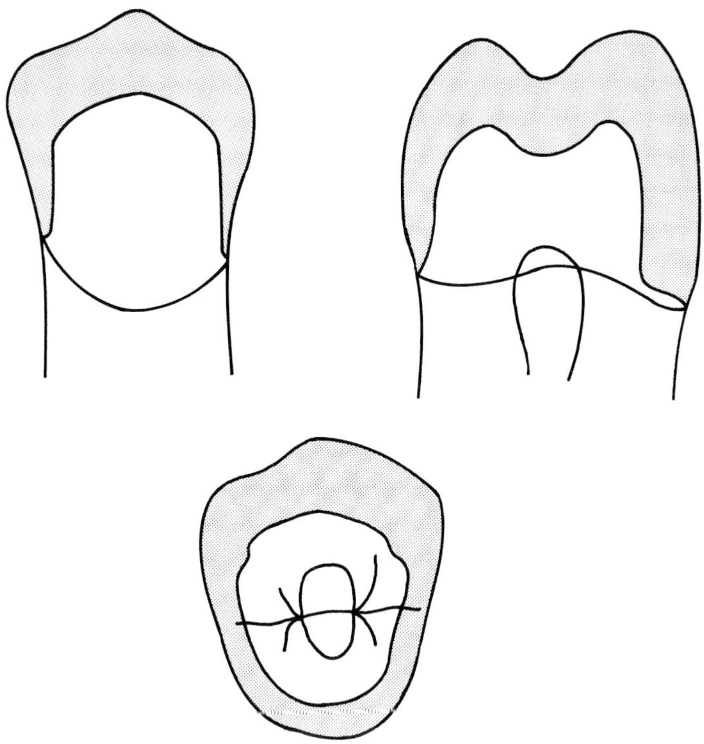

Fig 4–1.—Tooth preparation should be envisioned to determine the necessity of retaining or removing suspect tooth structure and proper location for retentive pins.

necessary.[1] All vertical walls in the preparation should be made parallel[5] or with a slight convergence occlusally. Boxes and grooves are cut, wherever possible, with definable opposing parallel walls.[5] Small rectangular channels or grooves can be placed in dentin at the gingival seat of proximal boxes or mesiodistally at the reduced cusp area (Fig 4–4).[2] This can be done with an inverted cone bur inserted to the depth of its head. Supplementary mechanical retention through the use of pins may be necessary if little sound retentive tooth structure remains.[6, 7] Pins should be used with discretion because they can potentially damage the tooth and

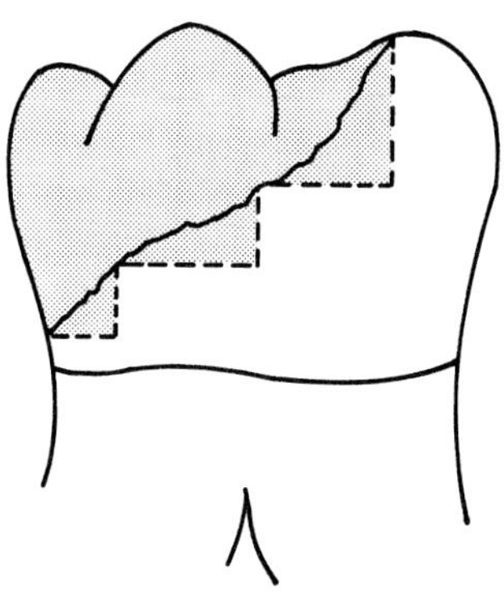

Fig 4–2.—Sloping surfaces of the cavity are converted to horizontal and vertical to improve resistance and retention.

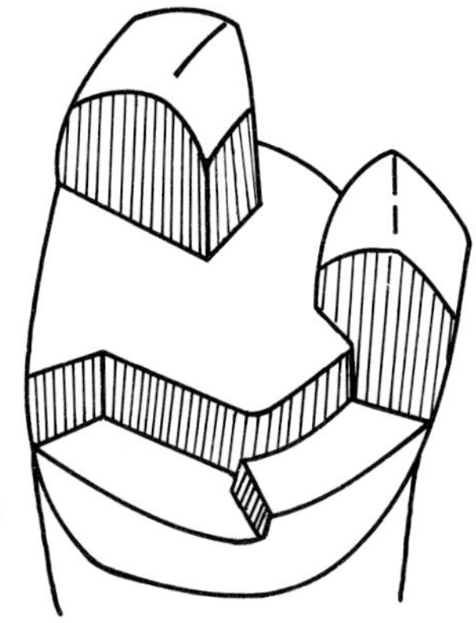

Fig 4–3.—Cavity floors should be made perpendicular to the anticipated occlusal forces to improve resistance. There is no attempt to make the floor on one level. Multiple levels conserve tooth structure and improve retention.

weaken restorative materials.[6, 8] The selection and placement of pins should be done only after their potential, rather than their convenience and availability, is understood.

PIN SELECTION

Type—Cemented vs. Noncemented Pins

As retention is the only reason we use pins, self-threading (noncemented) pins are chosen because they provide the greatest possible retention.[6] However, they also cause high installation stresses that may cause dentinal crazing if used closer than 0.5 mm from the dentinoenamel junction and in endodontically treated teeth.[8, 9] Cemented pins are useful in cases where high stresses are anticipated.

Size—Diameter

Pins are available in sizes ranging from .015 in. to .031 in. Larger diameters are stronger and provide more retention but cause higher stresses. We recommend the use of pin size .019 in. such as minikin pins (Whaledent) for anterior teeth and size .023 in.-.025 in. for premolars and molars. The larger size pins (.030 in.-.031 in.)

Fig 4–4.—Small rectangular channels in dentin at the reduced cusp area can supplement retention.

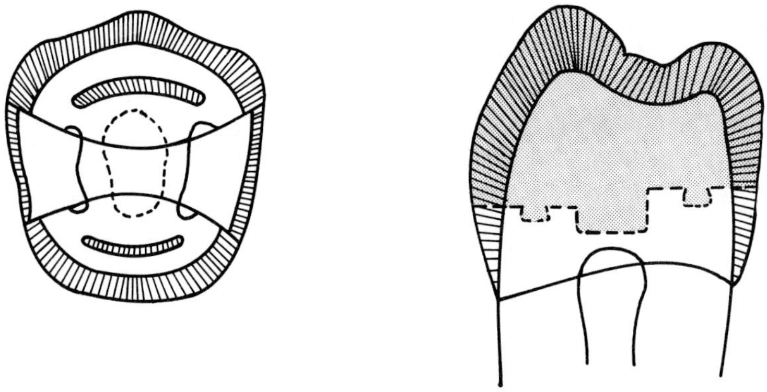

should only be used for large molars. The very small .015 in. such as minuta pins (Whaledent) are not useful for crown buildups because of their minimal strength.

Length

Optimal pin depth in dentin is 2 mm. Pin extension in restorative materials should be kept within 2-3 mm.[6, 7, 10]

Number

The rule of thumb is to replace each missing line angle or wall with one pin.[7] No more than 4 to 5 pins are needed for a complete crown foundation.

PIN CHANNEL PREPARATION AND THREADED PIN INSERTION

Careful examination of the diagnostic radiographs and familiarity with dental anatomy are necessary to avoid penetration into the periodontal tissues or pulp.[8]

Pin Location

Pins should always be located in dentin preferably midway between the dentino-enamel junction and the pulp.[6–8] The pin is placed as far as possible inside the projected preparation depth to avoid exposing the pin or weakening the restorative material that covers it during crown preparation. It is much easier and more reliable to treat pulpal perforation than root perforation or dentinal cracking that occurs as a result of pin insertion. Pins are best located at the line angles, proximolabial or proximolingual. A second choice location is between the line angles, avoiding furcation areas in molars and deep concavities in proximal surfaces such as the mesial aspect of maxillary first premolars.

Pin Angulation

Pin channels should be prepared parallel to the tangent of the external root surface to avoid pulpal or root perforation (Fig 4–5). Retention is improved if pins are not placed parallel to each other.

Pin Channel Preparation

Preparation should be done with a very slow speed handpiece. Initially, an indentation with a no. 1/2 round bur is made at the selected site to prevent skidding of the twist drill. The twist drill is held tangent to the external root surface and

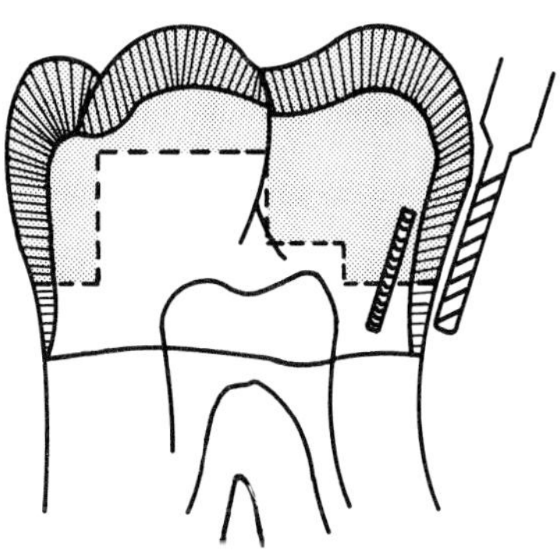

Fig 4–5.—Pins should be placed parallel to the external adjacent root surface area to prevent pulpal or root perforation.

moved to the indentation maintaining the angulation. The channel is prepared with one or two steady vertical strokes until the drill reaches the predetermined depth. Self-limiting drills are recommended whenever possible. Multiple entries should be avoided to prevent an oversizing and flaring of the pin channel that will unfavorably affect the retention of the pin.

Pin Insertion

Mechanical insertion of pins is both easier and faster than manual. Although mechanically seated pins may not reach the fundus of the pin channel, its retention is not significantly affected. If self-shearing pins are used, then the pin length will be automatically adjusted. Otherwise, the pin should be cut to 2 mm. above the tooth structure. The pin should then be slightly bent toward the center of the tooth to improve retention and to keep the pin within the coronal contour of the crown build-up after the crown preparation.

CEMENTED PINS

Cemented pins are recommended for endodontically treated teeth and in teeth where self-threading pins might cause cracks or high stresses.

Because the retention of cemented pins is much less than self-threading pins, more pins and deeper pin channels may be necessary to secure good retention.[9] Cemented pins should therefore be inserted 2 to 4 mm. in dentin.

Three luting agents are commonly used to cement pins. Zinc phosphate is the most retentive, cyanoacrylate is the least, and polycarboxylate is intermediate.[7] However, if copal varnish is used to protect the pulp from the acidity of zinc phosphate, retention drops significantly.[6] Cyanoacrylate is easy to manipulate, but because it may be biodegradable it is not reliable. Therefore, polycarboxylate cement is recommended for vital teeth, and zinc phosphate cement is preferred for endodontically treated teeth. The cement should be mixed to a consistency similar to that used in cementing castings. It is carried to the pin channel by a lentulo spiral in a slowly rotating contra-angle handpiece. The base of the pin is coated with cement and immediately seated in the pin channel. It should be left undisturbed until the cement is fully set, and then excess cement should be removed. It is not recommended to cement more than one or two pins at a time to allow for sufficient working time and proper consistency of cement.

PULP PROTECTION

The protection of the pulp from thermal, chemical, and/or mechanical irritation caused by dental procedures and materials is necessary. Pulp protection is best provided by the thickness of the remaining dentin. According to Going,[11] whenever the remaining dentin thickness falls below 2 mm., an intermediary liner and/or base is needed. Calcium hydroxide is recommended for deep cavities with a protective base of reinforced zinc oxide eugenol or polycarboxylate cement. The thickness of any base or liner should be kept to a minimum to allow a sufficient bulk for strength of the restorative filling material.

If amalgam is being used, a double coat of cavity varnish should be used to coat the cavity walls thereby minimizing the initial microleakage.[12]

If composite resin is selected, zinc oxide eugenol cement and cavity varnish are not to be used.[11]

THE MATRIX

Any restoration of two or more surfaces requires the use of a matrix. There are several designs and methods available, but the selection depends not only on the operator's preference but, more importantly, on the extent and size of the preparation and the restorative material to be used.

Regardless of the extent of preparation and the matrix selected, matrices should provide:

1. A wall against which the restorative material can be confined and condensed;
2. Rigidity to allow condensation of the restorative material without distortion;
3. Accurate fit (collar-like) at the cervical portion of the preparation;
4. Opportunity for restoration of proximal and occlusal contacts and axial contour if so desired; and
5. Stability and the optional use of gingival wedges.

Matrices can be grouped into several categories:

1. Conventional stock matrix band and mechanical retainer such as Tofflemire, Ivory, or Caulk;
2. Custom spot welded bands made from strip matrix band metal;
3. Copper bands or tubes; and
4. Preformed temporary crowns.

A conventional matrix band and retainer is useful whenever enough tooth structure is present to stabilize it. However, many of the teeth requiring crown foundations are so extensively damaged that a custom spot welded band or copper band is necessary.[13] If a spot welded band is chosen, a strip of band material is placed around the tooth and a mark is made to spot weld it before the tooth is prepared. This is set aside until the preparation is completed. The band is then festooned and contoured to fit the preparation and it's proximal walls are burnished against the adjacent teeth to secure proximal contact, if desired.

If a copper band is to be used, one that closely fits the cervical portion of the tooth should be selected.[3] The band is softened over a flame and allowed to cool. Gingival festooning and contouring is done with curved crown scissors and contouring pliers. The axial wall of the band is reduced slightly out of occlusal contact and to the level of the adjacent marginal ridges.

Preformed temporary crowns can be used in a similar manner to copper band.[14] Selection, festooning, and contouring is essentially the same. The occlusal surface of the temporary crown is completely removed if it is to be used for amalgam. If composite resin is selected, then only a hole is made in the occlusal surface to vent the composite resin. Polycarbonate crowns can be used for anterior teeth in a similar manner. Clear crown forms, both anterior and posterior, can be prepared similarly for composite crown foundations.

RESTORATIVE MATERIALS

Materials used for crown build-ups should be permanent in nature and should possess strength values equal to or exceeding those of tooth structure. They should resist breakdown in oral fluids and allow minimal or no microleakage.

The materials suitable for crown build-ups are silver amalgam and composite resin. Unfortunately, cements are commonly used to "base" cavities in lieu of amalgam or composite resin. This practice is not recommended because cements are weak, soluble in saliva and have microleakage.[11] Cements can only be used to fill small defects that are located away from the finish line of the crown preparation and only if the casting is entirely and adequately supported and retained by tooth structure.

Gold was used to form cores underneath crowns, but its use has diminished lately because of high costs and the improved physical properties of silver amalgam and the use of pins for retention. Furthermore, gold requires complicated and lengthy clinical and laboratory procedures to fabricate the foundation. It also adds another casting-cement interface that is the weakest link in all cast restorations. On the other hand, if sufficient tooth structure exists to support and retain a gold casting, it can be used to retain the final restoration.

Silver amalgam is definitely the first choice of materials for crown foundations. Amalgam is considered cariostatic because the margins seal themselves after a period because corrosion products are produced at the tooth interface.[15] The initial microleakage of amalgam can be significantly reduced by the application of multiple coats of a dentinal tubule sealer.[11, 12, 15] The material is radiopaque and, therefore, allows for the radiographic detection of secondary caries. The surface can be easily finished and polished. The color contrast between amalgam and tooth structure permits fine finishing of its margins and facilitates the placement of gingival margins of crown preparation on tooth structure. Ideally, all margins of cast restorations should be placed on sound tooth structure. However, if that is not possible for any reason, the margin can be left on amalgam.

Composite resin, on the other hand, must be covered by the crown margins because of its microleakage[16, 17] and hydrophilic nature.[18] Its surface can not be finely finished and polished because of its fillers,[19] thus encouraging plaque formation. Because the majority of available materials are not radiopaque, the detection of recurrent caries is difficult or impossible. Composite resin that is used for crown foundations should not be tooth colored so that the resin-tooth interface will be recognizable.

The major advantage of composite resin over amalgam is that the preparation of the crown can be done shortly after the material has set. Its placement is quick and easy. If time is not critical, it is still preferable to use the well proven and time tested silver amalgam.

FILLING OF THE CAVITY

Amalgam

The amalgam should be carefully condensed around the pins and along the gingival margins of the preparation first. The remainder of the foundation is condensed in the usual manner. If the final crown preparation is to follow the foundation, elaborate carving it not necessary. Instead, simple carving depicting the basic tooth form both occlusally and axially is done. However, if the final crown preparation is not planned in the near future, the foundation should be finished in harmony with the rest of the teeth in contour and occlusion. The restoration should then be smoothed and polished at a subsequent visit.

If customized matrix, copper bands, or a preformed temporary crown was used as a matrix, initial carving of the occlusal embrasure is done with an explorer. Then the matrix is removed by slitting it with a trimmer or with a bur. Occlusal, axial, and interproximal carving is completed afterwards. In some of these situations the matrix may be left in place and the occlusion established in the amalgam. The matrix may then be removed when the crown preparation is made.

Composite Resin

It is virtually impossible to clearly distinguish tooth colored composite resin from tooth structure, especially subgingivally. As it is imperative that the final preparation margin be on tooth structure, only tinted composite resin material should be used for crown foundations.

If a band and mechanical retainer, customized matrix, or copper band are to be used, they are adjusted, wedged, and stabilized on the tooth. The composite resin is mixed according to the manufacturer's directions. A composite resin syringe is recommended to carry the material into the cavity, especially around pins and other retentive features. The composite resin is lightly condensed, the cavity is overfilled, and the resin is held under pressure until it sets.

If a preformed temporary crown is to be used as a matrix, the composite is injected around the pins first, then the matrix is filled and seated on the preparation where it is held under pressure until it sets. The vent made in the matrix should not be blocked while the loaded matrix is being seated on the preparation. After the material sets, the matrix is removed and the tooth preparation is finalized.

REFERENCES

1. Shillingburg H.T., Hobo S., Whitsett L.D.: *Fundamentals of Fixed Prosthodontics.* Chicago, Quintessence Publishing Co., 1978.
2. Charbeneau G.T., et al.: *Principles and Practice of Operative Dentistry.* Philadelphia, Lea & Febiger, 1975.
3. Gilmore H.W., Lund M.R.: *Operative Dentistry*, ed. 3. St. Louis, C.V. Mosby Co., 1977.
4. Preston J.D.: Rational approach to tooth preparation for ceramometal restorations. *Dent. Clin. North Am.* 21:683, 1977.
5. Birtcil R.F., Venton E.A.: Extracoronal amalgam restorations utilizing available tooth structure for retention. *J. Prosthet. Dent.* 35:171, 1976.
6. Collard E.W., Caputo A.A., Standlee, J.P.: Rationale for pin-retained amalgam restorations. *Dent. Clin. North Am.* 14:43, 1970.
7. Caputo A.A., Standlee J.P.: Pins and posts: Why, when, and how. *Dent. Clin. North Am.* 20:299, 1976.
8. Dilts W.E., Mullaney T.P.: Relationship of pin hole location and tooth morphology in pin retained silver amalgam restorations. *J. Am. Dent. Assoc.* 76:1011, 1968.
9. Caputo A.A., Standlee J.P., Collard E.W.: The mechanics of load transfer by retentive pins. *J. Prosthet. Dent.* 29:422, 1973.
10. Janis J.H., Lugassy A.A.: Pin-retained composite resin buildup for extensively broken down vital teeth. *J. Am. Dent. Assoc.* 85:346, 1972.
11. Going R.E.: Intermediary bases and liners, in Clark N.J. (ed.): *Clinical Dentistry*, vol. 4. Hagerstown, Harper and Row, 1977.
12. Phillips R.W.: Cavity varnishes and bases, *Dent. Clin. North Am.* 159, March, 1965.
13. Birtcil R.F., Starr J.M.: Individualized matrix bands for amalgam restorations. *J. Prosthet. Dent.* 33:547, 1975.
14. Chapman K.W.: A matrix band technique for large amalgam cores. *J. Am. Dent. Assoc.* 102:56, 1981.
15. Christensen G.J.: Amalgam restorations, in Clark N.J. (ed.): *Clinical Dentistry*, vol. 4. Hagerstown, Harper and Row, 1977.
16. Christensen G.J.: Tooth-colored restorations, in Clark N.J. (ed.): *Clinical Dentistry*, vol. 4. Hagerstown, Harper and Row, 1977.

17. Hormati A.A., Denehy G.E.: Microleakage of pin-retained amalgam and composite resin bases. *J. Prosthet. Dent.* 44:526, 1980.
18. Pearson G.J.: Long-term water sorption and solubility of composite filling materials. *J. Dent.* 7:64, 1979.
19. Ryge G.: Composite resin restorative materials, in Clark, N.J. (ed.): *Clinical Dentistry*, vol. 4. Hagerstown, Harper and Row, 1977.

CHAPTER 5

Preparations

KEITH E. THAYER, D.D.S.

PREPARATION SELECTION, design, and tooth reduction is extremely important to the success of any fixed restoration. The selection between full and partial coverage or between full cast and esthetic veneer restorations depends on the esthetic requirements of the patient, the condition of the teeth being prepared, and the nature of the fixed restoration being constructed. The design of the selected preparation may need to be modified to satisfy retention and resistance requirements for the individual case. Periodontal conditions may modify margin placement and geometry. Finally, the actual tooth reduction technique must be carefully planned. Appropriate cutting instruments must be selected to accurately and efficiently carry out the mechanics of tooth reduction and preparation.

RETENTION AND RESISTANCE FORM

Retention and resistance form of the preparation, coupled with the fit of the casting and the effect of the luting agent used for cementation, determines the amount and direction of force needed to unseat a restoration. In general, retention form guards against unseating in a vertical direction, whereas resistance form guards against unseating from lateral or horizontal loads. The two are not totally independent, however, as they compliment each other to produce a maximum holding power.

Retention and resistance are enhanced by a number of factors. These include a reduced convergence angle or more parallel walls, greater length and circumference of the preparation that controls the area of contact of casting to tooth, and use of auxiliary aids such as grooves, boxes, and pins.[1]

The convergence angle or taper of the preparation is primarily a result of the skill and preference of the operator. The anatomy and position of the tooth, in the case of a fixed bridge abutment, may be a factor in the resultant taper as there must be no undercuts on individual preparations and abutment teeth must be prepared with a common path of insertion for the eventual restoration. Location, inclination, and position of contact points of adjacent teeth may also effect the parallelism that can be accomplished in preparations.

The circumference of the tooth, including the range in size of individual teeth as well as the variation in size between molars and mandibular central incisors, is beyond the control of the operator. The operator can affect the circumference of the preparation with full instead of partial coverage. The length of the tooth is an anatomic given but the choice of subgingival or supragingival margin placement will affect the length of the preparation.

Anatomic axial and occlusal grooves should be maintained in the preparation. They provide antirotational effect, increase surface area for added retention and give good anatomical form and size. They allow a uniform thickness of the finished restoration. If special resistance and retention needs are anticipated, either because of the expected load on the restoration or because of a short, small, or overtapered preparation, auxiliary retention grooves, boxes, or pins may be used. These are positioned in the preparation to resist the anticipated functional loads. Grooves and boxes are usually recorded accurately with any final impression procedure. If pin holes are made in the preparation, special impression techniques are required to properly record them and ensure their desired effect.

Parallelism, length, and surface area are primary factors in retention and resistance form.[2] Parallelism is the factor that receives the greatest attention as the taper of the preparation is more under the control of the operator than the surface area and length of the teeth. The degree of taper and its effect on retention has been widely researched and published in the dental literature. These studies have ranged from laboratory bench studies with precise and controlled conditions[3, 4] to measuring the taper of dies sent to commercial dental laboratories for fabrication of fixed restorations.[5] This study[5] concluded that, even though recommended taper of prepared surfaces and walls range from 2 to 7 degrees, it is difficult to determine visually that a preparation is clinically free of undercuts at less than approximately 17° of taper. This degree of taper, in many instances, results from the need to reduce additional tooth structure to assure a common path of insertion for the fixed partial denture. This degree of taper was judged acceptable by measurements of dies of clinically successful restorations. Another study[6] measured convergence angles of crown preparations on vital and nonvital teeth. Microscopic measurements were made on 190 stone dies; the convergence angles, which seemed to be appropriate for single crowns, varied from 12 to 37 degrees.

This does not mean that all restorations should be prepared with severe tapers. We know that the more parallel the preparation the more retentive it is and that we cannot always accurately predict the maximum load a restoration will be subjected to. Reducing the taper of the preparation reduces the margin of error!

Retention and resistance form is primarily concerned with enabling the restoration to resist the forces placed on it. It must at the same time satisfy additional principles of preparation design, including strengthening remaining tooth structure, satisfying outline form, providing a workable margin design, and sufficient reduction to enable the restoration to resist deformation.[7]

GINGIVAL MARGINS

Two major decisions must be made regarding the gingival margin of every tooth to be prepared for a crown. One is the position of the margin relative to the gingiva. Should it be placed at the crest of the gingiva, subgingivally or supragingivally, and if so, how far? The second decision regards the design or geometry of the margin. This decision usually relates to the type of restoration being fabricated and the materials and techniques being used.

Position of the Gingival Margins

Subgingival margins were once the standard for all full coverage restorations regardless of location in the mouth or conditions present. Most current philosophies agree that supragingival margins are preferred unless there is a reason, on an individual tooth basis, to place a preparation margin subgingivally.

A major reason for this change in philosophy regards periodontial concerns and considerations. Numerous studies have been carried out relative to gingival irritation and inflammation from subgingival crown margins. A study of 66 crowned anterior contralateral teeth with subgingival margins reports significantly more gingival irritation the deeper the margin is placed subgingivally.[8] In addition, the closer the margin to the base of the crevice or the gingival attachment the greater the inflammation. The study[8] recommends the margin be at the crest of the gingiva or only slightly subgingivally if esthetic appearance demands.

Another study[9] is reported where crowns were made on 12 mandibular first molars with half the buccal margin placed supragingivally and half subgingivally. In three of the 12 cases the subgingival margin produced mild inflammation. The two margin placement positions resulted in no difference in sulcus depth, gingival contour, or plaque formation between the halves of the buccal surface of the crowned tooth or with other teeth. The fit and finish of the restoration and the margin was as significant or more significant than the location of the margin.

In addition to periodontal considerations, numerous other advantages occur from supragingival margins. Supragingival margins are easier for the dentist to prepare and examine for accuracy, easier or unnecessary to retract for impression making, easier to fit, finish, and examine accuracy of the restoration margin, and easier to examine at recall. Supragingival margins are easier for the patient to brush, floss, and maintain on a daily basis.

There are, however, reasons that remain for placing crown margins subgingivally. One of major concern to many patients is esthetic appearance. Subgingival margins, especially when a metal collar is used on a porcelain-fused-to-metal restoration, have a better esthetic appearance. The attitudes of patients and dentists of such placement are interesting.[10] In a survey, 83% of the dentists indicated that they analyzed tooth visibility when deciding on esthetic appearance or margin placement. Obviously, if a gingival margin is not visible during speech or laughter, the margin placement is of no esthetic concern. Every dental examination should include a record of the teeth that show gingiva, both maxillary and mandibular, during conversation or laughter. It is interesting to note on this survey[10] that only 64% of the dentists assessed the patient's desires before arriving at their decision about margin placement. Some patients will accept supragingival margins even if they are visible, and many patients will choose the optimum gingival health prognosis of a supragingival margin over the optimum esthetic results of a subgingival margin, if given the choice.

An additional reason for subgingival margin placement is in teeth where caries, restorations, or fractures have extended subgingivally.[11] In most of these cases a supragingival margin would result in a restoration to foundation margin followed by a foundation to tooth margin subgingivally. This is seldom advantageous over a single restoration to tooth margin subgingivally.

Teeth where only insufficient or questionable retention can be gained from supragingival margins may be indicated for subgingival placement. This affords greater length, surface area, and sometimes more parallelism for increased retention. On some such teeth the use of auxiliary retentive grooves, boxes, or pins are an alternative to subgingival margin placement.

Subgingival margin placement may also be indicated where root sensitivity is a major problem. This may only be a temporary solution if gingival recession continues. However, it may well carry the tooth past the acute sensitive period. Cases where cervical erosion is present often need subgingival placement to control continued erosion.

The pros and cons of subgingival versus supragingival margin placement have been discussed thoroughly. No mention has been made of placement at the crest of the free gingiva or equagingivally. This level has been reported as an acceptable location.[8] Regardless of the factors that lead to the final decision of placement the dentist should not forget that the margin does not have to be placed at the same level around the entire circumference of the tooth. If caries or restorations require interproximal subgingival margins, it is not mandatory that facial and lingual margins be placed at that level. Similarly, if facial margins are placed subgingivally for esthetic reasons the lingual margin of that preparation may be held supragingivally if all other requirements for the preparation are satisfied at that level.

Finally, the degree of margin variation from the gingival crest must be emphasized. A gingival margin placed .2 mm supragingivally usually accrues all of the supragingival advantages of a margin placed 2.0 mm supragingivally. Obviously, the closer to the gingival crest the greater the opportunity for maximizing the retention and resistance form of the preparation through greater surface area coverage and greater preparation length. The optimum subgingival placement is no more than half the depth of the sulcus, which is the distance from the free gingival crest to the periodontal attachment. It is widely agreed that the closer the margin encroaches on the periodontal attachment the greater the incidence of irritation and periodontal inflammation.[8]

Design of Gingival Margins

The design of the gingival margin results from the amount and the configuration of the tooth reduction in the margin area (Figs 5–1,A–F). There are varying terminologies that are applied to margins. We will use six basic terms and consider variations and modifications of some of them. They are the feather edge, knife edge, chamfer, bevel, beveled shoulder, and shoulder.

The feather edge margin as diagramed (Fig 5–1,A) is not recommended for any fixed restoration margin. It is the most conservative in terms of tooth reduction but because the tooth reduction is so minimal for such a great distance from the margin it nearly always results in an overcontoured restoration. The convexity of the preparation in the gingival aspect invites opposing undercuts.

The knife edge, chisel, or slip joint preparation is the most conservative preparation that will satisfy the requirements for a cast metal margin (Fig 5–1,B). It provides a distinct junction between prepared and unprepared tooth structure and sufficient axial reduction to provide space for a normally contoured casting. The taper of the walls can be controlled easily for optimum retention. Obviously, the reduction is not adequate for any kind of an esthetic veneered restoration. It is best established with a tapered or pointed diamond cutting instrument.

The chamfer is a versatile margin design (Fig 5–1,C). The light chamfer is only slightly different and slightly more severe than the knife edge and is an ideal design for metal margins. A heavy chamfer is adequate for porcelain-fused-to-metal restorations with a thin metal collar. A light chamfer may be established with a flame-shaped diamond whereas a heavy chamfer can best be developed with a rounded end tapered diamond instrument.

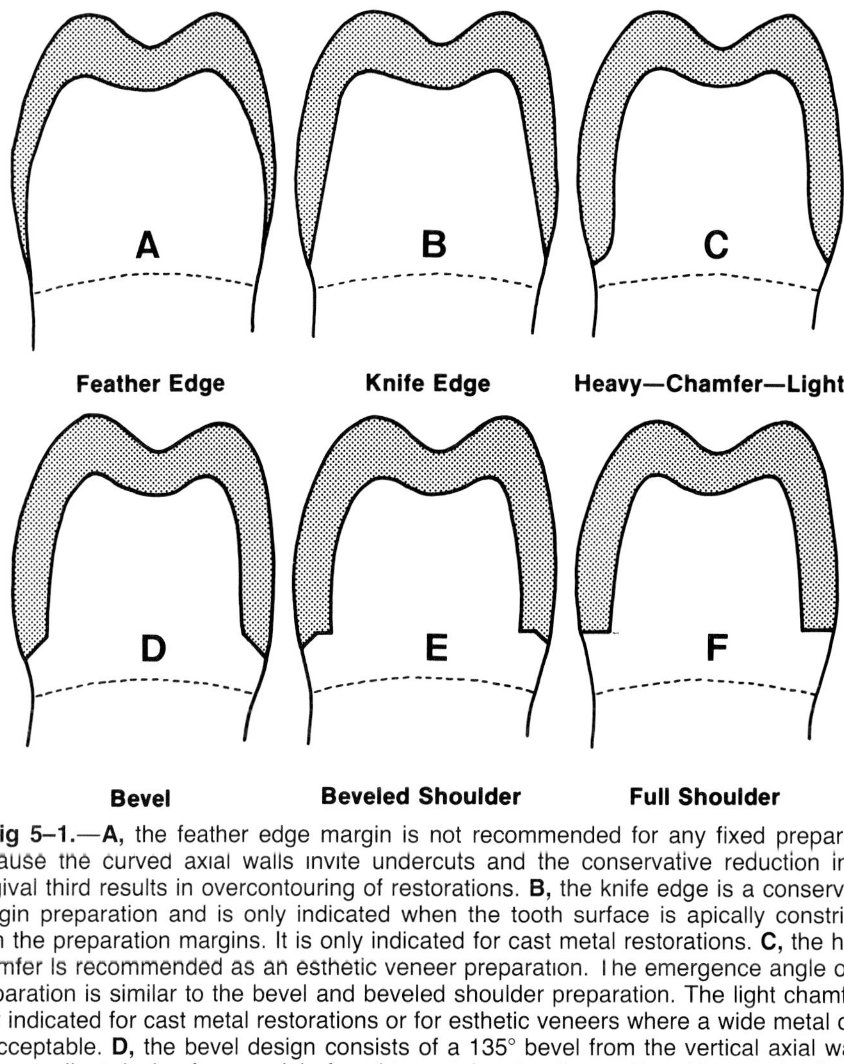

Fig 5–1.—**A,** the feather edge margin is not recommended for any fixed preparation because the curved axial walls invite undercuts and the conservative reduction in the gingival third results in overcontouring of restorations. **B,** the knife edge is a conservative margin preparation and is only indicated when the tooth surface is apically constricting from the preparation margins. It is only indicated for cast metal restorations. **C,** the heavy chamfer is recommended as an esthetic veneer preparation. The emergence angle of the preparation is similar to the bevel and beveled shoulder preparation. The light chamfer is only indicated for cast metal restorations or for esthetic veneers where a wide metal collar is acceptable. **D,** the bevel design consists of a 135° bevel from the vertical axial wall. It is an excellent design for porcelain-fused-to-metal restorations with a thin metal collar and is also indicated for full cast restorations. **E,** the beveled shoulder is an ideal design for esthetic veneer preparations. The bevel is at a 45° angle from the horizontal shoulder and allows a thin metal collar on porcelain-fused-to-metal units. Its double angular design allows optimum resistance to metal distortion during firing. The preparation is also recommended for cast metal restorations. **F,** the shoulder preparation is not generally recommended for full cast restorations or porcelain-fused-to-metal restorations. Some dentists do use the design for full cast crowns as well as porcelain-fused-to-metal with a full porcelain shoulder on the facial. The design is necessary for porcelain jacket crowns including twinfoil restorations. It is also recommended for the Cerestore crown—the latest development in porcelain restorations.

The bevel preparation (Fig 5–1,D) is made at a 135° angle from the vertical axial wall.[12] This results in the same emergence angle as the beveled shoulder. The shoulder is 90° from the vertical and the bevel is an additional 45°. This preparation is recommended for esthetic veneers and provides an angular stiffening of the casting that assures more resistance to distortion during firing than the chamfer.

The beveled shoulder, along with the bevel, is perhaps the most popular and best margin design for porcelain-fused-to-metal restorations with a metal collar (Fig 5–1,E). The shoulder aspect of the preparation provides the reduction necessary for an esthetic veneer. The beveled aspect provides for a thin metal collar that may be placed subgingivally for a good esthetic appearance. The bevel provides an angled marginal fit to tooth structure that, with most techniques, results in a better marginal fit than a butt joint relationship. The double angular nature of the preparation margin imparts rigidity to the metal coping and optimum resistance to distortion of the coping during porcelain firing procedures. The beveled shoulder design is also recommended for full cast restorations.[13]

The shoulder preparation is recommended for all porcelain jacket crown restorations (Fig 5–1,F). Porcelain strength at the margin is increased with bulk. Thin edges of procelain on bevels in this margin area will not withstand the functional stresses.

There is considerable discussion in the literature about the merits of the slip joint versus the butt joint regarding the accuracy of the casting to tooth relationships or the marginal fit. A slip joint margin, such as that accruing from a knife edge margin design results in the most geometrically predictably accurate fit.[14] Other studies[15] report the most accurate marginal fit with a shoulder preparation and a slightly over-sized casting. A variation in the casting technique may then reduce the geometrical advantages of a beveled margin.[16]

The geometrical advantage of a beveled margin does not become clinically significant until it reaches a 70–80-degree angle from the horizontal.[12] Hence, beveled margins of 30–45 degrees do not provide significantly better marginal fits than a full shoulder but they may provide a better fit resulting from angular reinforcement of the coping to resist distortion during firing of porcelain fused to metal units, and provide for a metal collar that may be helpful in fitting and finishing the margin.

Many factors are involved in marginal fit accuracy. In addition to margin design, the expansion factors of die stone, wax, investment, and casting metals have a significant influence on the resultant marginal fit. In fact, these factors may have a greater effect on the clinical result than the variation in finish lines.[14]

PRINCIPLES OF TOOTH REDUCTION

Careful attention must be given to the preparation of teeth for fixed restorations. Because of the volume of tooth structure being removed, cutting with the aid of a water spray is mandatory. The spray acts as a coolant for vital teeth and as a lubricant for the cutting instrument. Hence, the water spray is recommended for nonvital and vital teeth. The water lubricated cutting instrument, diamond or carbide, will cut faster and more efficiently and will have a longer life than when cutting is done dry.

The diamond cutting instrument is used for most fixed preparations. They cut rapidly and efficiently and are available in a variety of sizes, shapes, and grits to meet individual preferences and choices. Some operators prefer carbide instruments, especially for finalizing margins and sometimes for partial veneer crown preparations.[17]

Tooth preparation for fixed restorations must be done systematically for operator efficiency and to secure the optimum final preparation. This involves a set series of

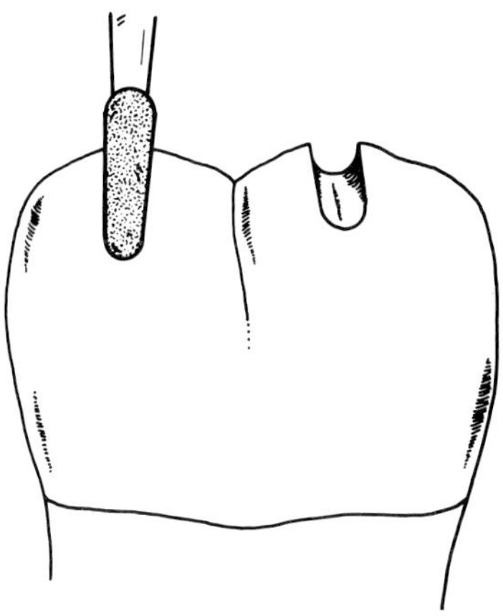

Fig 5–2.—The reduction for the full cast crown preparation is begun by establishing depth guide grooves of one to one and a half mm in depth on the functioning cusps with a diamond cylinder.

steps for each preparation. Such a system reduces oversights relative to taper, occlusal clearance, line of draw, and preparation contour in the preparation design.

The most popular step sequence for full cast crown preparation is occlusal reduction, axial surface reduction, rounding of line angles, rounding of occlusoaxial angles, finalizing gingival margin geometry, finalizing cavosurface margins, and contouring and smoothing preparation. The first two reductions are easily interchanged to satisfy individual operator preferences. Each operator should decide on step sequencing preferences and follow them routinely for optimum results and maximum efficiency.

The following is a discussion of the more common individual crown and abutment retainer designs used in fixed restorations.

Full Cast Metal Crown

The full cast crown (Figs 5–2 to 5–9) is the strongest, most durable, and most retentive and resistant fixed restoration.[18] Porcelain-fused-to-metal crowns have the same retention and resistance but porcelain is susceptible to fracture. All partial veneers have significantly less retention and resistance given the same ideal taper and groove design. Addition of grooves or boxes to full crown preparations and

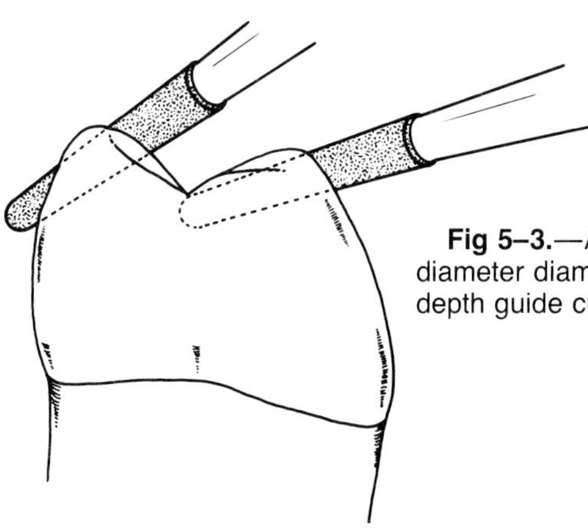

Fig 5–3.—A cross-sectional view of a 1 mm diameter diamond illustrates the desired depth of all depth guide cuts.

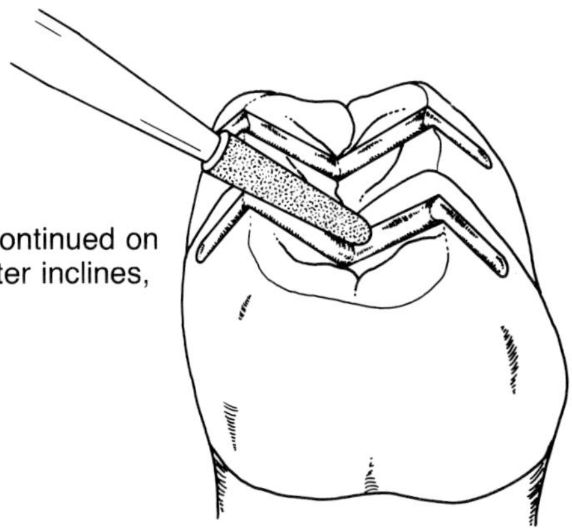

Fig 5–4.—The depth guide grooves are continued on the nonfunctioning cusps, both inner and outer inclines, and are added to the grooves, if desired.

gingival extension of the margin of the preparation produce small increases in retention but significant increases in resistance values.[18] Addition of grooves can adversely effect the full seating of cast crowns and further complicate cementation by increasing hydrodynamics.[19]

It must be remembered that there is always more than one factor involved in the retention and resistance of a restoration. If the tooth is short, special attention must be given to the taper, or the margin must be carried subgingivally or grooves added. At least some of the retentive factors must be optimized.

Three Quarter Crown

Three-quarter crowns are the most commonly used partial veneer crown. The preparation is adaptable to both anterior and posterior teeth (Figs 5–10 to 5–21). They are most ideally suited for virgin teeth that are being prepared for fixed partial denture abutments. Teeth that are involved with prior caries, restorations, or fractures can affect the esthetic appearance of the three-quarter crown and may also significantly reduce the retention and resistance form that could be attained. Frequently, preparation modifications can be made to overcome these disadvantages.[20] The groove system is important in making the casting attain the required structural

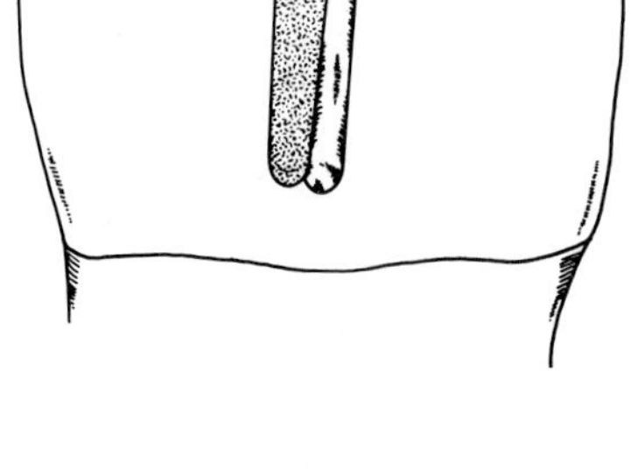

Fig 5–5.—The reduction in the buccal and lingual grooves is also established at this time, as maintaining their depth and position in the preparation is extremely important in assuring the proper anatomy and contour of the finished crown.

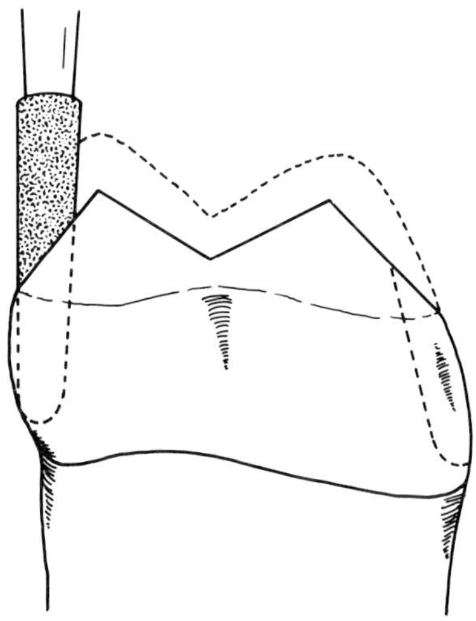

Fig 5–6.—After the buccal and lingual groove reduction is completed the same diamond is used to continue the reduction of the occlusal surface and the axial surfaces to the depth of the guide grooves.

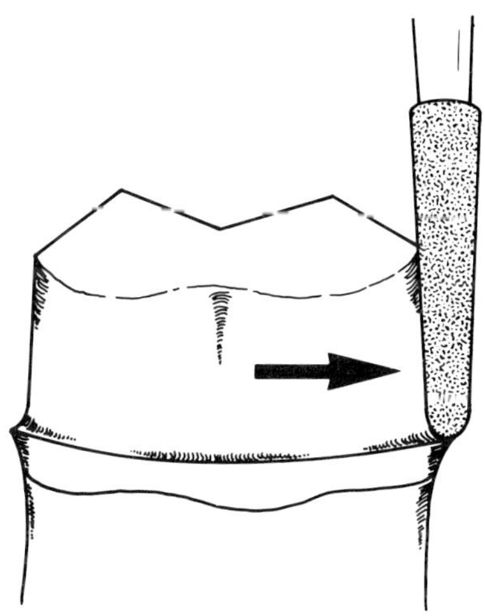

Fig 5–7.—The axial surface reduction is completed to establish a chamfer. Depending on tooth size and other factors a smaller diameter diamond may be selected for interproximal reduction.

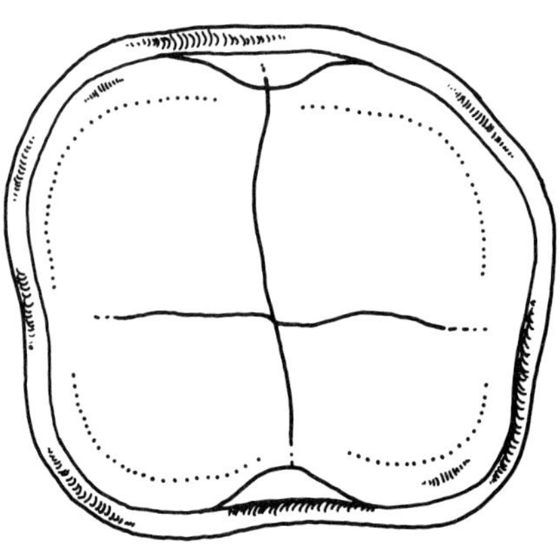

Fig 5–8.—The occlusal view of the preparation at this point should show a definite chamfer around the entire circumference. The occlusal grooves, cusps, and buccal and lingual grooves should be maintained, thus leaving the prepared tooth as a miniature of the original anatomy.

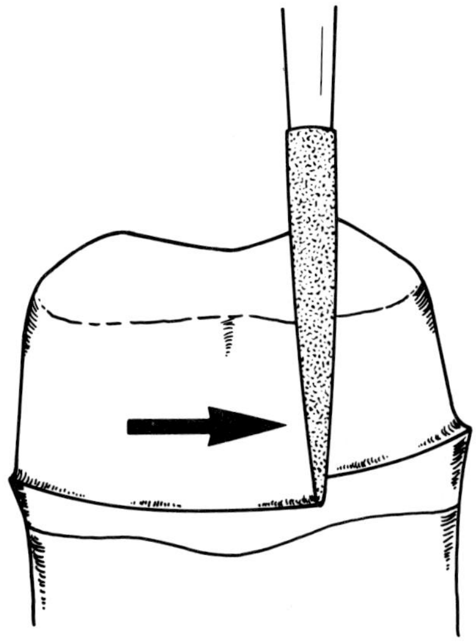

Fig 5–9.—The gingival margin is established to the desired chamfer or knife edge and to the desired position relative to the gingiva. Any remaining sharp areas on line angles, occlusoaxial angles, marginal ridges, or cusp tips are rounded and smoothed. This helps to reduce dimensional errors in the numerous materials and steps used in the fabrication of the restoration from impression to finished product.

strength. Proximal grooves that are joined with occlusal or incisal grooves form a continuous horseshoe or staple that greatly increases the strength of the casting. The resistance to deformation or spreading at the gingival margins under functional loading is also enhanced.

Three-quarter crowns are commonly considered to be more difficult to prepare than full coverage crowns. A major factor in this conception is that the operator usually has less experience in three-quarter crown preparations and thus less confidence in making the preparation. With proper case selection the three-quarter

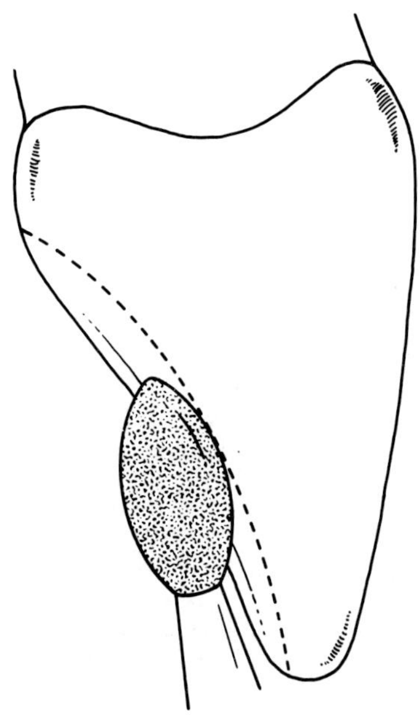

Fig 5–10.—The lingual reduction for an anterior three-quarter crown preparation is done with a football-shaped lingual contouring diamond. The prepared surface should clear the opposing teeth by a half to 1 mm.

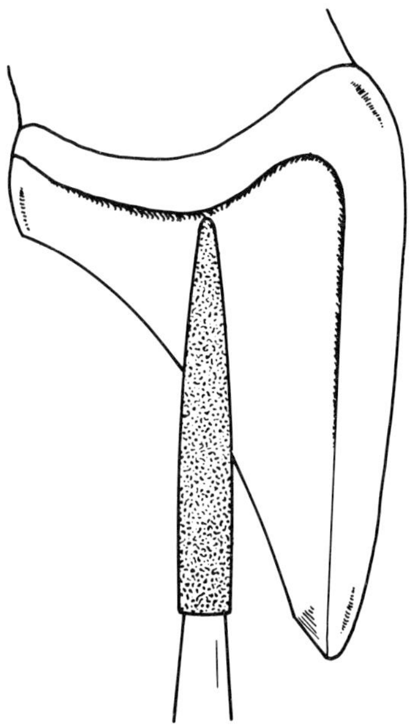

Fig 5–11.—The proximal surfaces and cingulum are prepared with a tapered, flame-shaped diamond. The facial outline form is established parallel to the incisal two-thirds of the facial surface.

crown is not difficult. Badly broken down teeth should be avoided. Short posterior teeth are contraindicated as are short or thin anterior teeth. With proper case selection both esthetic and mechanical requirements can be met quite adequately.

Porcelain-fused-to-metal Crowns

The porcelain-fused-to-metal restoration, both as a retainer and as an individual unit, is now the esthetic restoration used by the vast majority of dentists (Figs 5

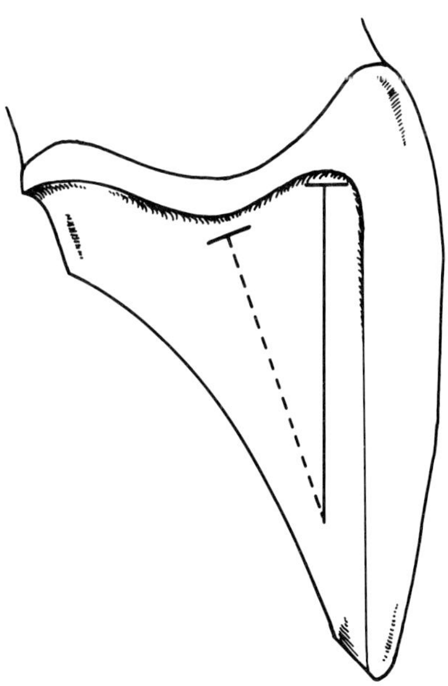

Fig 5–12.—The proximal groove is started parallel to the incisal two-thirds of the facial surface. If the groove were placed in the long axis of the tooth as indicated by the broken line, it would be much shorter. This would reduce its retention and leave less tooth structure lingual to the groove reducing its resistance form.

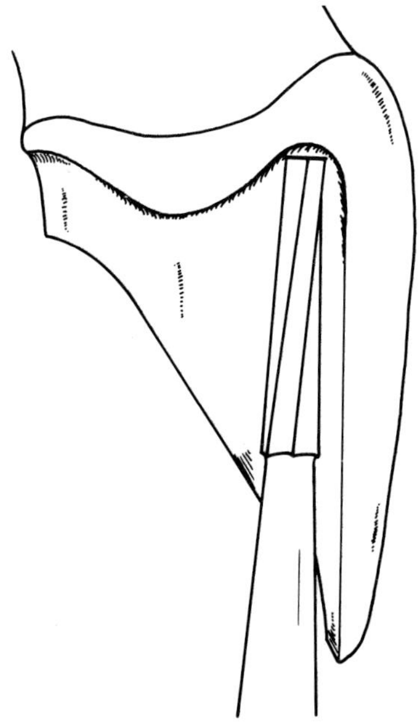

Fig 5–13.—The proximal groove is finished with a tapered fissure bur slightly short of the proximal reduction and parallel to the incisal two-thirds of the facial surface.

22 to 5–30). There is a limited use of acrylic as a veneer material, but it has nearly been replaced by porcelain.

The preparation features that are most important are, first, the adequate reduction of the facial surface to allow sufficient space for metal and porcelain, and, second, the geometry of the facial gingival margin. This casting margin tends to distort during the porcelain firing process if it is not properly designed. This distortion, which takes place more easily as the temperature of the metal rises to

Fig 5–14.—The incisal groove is established with an inverted cone bur. The depth of the incisal groove is prepared continuous with the proximal grooves to maximize casting rigidity. A cingulum ledge may be prepared with a pinhole parallel to the proximal groove if additional retention and resistance form is needed.

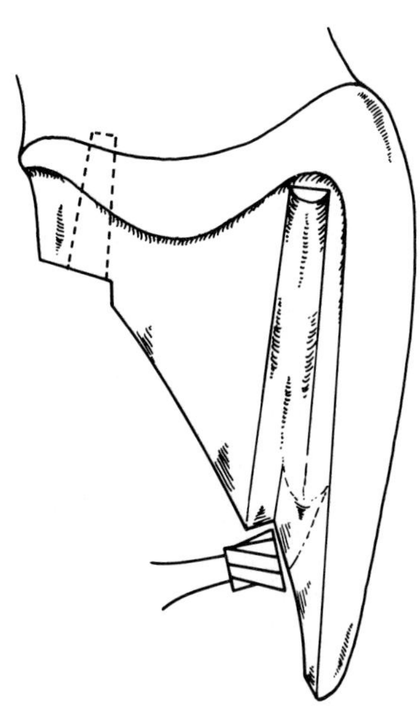

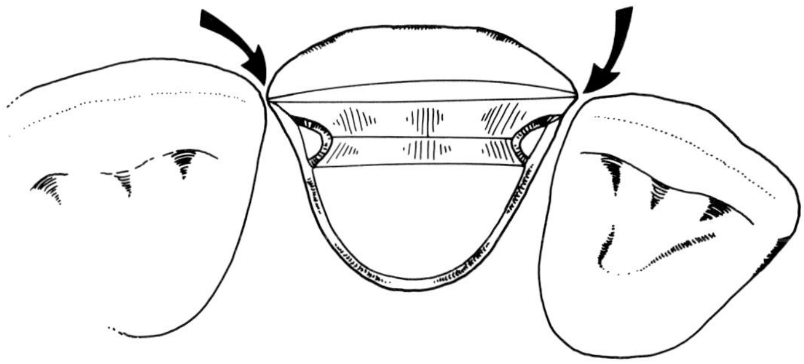

Fig 5–15.—The facial proximal extension is determined by esthetic appearance requirements. The proximal grooves should be deep enough to provide resistance to lingual displacement. The incisal groove should be definite and continuous with the proximal grooves.

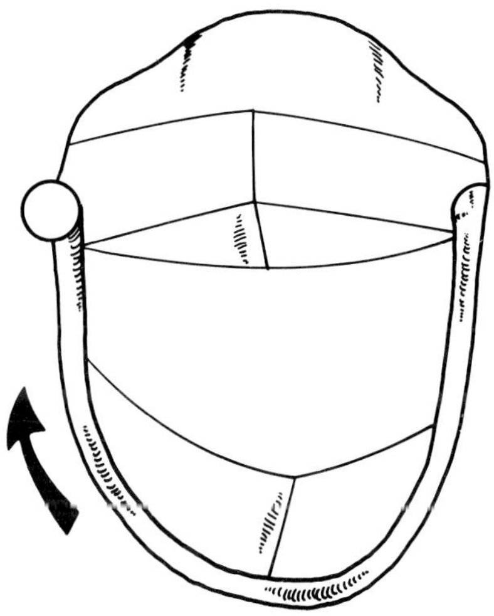

Fig 5–16.—After occlusal clearance, the proximal and lingual reduction of the premolar three-quarter crown preparation is accomplished with a tapered, flame-shaped diamond.

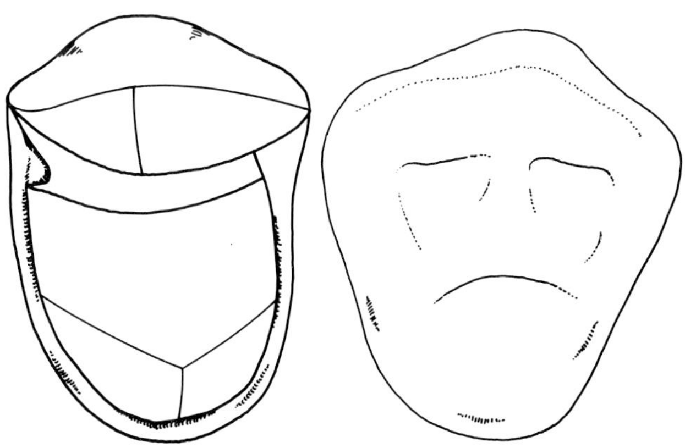

Fig 5–17.—The desired proximal preparation design is established. Two designs are illustrated. The two may be used together as shown or the same design may be used for both grooves. The mesial preparation establishes a somewhat triangular gingival seat that, along with the buccal wall, resembles the buccal portion of an MOD inlay preparation. This blends to a full crown design preparation at the lingual line angle. The buccal extension on the mesial is an important esthetic consideration. The distal preparation is the conventional definite groove design.

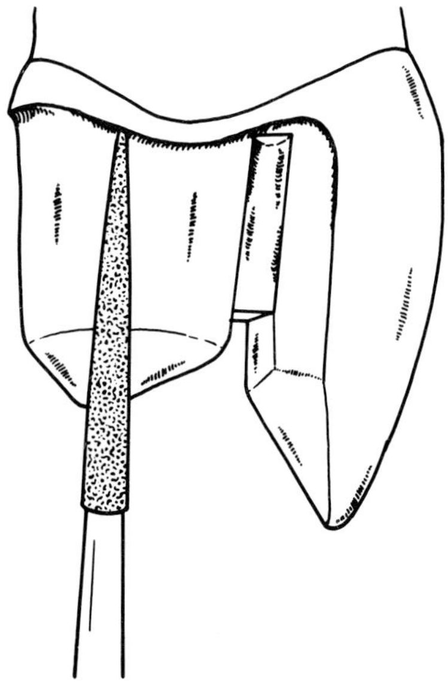

Fig 5–18.—When a definite proximal groove is used an occlusal groove is recommended to stiffen the casting and increase retention and resistance form. The flame-shaped diamond is used to establish the gingival margin.

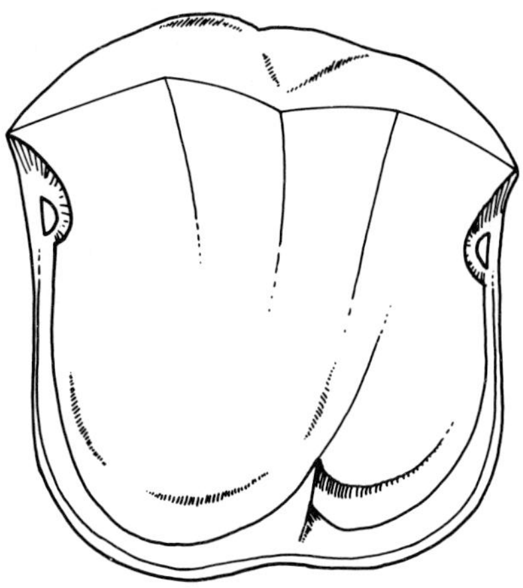

Fig 5–19.—The molar three-quarter crown preparation is similar to the premolar preparation. Proximal grooves may be used on intact teeth.

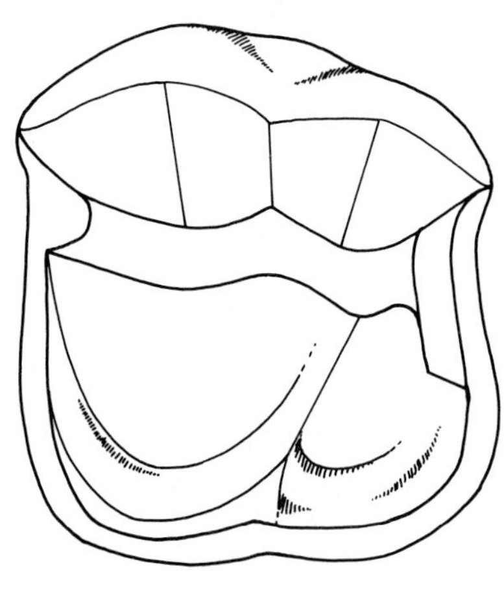

Fig 5–20.—When there are existing proximal caries or Class II restorations, the groove may be replaced with a box preparation.

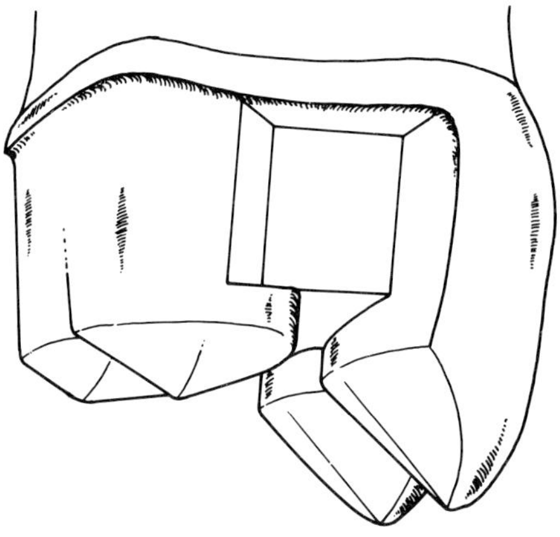

Fig 5–21.—The proximal box preparation resembles a Class II inlay proximal preparation design. An occlusal groove preparation is important to any three-quarter crown preparation.

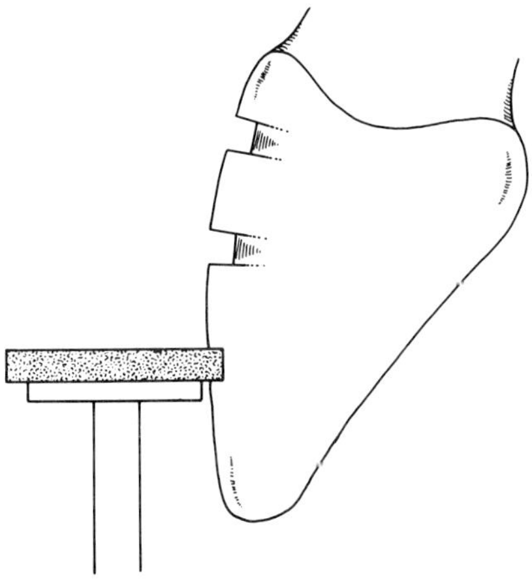

Fig 5–22.—A 1 mm depth gauge diamond wheel is used to channel the facial surface of the tooth for a porcelain-fused-to-metal preparation. The cuts are made in the gingival, middle, and incisal third of the tooth. This assures the uniform removal of more than 1 mm of tooth structure when the facial surface is reduced to eliminate the channels.

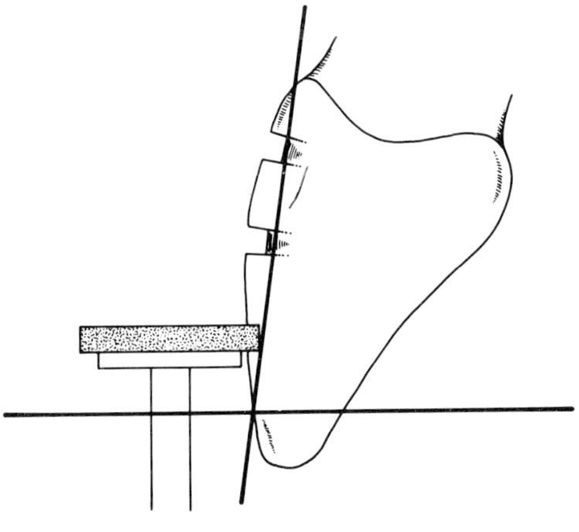

Fig 5–23.—The straight lines illustrate the effect of reducing the facial and incisal in flat planes. Even with the middle third of the surface overreduced the labioincisal angle has no reduction and the gingival margin reduction is insufficient. This emphasizes the importance of uniform labial reduction to the same curvature as the natural tooth.

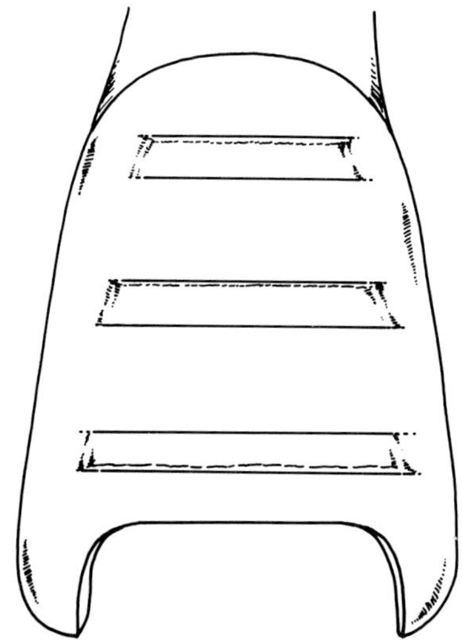

Fig 5–24.—After labial channeling the incisal edge is reduced approximately 2 mm leaving the incisal angles intact as a gauge.

within a few hundred degrees of its melting point, results in marginal fit discrepancies. Thickness of metal and/or angulation or shape of the metal in this area imparts the needed resistance to distortion.[13]

A butt joint porcelain to prepared tooth junction may be designed. The more popular design involves an exposed subgingival thin metal collar. Properly fabricated, this provides the best marginal fit and restoration-to-tooth contour. Metal rigidity can be attained with several margin designs. These include the shoulder, heavy chamfer, beveled shoulder, and 135° bevel, which has the same emergence angle as a shoulder with a 45° bevel. Any of these designs can provide adequate metal for strength, provided there is adequate depth of tooth structure removed

Fig 5–25.—A round-end tapered diamond is used to reduce the facial surface, thereby eliminating the channels. The labial curvature is maintained with special care for adequate reduction at the labioincisal angle and at the gingival margin.

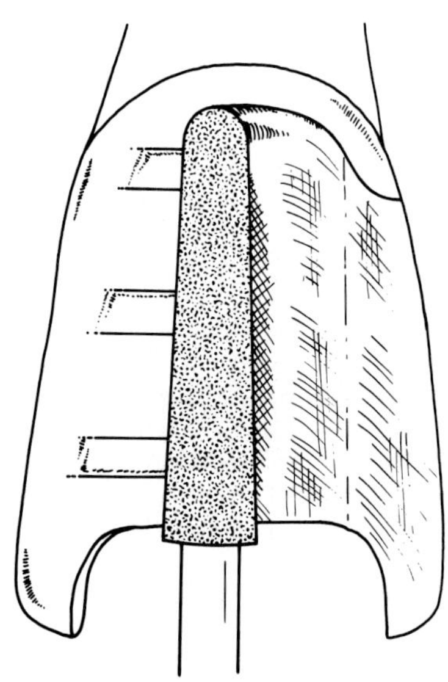

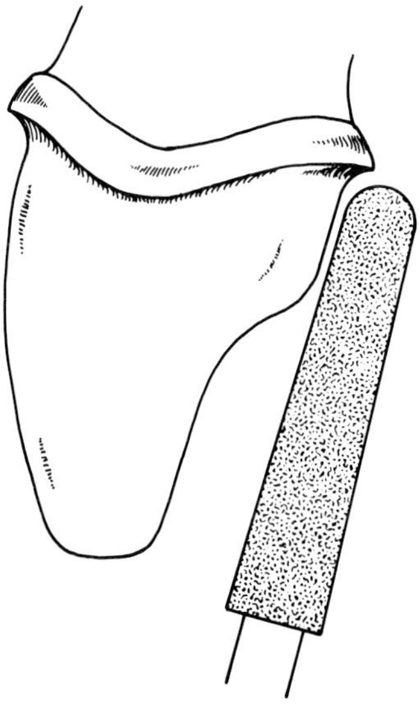

Fig 5–26.—The same diamond is used to prepare the cingulum. With smaller teeth is may be necessary to use a smaller diameter diamond for the reduction of the proximal surfaces.

in the preparation. If esthetic appearance is important in the gingival region, the gross preparation reduction must be carried subgingivally. Extremely long bevels in the 70° range are counterproductive with porcelain-fused-to-metal though they may be effective for the full cast restorations. They are susceptable to distortion during firing and result in a much wider metal collar that requires a deeper sulcular margin or a compromise of the esthetic appearance with an exposed gingival collar.

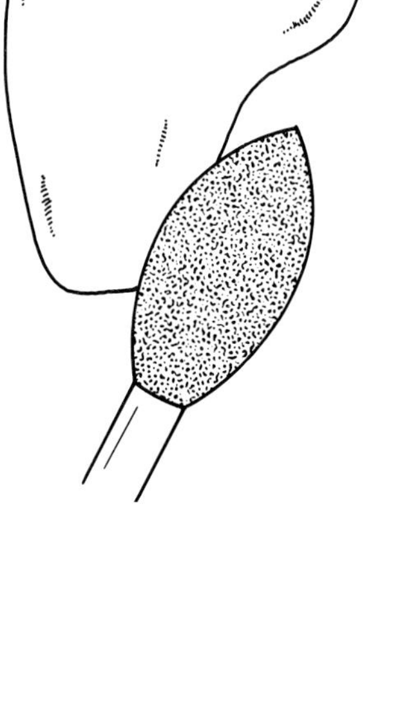

Fig 5–27.—The lingual contouring diamond is used for lingual reduction. Half to 1 mm of lingual clearance is mandatory.

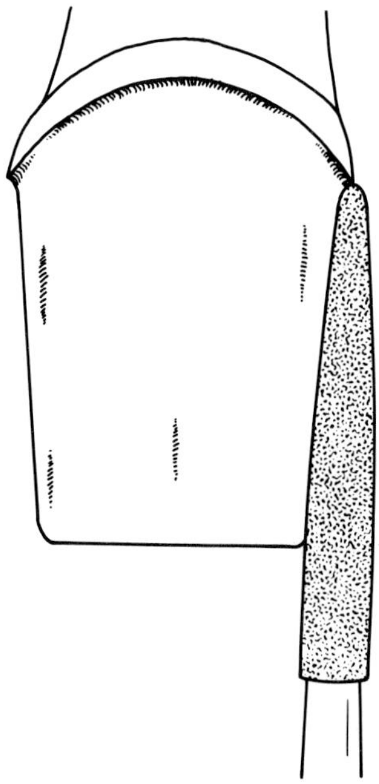

Fig 5–28.—The smaller diameter flame-shaped diamond may be used to establish a light chamfer on the proximal. It provides a greater margin of safety from damaging contacts of adjacent teeth and over-preparing or over-tapering the proximal surfaces.

RESTORATION DESIGN MODIFICATIONS

Restoration design modifications are limited only by the imagination of the operator. Three commonly used modifications are the seven-eighths crown, mesial half crown, and MOD onlay.

Seven-eighths crowns are usually applicable only to maxillary first molars where the esthetic appearance of the mesiobuccal surface is important and when that cusp

Fig 5–29.—The flame-shaped diamond can be used to finalize the position of the gingival margin with minimal abrasion of gingival tissue. A fine grit diamond is usually preferred for this reduction.

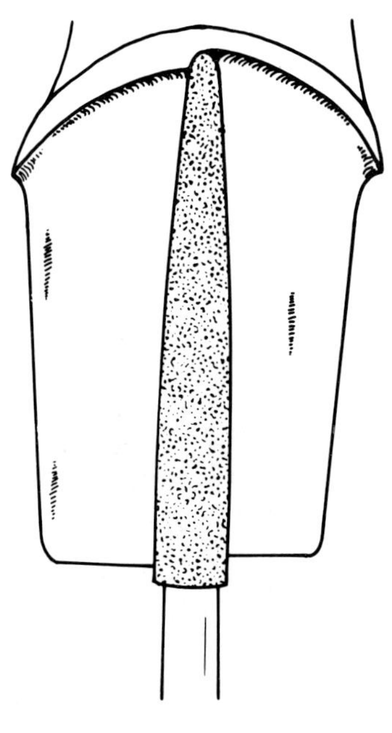

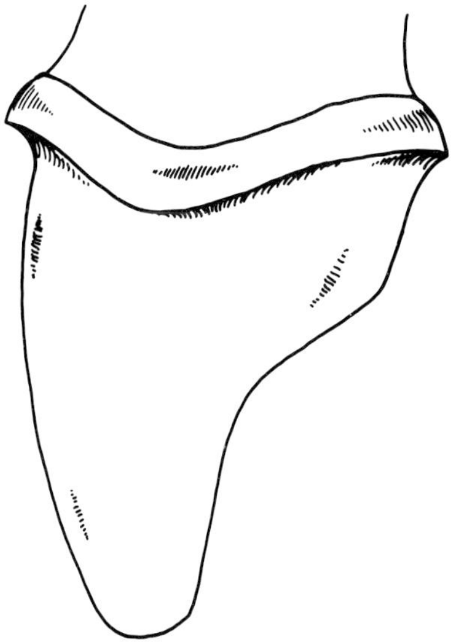

Fig 5–30.—The finished preparation on the labial shows a heavy chamfer with a sharper emergence angle, whereas the lingual reduction illustrates a light chamfer.

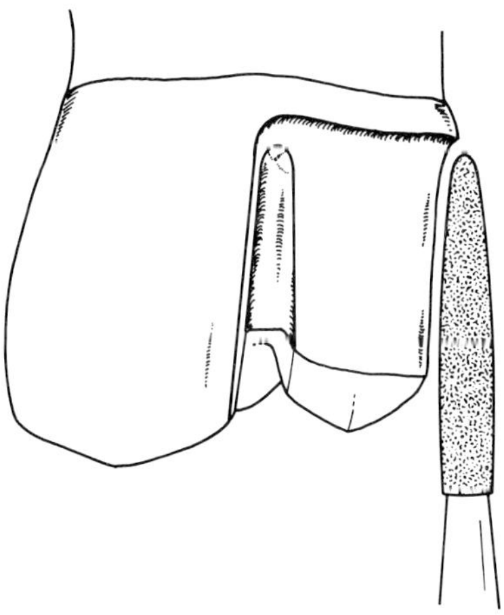

Fig 5–31.—The seven-eighths crown is prepared on the distal the same as a full crown. The buccal groove is deepened on the buccal surface. The buccal groove is carried into the occlusal groove.

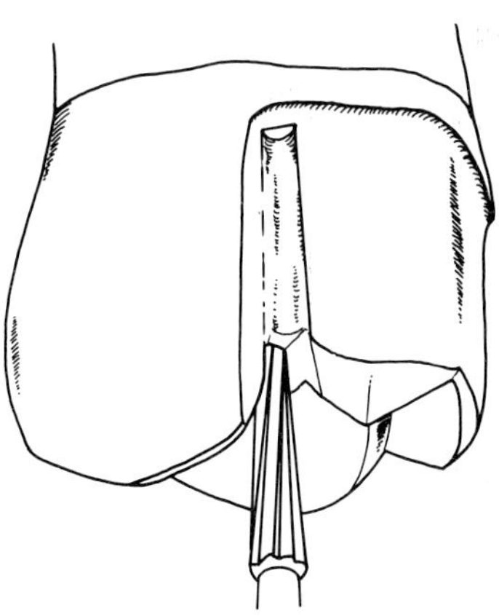

Fig 5–32.—The buccal groove is prepared with a fissure bur to definite retention and resistance form. The definite groove system is extended to the occlusal surface.

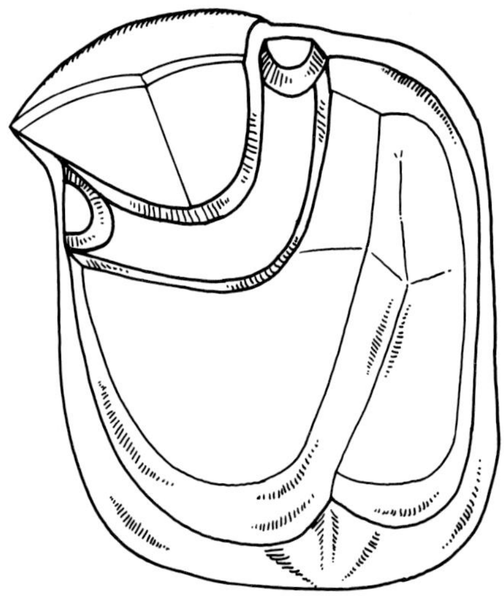

Fig 5–33.—The occlusal view of the finished seven-eighths crown preparation shows the definite buccal and mesial grooves with the occlusal groove preparation connecting the two. The distal and lingual reduction is the same as for a full cast crown. The buccal cusp is capped to protect it from fracture during the occlusal loading.

is intact and not undermined by caries (Figs 5–31 to 5–33). It can be used as an individual restoration or as a retainer. A preparation design of a full cast crown on the distal combined with a three-quarter crown mesial preparation and a three-quarter crown type groove on the buccal results in a retentive and esthetically pleasing restoration.

The mesial half crown (Fig 5–34) is an especially useful design modification for mesially inclined mandibular molars that are being prepared as fixed partial denture abutments. This is especially true if the second molar is present and the distal of the first molar is noncarious and nonrestored. The mesial surface of the first molar is prepared with a full cast crown design to a common line of draw with the pre-molar preparation. Three-quarter crown design grooves are placed on the buccal and lingual surfaces of the inclined molar to the same line of draw. The remainder

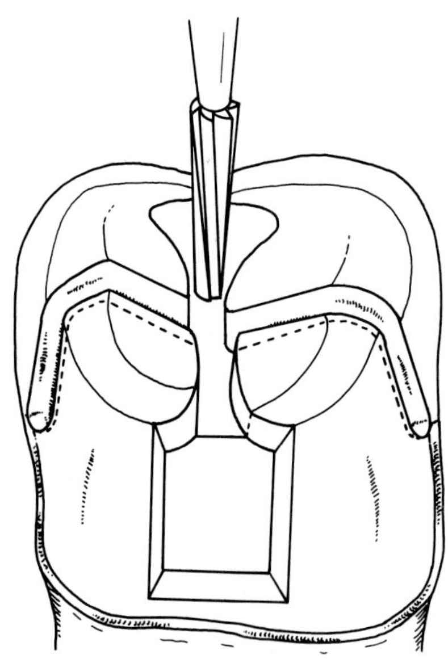

Fig 5–34.—The mesial half crown incorporates an inlay type box preparation on the mesial with three-quarter crown type retentive grooves on the buccal and lingual. The occlusal is reduced on the distal half to cap both distal cusps. A definite occlusal groove preparation is made including a distal occlusal dovetail for retention and resistance.

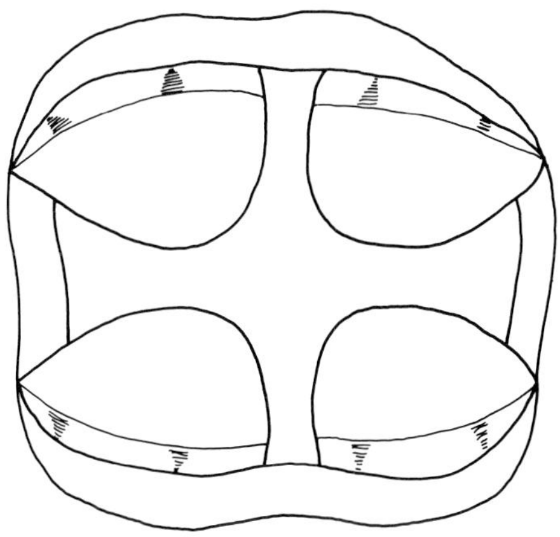

Fig 5–35.—The onlay preparation is the least retentive of the preparations discussed. Its only axial retention is from the proximal box preparations. There is no buccal or lingual axial retention. The deeper and more precise the occlusal groove pattern, the more retentive will be the casting.

of the occlusal surface is reduced to allow full occlusal coverage to resist masticating forces. The distal margin can be held occlusally to the proximal contact with the second molar because the tipping usually results in the contact between the two molars moving gingivally. The mesial proximal box is then added along with the distal occlusal dovetail for increased resistance and retention form.

The MOD onlay preparation (Fig 5–35) is most indicated for individual restorations where the plane of occlusion or the occlusal scheme is being altered. The preparation combines the box type three-quarter crown preparation on the proximals with a heavier occlusal channel and heavier occlusal capping of all cusps. The major difference in this design from the three-quarter crown is that the lingual surface of the preparation is not carried gingivally. This results in a staple design casting. The restoration may be used as a fixed retainer but is contraindicated if heavy occlusal loading is anticipated as it is more susceptible to flexing than the three-quarter crown.

REFERENCES

1. Gilboe D.B., Teteruck W.R.: Fundamentals of extracoronal tooth preparation. Part I. Retention and resistance form. *J. Prosthet. Dent.* 32:651, 1974.
2. Eames W.B., et al.: Techniques to improve the seating of castings. *J. Am. Dent. Assoc.* 96:432, 1978.
3. Abdullah S.I., Mohammed H., Thayer K.E.: Factors in the failure of cemented full crowns. *J. Can. Dent. Assoc.* 40:721, 1974.
4. Woolsey G.D., Matich J.A.: The effect of axial grooves on the resistance form of cast restorations. *J. Am. Dent. Assoc.* 97:978, 1978.
5. Mack P.J.: A theoretical and clinical investigation into the taper achieved on crown and inlay preparations. *J. Oral Rehabil.* 7:255, 1980.
6. Ohm E., Silness J.: The convergence angle in teeth prepared for artificial crowns. *J. Oral. Rehabil.* 5:371, 1978.
7. Douglass G.D.: Principles of preparation design in fixed prosthodontics. *J. Acad. Gen. Dent.* 21:25, 1973.
8. Newcomb G.M.: The relationship between the location of some gingival crowns margins and gingival inflammation. *J. Periodontol.* 45:151, 1974.
9. Richter W.A., Oeno H.: Relationship of crown margin placement to gingival inflammation. *J. Prosthet. Dent.* 30:156, 1973.
10. Watson J.F., Chrispin B.J.: Margin placement of esthetic veneer crown. Part III. Attitudes of patients and dentists. *J. Pros. Dent.* 45:499, 1981.

11. Berman M.H.: The complete coverage restoration and the gingival sulcus. *J. Prosthet. Dent.* 29:301, 1973.
12. McLean J.W., Wilson A.D.: Butt joint versus beveled gold margin in metalceramic crowns. *J. Biomed. Mater. Res.* 14:239, 1980.
13. Gilboe D.B., Thayer K.E.: Beveled shoulder concept: Full gold crown preparation. *J. Can. Dent. Assoc.* 46:519, 1980.
14. Gavelis J.R., et al.: The effect of various finish line preparations on the marginal seal and occlusal seat of full crown preparations. *J. Prosthet. Dent.* 45:138, 1981.
15. Pascoe D.F.: Analysis of the geometry of finishing lines for full crown restorations. *J. Prosthet. Dent.* 40:157, 1978.
16. Rosenstiel E.: To bevel or not to bevel? *Br. Dent. J.* 138:389, 1975.
17. Lustig L.P., et al.: A rational concept of crown preparation. *Quint. Int.* 3:35, 1972.
18. Pots R.G., Schillingburg H.T., Duncanson M.G., Jr.: Retention and resistance of preparations for cast restorations. *J. Prosthet. Dent.* 43:303, 1980.
19. Tjan A.H., Sarkissian R., Miller G.D.: Effect of multiple axial grooves on the marginal adaptation of full cast gold crowns. *J. Prosthet. Dent.* 46:399, 1981.
20. Tjan, A.H., Miller, G.D.: Biogeometric guide to groove placement on three-quarter crown preparations. *J. Prosthet. Dent.* 42:405, 1979.

CHAPTER 6

Porcelain-Fused-to-Metal Restorations

ROBERT J. CONNOR, D.D.S.

THE PREPARATION of a tooth that will receive a ceramo-metal restoration differs little from preparations required for other full coverage crowns and fixed partial dentures. The specific metal design and minimal thickness of porcelain are special requirements necessary to obtain good structural and esthetic results. The tooth preparation for porcelain-fused-to-metal crowns is of special interest because this treatment is widely used. The design of the tooth preparation can have a direct correlation with the success of the porcelain-fused-to-metal restoration.

RESTORATION CONSIDERATIONS

The suggested thickness of metal copings is 0.5 mm. This may be reduced to 0.2 mm when it is necessary to provide space for the required thickness of porcelain. The porcelain veneer should have a thickness of 1 mm axially and 1½ mm incisally and occlusally. A greater thickness could result in a structural weakness, and a lesser thickness of porcelain could create problems in obtaining a satisfactory shade.

Axial Designs

Three common problems in the preparation of anterior teeth are:

1. Preparations where the labioincisal area has not been reduced enough. This will result in either an overcontoured crown or poor shade match (Fig 6–1);
2. Preparations with inadequate incisal reduction will result in weakened porcelain and/or poor shade matching (Fig 6–2); and
3. Preparations with inadequate lingual reduction will greatly hinder the technician in achieving proper metal design (Fig 6–3).

Margin Designs

The efforts to provide both strength and a good esthetic appearance have led to the design of several finish lines for the porcelain fused to metal restoration. The labial margin is the area where the most controversy exists because the thickness of the metal is limited by esthetics and because it is the most prone to distortion. These problems are not encountered on the lingual and proximal margins.

The generally accepted labial margin finish lines are the chamfer (Fig 6–4), heavy chamfer with a bevel (Fig 6–5), shoulder (Fig 6–6) and shoulder with a bevel (Fig 6–7).

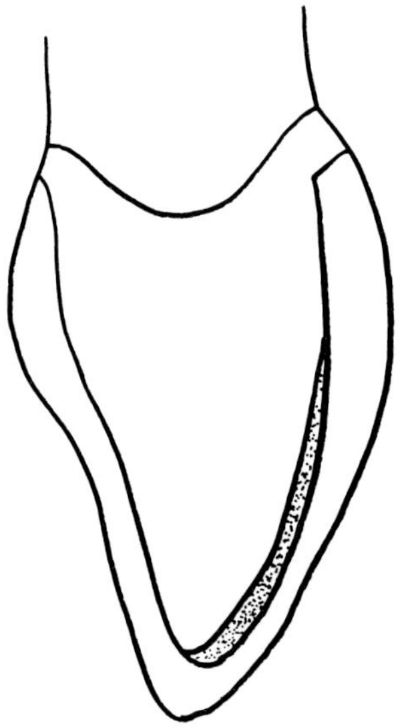

Fig 6–1.—Inadequate labioincisal reduction.

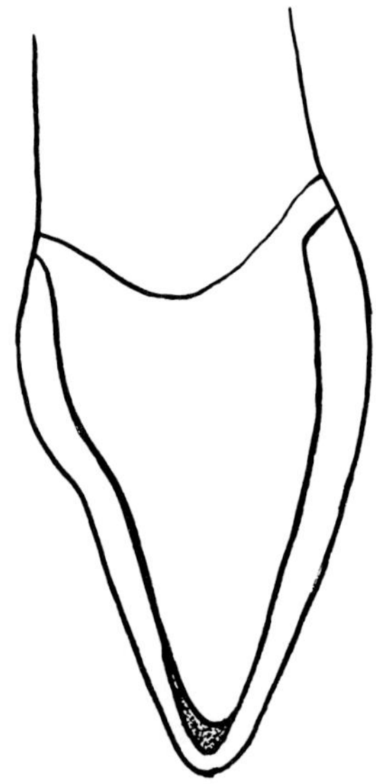

Fig 6–2.—Inadequate incisal reduction.

The chamfer has been used as a finish line for full cast gold and ceramo-metal restorations. Some dentists have advocated a heavy chamfer with a bevel. The shoulder, as used on a porcelain jacket preparation or a shoulder modified with a bevel can also be used. At this time the preparation accepted by the majority of operators is a beveled shoulder on the labial aspect carried interproximally with a chamfered lingual aspect. The beveled shoulder has also been shown to produce the least distortion during the firing cycle.[1]

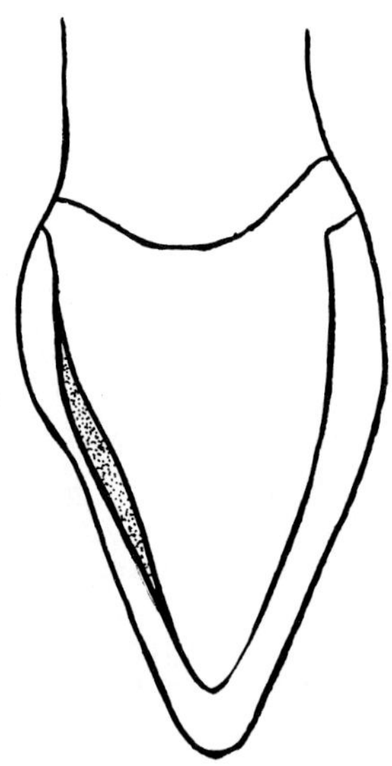

Fig 6–3.—Inadequate lingual reduction.

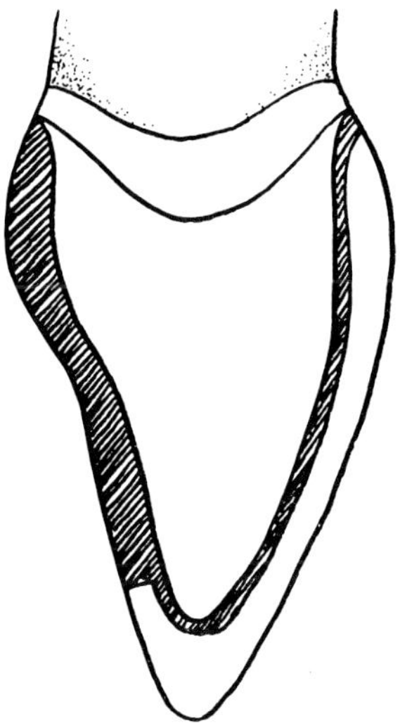

Fig 6–4.—Chamfer.

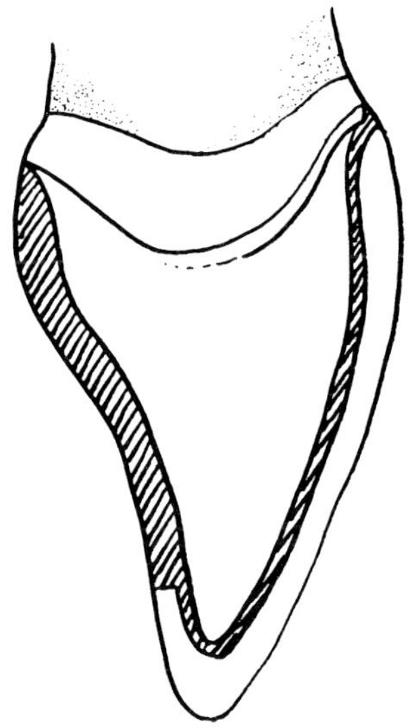

Fig 6–5.—Heavy chamfer with a bevel.

FRAMEWORK DESIGN

Anterior Teeth

The design for anterior porcelain-fused-to-metal substructure can vary considerably and is effected by the relationship of maxillary to mandibular teeth. Full arch models should be articulated and studied to determine the design of the anterior substructure for single or multiple units.

In the design of the anterior ceramo-metal restoration the junction of the porcelain to metal on the lingual surface must not have centric or excursive contact.

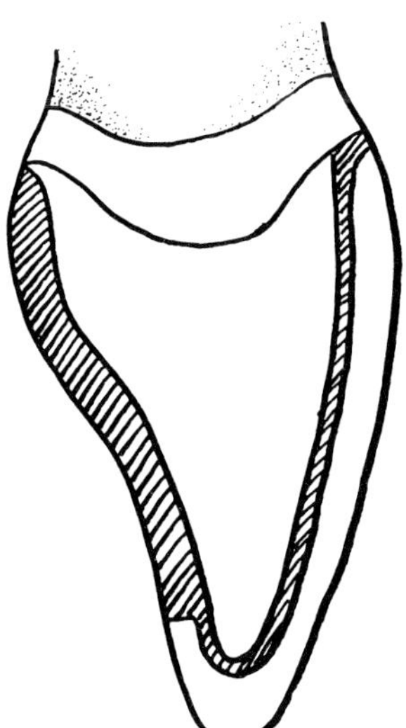

Fig 6–6.—Shoulder.

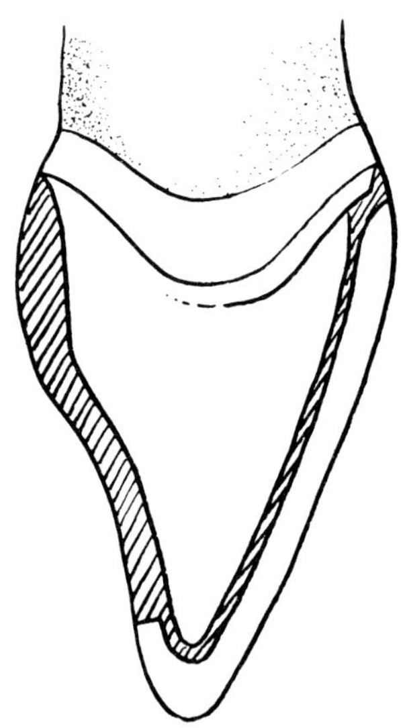

Fig 6–7.—Shoulder with a bevel.

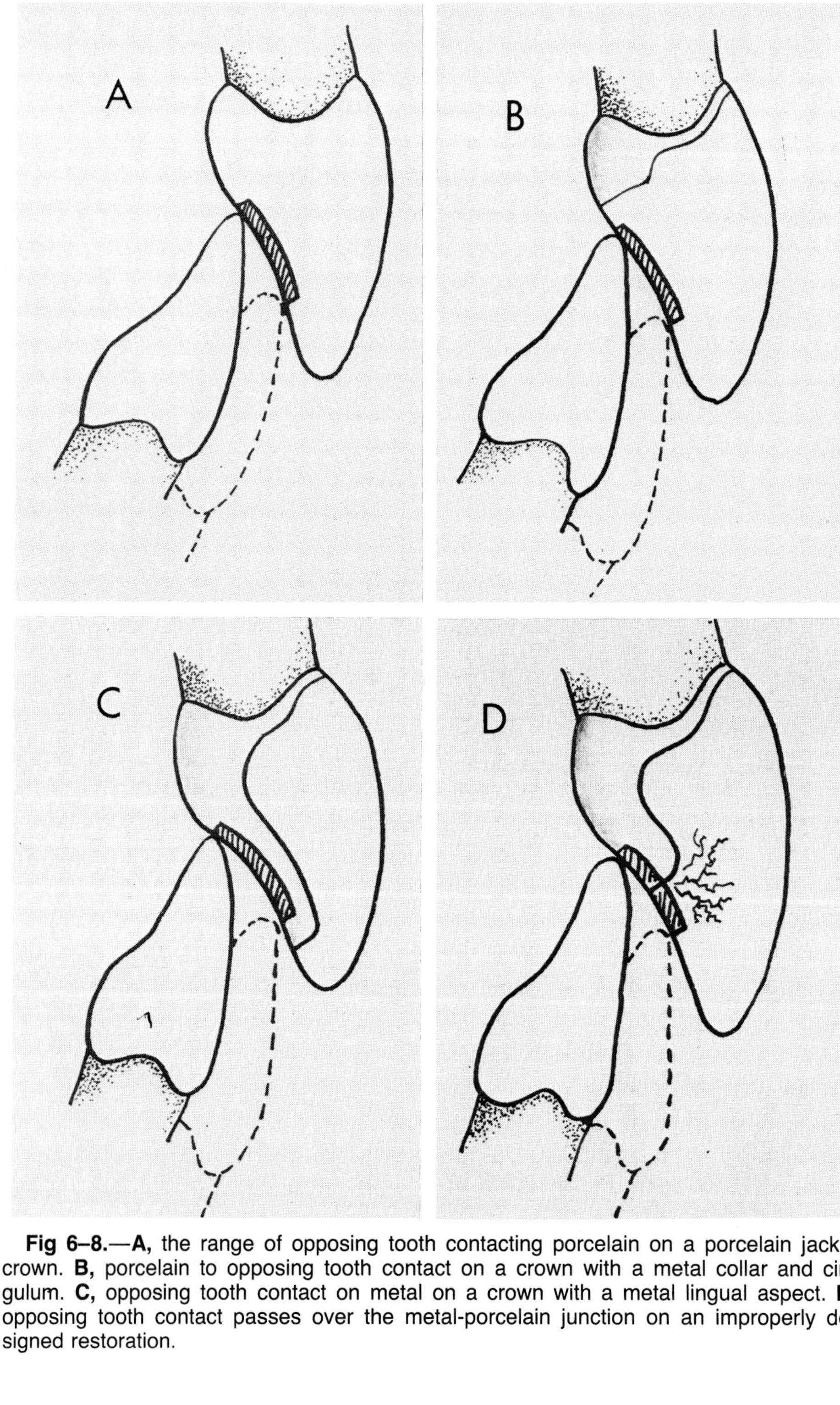

Fig 6–8.—**A,** the range of opposing tooth contacting porcelain on a porcelain jacket crown. **B,** porcelain to opposing tooth contact on a crown with a metal collar and cingulum. **C,** opposing tooth contact on metal on a crown with a metal lingual aspect. **D,** opposing tooth contact passes over the metal-porcelain junction on an improperly designed restoration.

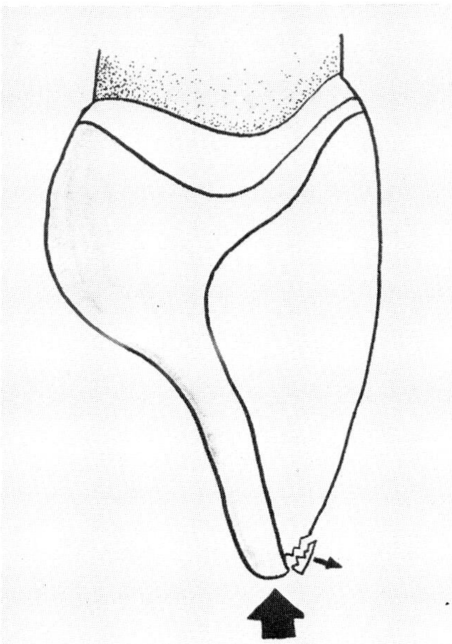

Fig 6–9.—Metal-porcelain junction on the incisal edge. This design invites distortion of metal in any functional contact that results in chipping or fracture of the porcelain.

The contact of the opposing tooth in its excursive path must be entirely on the porcelain or entirely on the metal, but not contacting or terminating on the porcelain-to-metal junction. The stress placed on the porcelain metal junction can result in a distortion of the metal and fracturing or shearing of the porcelain.[2]

If no centric contact or excursive contact exists the design of the framework can be left to the discretion of the technician. One design that is not recommended, even when there is no centric contact, is a porcelain-metal junction on the incisal edge (Fig 6–9). This is a common reason for an anterior porcelain fused to metal restoration to fail. Porcelain has excellent compressive strength, but little shear strength. This design does not have a metal step or support under the porcelain, and any incisal stresses can result in shearing of the labial porcelain.[3]

Posterior Teeth

The design of the framework on posterior teeth is determined by the amount of reduction, tooth to tooth relationship, and excursive movements. As with anterior restorations the junction of the porcelain and metal must not have centric or excursive contact (Fig 6–10).

The design of the posterior porcelain-fused-to-metal framework must be determined by studying the centric contacts and excursive movement of correctly articulated casts.[4] Frameworks may be designed for full porcelain coverage or for metal occlusal surfaces (Fig 6-11,A,B).

Bridge Pontics

The pontic should be contoured to be a miniature of the finished unit's size. This will ensure proper thickness and shade of the porcelain. Connectors on anterior bridges should be placed slightly lingual of center line from the incisal aspect (Fig

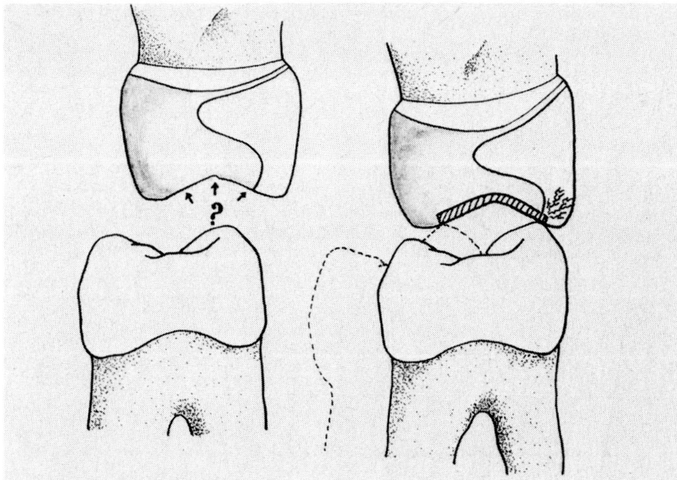

Fig 6–10.—Contact of the opposing functional cusp on the metal-porcelain junction leads to porcelain fracture in function.

6–12). This will ensure that the technician can make the proper depth cuts between the pontics and create the appearance of individual teeth.

Inadequate connectors have often caused failures in porcelain fused to metal bridges. Both anterior (Fig 6-13,A,B) and posterior (Fig 6-14,A,B) connectors between units, either soldered or cast, should be designed with the greatest possible dimension in a gingival-occlusal direction without distracting from the esthetic appearance or encroaching on the gingival embrasures. This will achieve the greatest strength with minimal metal.

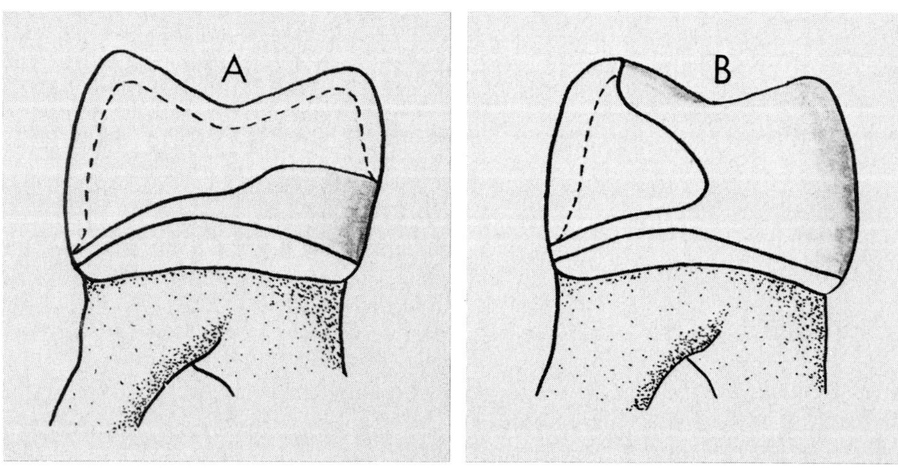

Fig 6–11.—**A,** design for full porcelain occlusal coverage provides maximum esthetic appearance. It requires more occlusal reduction of the preparation. In some cases it is contraindicated for occlusal wear and strength considerations. A metal collar is maintained around the entire gingival for porcelain support, contour, and marginal fit. **B,** it is easier to adjust and maintain occlusion with metal occlusal surfaces. If property designed, they provide better support for porcelain and reduce frequency of fracture.

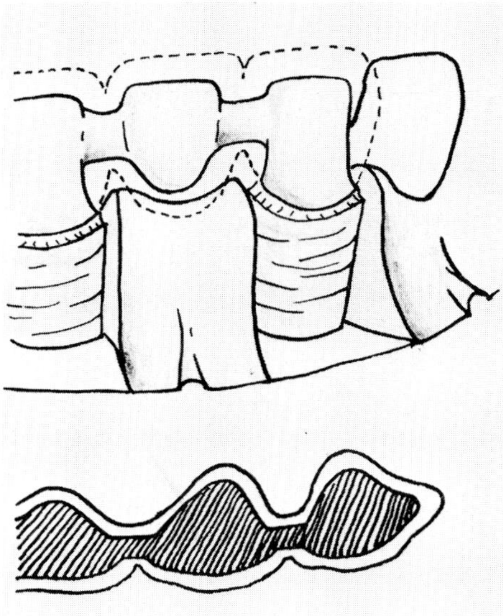

Fig 6–12.—Metal framework on dies showing pontic contour, connectors, and gingival clearance. Connectors are placed slightly lingual *(bottom)* to allow esthetic interproximal embrasures in porcelain.

THE METAL FRAMEWORK

Waxing

The casting can be no better than the wax pattern. The structural success of a porcelain fused to metal casting is based on the care and craftsmanship used in the fabrication of the wax pattern. At best, a rough wax pattern will produce a casting

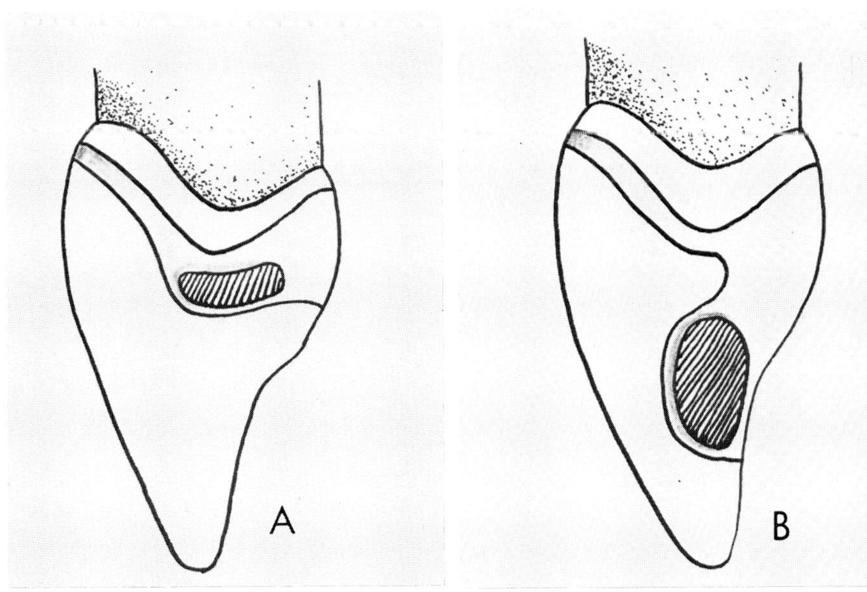

Fig 6–13.—**A,** improper size and placement for anterior connector. It is too near the gingival and too narrow incisogingivally. **B,** the larger and more vertical connector has a better esthetic appearance and is much stronger.

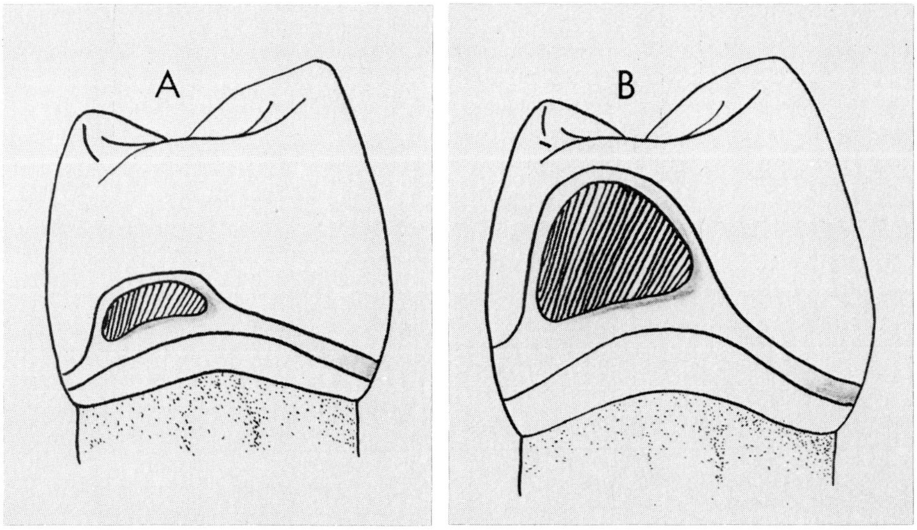

Fig 6–14.—A, the position, size, and direction of this posterior connector would encroach on the gingival embrasure and would not adequately resist flexure from occlusal loads. **B,** the larger, well-positioned connector is necessary for strength in posterior restorations.

that is extremely difficult to finish and polish. Realizing this, the finer the finish on the wax pattern, the less time that will be involved in polishing.

After the working model and the dies have been prepared, they should be thoroughly lubricated with a water soluble lubricant. The proximal surfaces of the teeth adjacent to the abutments, the occluding surfaces opposing the abutment, and the edentulous area should also be lubricated.

There are several ways to begin the adaptation of the wax pattern. Many modern laboratories will use a vacuum former to form as many as 20 copings at one time automatically. The copings are trimmed about 1 mm. short of the indicated margin. Wax can be flowed in the marginal areas, and lingual skirts can be waxed that will be ideal for full porcelain coverage.

An alternate method is to apply the molten wax to the lubricated die. The die is dipped into the melted wax to form a thimble of sufficient bulk. Fewer strains are set up in the wax in this method. After the bulk has been attained, the partially carved pattern is returned to the working model to establish the proximal contact areas and the occlusal contour. The abutments and pontics should be waxed to the full contour, making certain that contacts, occlusion, and anatomic form are correct in all respects.

The next step is to outline the areas that will be veneered with a pointed instrument. The factors that determine the outline of the veneered areas has been explained in the framework design section. To ensure a complete casting of thin sections, wax should be at least 0.5 mm. thick. This thickness may be reduced later by grinding the final castings.

Sprueing

Large diameter sprues and adequate reservoirs are absolutely essential to avoid casting failure. Small diameter sprues and a lack of sufficient reservoirs are the two major factors that cause porosity and miscastings.

If a reservoir sprue is used, the reservoir should be no more than one sixteenth inch from the unit to properly supply the casting during the cooling and shrinkage period. If a unit has more mass than the reservoir, the reservoir should be thickened so that its mass will be greater than the unit it supplies. Eighteen-gauge auxiliary escape vents may be used if desired.

The total length of the sprue from the button to each unit should be one quarter inch. If the spans are of considerable length or curvature, the button need not be round, but may follow the curvature of the span.

Units are always sprued so that the abutment openings are facing up to avoid trapping air during the investing procedures.

The length of sprues from the runner bar are adjusted to the sprue former so that a distance of approximately one quarter inch will remain from the top of the wax pattern to the top of the casting ring.

Investing and Burnout

The high fusing alloys that are in use today require specifically designed investments. The manufacturer's instructions for their use should be meticulously followed during investing, burnout, and casting. Only high quality phosphate bonding investments will ensure consistently satisfactory results.

The casting ring is lined with one or two layers of liner depending on manufacturer's instructions. The liner should be secured with wax. The casting ring is dipped in water and set aside to drain. The wet liner should not be compressed with the fingers as its effectiveness as an expansion medium will be decreased.

The special refractory investment used with porcelain-fused-to-metal alloys is mixed to the manufacturer's suggested water-powder ratio.

The majority of investments have a ratio of 14 to 15 ml of liquid mixture combined with 100 gm of investment. These may be mechanically spatulated for 20 seconds or hand spatulated for approximately 40 seconds. Hand spatulating should be done on a vibrator to help expel included air.

The casting ring is carefully filled with the investment. The maximum thickness of the investment should be approximately one quarter inch between the highest point of the wax pattern and the top of the casting ring. Too much thickness of investment over the patterns will prevent the rapid escape of mould gases during the casting process.

The ring should be slightly overfilled rather than underfilled. The invested ring should be allowed to set approximately 45 to 60 minutes before burnout.

The recommended procedure before burnout is to submerge the invested ring in water for approximately 5 seconds. If the ring has been invested for several hours, a 5-minute soak in room temperature water is recommended. The crucible former and any metal sprues are removed before burnout. The casting ring is placed in the room temperature furnace and the control set for 1,400–1,500°F for a 90-minute heat soak.

Casting Procedures

The alloys may be melted by induction or by gas fuel techniques. Generally, ceramic alloys are melted with a gas-oxygen torch. When the alloy appears to roll in the crucible, it is ready to cast. A gas-oxygen torch produces a flame hot enough to melt the ceramic alloy and provides a protective and reducing atmosphere. A gas-air torch will not produce a hot enough flame to melt the ceramic alloys satisfactorily. The use of an oxy-acetylene torch is not recommended as it is too hot and difficult to control.

Buttons and new alloy may be melted together, but at least 50% new alloy is always used. Any buttons must be scrupulously clean and free of any oxide contamination.

The alloy is first heated without flux in a regular unlined casting crucible. A new crucible should be reserved for porcelain-fused-to-metal alloys only. The ring should be placed in the casting machine so that the units that are to be cast are trailing in the rotation direction of the spinning centrifugal arm.

The alloy is ready to cast when the dull surface on the hot metal disappears and the melt is completely liquid. The alloy is cast into the mold and allowed to bench cool until it reaches handling temperature. The investment will separate easily from the casting and scrubbing will remove most of the loose investment. To remove the final traces of investment the casting is soaked for approximately 15 minutes in warm 50% hydrochloric acid pickle solution.

Procedures for Finishing

The quality of any casting is in direct relation to the amount of effort and care in the development of the wax patterns and attention to sprueing, investing, burnout, and casting procedures.

The first step in finishing a ceramic casting is to cut the sprues and to blend these areas into the contours of the castings with a separating disc. For smoother cutting and blending, the separating disc is moved quickly back and forth with light pressure over the area that is being reduced. This should be confined to the sprue areas only.

Before seating the castings on their dies to verify the fit, any internal roughness, bubbles, or other inaccuracies must be removed. Any fitting procedure should be done with a great deal of care and with as little metal removal as possible to prevent these adjusted areas from becoming too thin.

All surfaces that will receive porcelain should be ground to ensure the removal of all casting debris. Coarse stones are used first, followed by aluminum oxide stones or carbide burs to finish those areas that will receive porcelain. This procedure will ensure that any debris that may have been trapped in the subsurface will be removed. Abrasives such as rubber or plastic wheels that have any organic binder are not recommended.

Any sharp angles on the areas that are to receive porcelain, whether positive or negative, must be removed. They should be rounded and blended into the adjacent areas. The areas where the porcelain is to be terminated should end in a butt joint and finished to a fine sharp line. The margins or other thin parts are not finished at this time if the case is to be soldered. Thin edges are left full so that they are not vulnerable to the high temperature of the soldering flame. The casting should not receive the final polish until the porcelain fabrication is completed.

Degassing

Degassing or heat treating of the finished casting performs three functions that are essential to the success of the porcelain-fused-to-metal restoration. The process:

1. Imparts maximum hardness to the alloy;
2. Degasses the alloy; and
3. Establishes a surface oxidation which is essential for bonding of the porcelain to the metal.

The molten alloy, during the casting procedure, will absorb considerable amounts of gas that will migrate to the surface of the casting during the porcelain firing cycle. If these gases are not expelled previously, blistering and stressing will result in the finished porcelain restoration. The casting must be raised to a temperature higher than any temperature in the porcelain firing cycle to expel gases and stabilize the alloy.

Before the degassing is begun the framework should be placed in hydrofluoric acid to eliminate any new gas formation from embedded abrasive particles. The casting should be placed in an oven of 1000°F or lower and the temperature raised at about 75 F per minute. If the porcelain glazes at 1850°F, the heat treatment or degassing should be slightly higher or about 1875°F. Long span bridges must be adequately supported. The casting is then removed from the oven and placed under a glass beaker and allowed to bench cool.

Soldering

Solder is a precious metal containing gold and palladium that is furnished in strip form. It will bond to porcelain fused-to-metal alloys to form strong joints. In addition, it will accept porcelain in the same manner as the casting alloy.

The technique for handling the solder is relatively simple:

1. Surfaces to be joined must be smooth, clean, and free of debris. The metal surfaces should be separated by approximately one quarter mm. for maximum accuracy;
2. A good quality, high-heat, all purpose soldering investment must be used. Never use a casting investment for soldering because it provides too much expansion for this purpose;
3. The castings are seated on their respective dies and assembled. An autopolymerized resin, or plaster core and sticky wax can be used to secure the relationship of the units to be soldered. After setting the castings are removed from the model and the joint to be soldered is checked to be sure that there are no voids;
4. The assembled units are invested in a soldering investment recommended for soldering ceramic high-fusing gold alloys. The metal units should be exposed as much as possible without weakening the investment. The investment is allowed to set for at least 30 minutes;
5. The invested cast units are placed in a cold burnout furnace and the temperature is raised to approximately 1100°F. The assembly is now ready to be soldered;
6. A gas-oxygen torch is used to burn off any remaining traces of resin and a small amount of soldering flux paste is placed on the joint. The torch heating should

be done in a relatively dark area so that when the color of the metal changes to red it is easily seen. When the gold is sufficiently heated to the required temperature it is ready to receive the solder. When the solder flows freely, the flame is immediately removed and the entire case is allowed to bench cool; and

7. The unit is placed under cold running water and the casting recovered from the investment. The fixed partial denture is next placed in a fresh dilute solution of hot hydrochloric acid to remove any trace of flux.

THE PORCELAIN APPLICATION

The opaque porcelain application and firing provides the intermediate base between the metal casting and porcelain structure. The opaque porcelain application performs three functions:

1. The opaque porcelain chemically combines with the metal surface oxide to produce a compatible balance and a cohesive bond;
2. It masks the metal substructure with a layer as thin as one tenth mm; and
3. It is pigmented in several colors to compliment the porcelain body shades.

There are several precautions that must be observed during the opaque application. After heat treatment, the castings must not be exposed to contamination, such as finger contact or airborne dust. The castings are kept covered until ready for opaque application. The casting must not have been inadvertently over-oxidized. Excessive oxidation may be caused by higher degassing temperatures than recommended or by prolonged heat soak. If recommended firing temperatures are followed accurately interference with the oxide diffusion phenomenon at the metal opaque interface will be controlled. Faulty applications of fired opaque may be removed by the use of hydrofluoric acid.

The opaque should be mixed with distilled water to a consistency of thick cream. Numerous opaquing mediums can be used to provide more control of the opaque. An even layer of opaque mix is applied to the casting in a light stroking application using a small camel or sable hair brush. The surface is blotted with a clean facial tissue to absorb excess moisture. Any overlap of opaque porcelain beyond the porcelain-to-metal junction is removed with a damp brush while being held in front of the furnace door.

Usually, one even application of opaque, one-tenth mm thick, is sufficient for single units. On more extensive restorations, two light applications will be required for a complete cover. The opaqued restoration is then placed on a suitable firing sagger tray, carried into the oven, and fired to the desired temperature.

Build-up and Contouring

The same procedure for mixing, which was detailed in the opaque porcelain application step, is repeated for the body and gingival porcelains. Distilled water or various commercial mediums are used to wet and mix the body porcelains. A soft tissue or gauze is held on the lingual side of the restoration and the porcelain is carried to the opaqued restoration with a brush or instrument. The porcelain application, vibrating, and blotting are repeated until the desired amount of porcelain has been applied to the substructure. The built-up porcelain can then be carved to full contour.

The body porcelain build-up is trimmed with a sharp instrument to allow for overlaying and blending of the enamel or incisal porcelains. The mesial and distal line angles are also slightly trimmed and beveled. The enamel porcelain is mixed to a thin consistency. If the previously applied porcelain has become dry, it should be moistened slightly before additional porcelain is applied. The enamel mix applied at the incisal or occlusal portion of the restoration should be overbuilt about three quarters mm to one mm longer than the adjacent teeth on the model to compensate for porcelain shrinkage. In most instances, the overlapping of the body color with the incisal porcelain will satisfy the color specification for that restoration.

A maximum condensation of porcelain powders is achieved by arranging the various particle sizes of the material in such a way as to minimize spaces or voids in the build-up of the restoration. This is accomplished by first bringing the contained liquid to the surface. As the liquid is brought to the surface of the porcelain and absorbed, the resultant spaces are simultaneously replaced by smaller size particles. This is usually done with some form of vibration. The vibration technique consists of tapping the work and quickly blotting until the deepest subsurface moisture gradually rises to the surface where it can be gently removed.

When the restoration has been carved and removed from the model for the placement of porcelain on the contacts and tissue side of pontics, the porcelain is further condensed and dried. This is done by holding the metal frame with a hemostat and lightly tapping the hemostat with an instrument until the moisture appears on the surface. The moisture is then immediately and gently blotted, and the tapping and blotting is repeated. The sequence is repeated until no moisture comes to the surface. There will be no loss of shape or contour if the procedure is done carefully. The results of a well-condensed porcelain include minimal shrinkage, greater strength, higher translucency, and color control.

Staining

Esthetic appearance has become an important consideration to the modern dental patient. Patients are no longer satisfied with an anterior restoration that merely restores form and function. They also insist that the restorations have a vital natural appearance that replaces or improves the original tooth.

Fortunately, dentistry now has the materials to satisfy these demands. However, the results achieved by these materials depend to a great degree on the skills and care of the dentist who uses them. The process of staining porcelain-fused-to-metal restorations does not involve complex or expensive equipment. As the setting of stains and glazing is done without vacuum, a simple air firing oven is all that is necessary. A staining kit consisting of stains, liquid medium, brushes, and palette is also essential.

Stains consist of precise quantities of colored mineral oxide pigments that are incorporated into a liquid medium. Stains can be applied to a smoothly ground porcelain surface or to natural glazed porcelain. One or more applications can be made.

When stains are applied before the glaze bake, the case should be anatomically and functionally correct with no further adjustments expected. The porcelain surface must be scrupulously clean and bone dry.

The porcelain restoration is held with locking tweezers and the tip of the staining brush is used to spread a thin film of liquid medium over the surface that is to be stained. This is done to simulate a glaze and to enable the dentist to judge the necessary corrections. Small quantities of the stains to be used are placed on a clean dry palette. Several primary colors or hues (red, blue, and yellow) are placed on one side of the palette and a blending instrument is used to make secondary colors (orange, green, purple) and to adjust them as necessary. Two or three small drops of the liquid medium are placed on the palette to clean the brush and dilute the colors.

With a brush, the colors that are required are transferred to the working area of the palette. They may be blended and diluted as necessary to achieve the desired result. When the newly blended color seems correct, a generous amount is lifted with the end of the brush and transferred directly to the center of the area to be stained. The staining brush is then wiped on a tissue or cloth until it is semi-dry and highly absorbent. As the tip is passed over the just stained area, using light feathery strokes, it will absorb the excess stain and medium. This may be repeated as often as necessary until the desired effect is achieved. If the shade is incorrect, the restoration can be wiped clean with tissue and the process repeated until both the dentist and patient are satisfied.

When the shade is correct, the stain may be fixed by holding the restoration in front of the open furnace at 900 F until the liquid medium evaporates and a powdery film is seen covering the stained surface. At this point, the restoration is ready to be glazed.

Glazing

The final step in the construction of a porcelain-fused-to-metal restoration is the glaze. A glazed or vitreous condition is given to the surface of the restoration to make it hard and impermeable. There are two types of glazes common to dental porcelain restorations. The first is a natural or self-glaze and the second is an applied or overglaze.

A natural glaze is self-formed as a result of the correct firing of dental porcelain. The glaze is done by rapidly firing the ceramic body to a relatively high temperature or by holding a high temperature for a short period until the porcelain surface becomes molten.

An applied or overglaze is a thin, transparent continuous coating made of fine particles of porcelain mixed in a liquid medium. Ceramic materials use glass as a flux. The glaze or glass begins to melt at a fairly low temperature thereby causing the porcelain to form more glass of its own. Overglaze is applied with a brush and fired onto the surface of the dental porcelain. Overglaze is hard and insoluble, and effectively seals the surface of ground porcelain.

Staining After Glazing

A restoration can be stained after glazing. There are two ways to proceed. The first is with a natural glaze. This is accomplished by firing the restoration rapidly (100°F per minute) to the glazing temperature of the porcelain being used and maintaining it there until its surface becomes molten. Most porcelains used with metal glaze at about 1850°F. When ceramic stains are applied to the biscuit-bake surface and fired, they are incorporated into the molten surface.

The second method is with the overglaze. When using this technique, the stains must be fixed after they are applied to the biscuit-baked porcelain by bringing the restoration up to 1500°F in the oven. This will fix the stain into the surface of the porcelain so that when the liquid overglaze is applied there will be no running or discoloration of the stain. Now the overglaze can be applied to the surface of the porcelain.

A glaze will increase the strength of the porcelain and render it impermeable to liquids. It can be readily cleaned and covers small blemishes. It also wets the dull surface of the porcelain, thereby restoring the property of light penetration and permitting the true shade of the restoration to be clearly visible.

REASONS FOR FAILURES

Failures of an esthetic or functional nature result mostly from poor planning and implementation of the actual restoration. The material used accounts for only a small fraction of the failures. A dentist should arrive at the design of the restoration only after careful planning on the basis of models mounted in centric relation, radiographic diagnosis, and the clinical examination. Dentists must bear the responsibility for not only their part of the treatment but also that of the laboratory technician and the assistant.

Successful bonding of porcelain to metal alloys is not only dependent on the handling of materials in the dental laboratory, but also on the design of the preparation and the metal framework. The bonding of porcelain to metal eliminates many flaws that unsupported porcelain restorations can present. The metal substructure helps the brittle porcelain achieve its theoretical strength.

The most common causes of porcelain-fused-to-metal restoration failures can be attributed to the basic designs of the prepared abutment teeth. Insufficient or uneven reduction of the preparation will result in insufficient or uneven amounts of porcelain. This will set up residual stresses in the porcelain itself and make it more subject to fracture. The metal substructure design will cause fractures when there are sharp corners or angles.

The location of the porcelain to metal junction, if the junction coincides with a centric or excursive path contact, can cause a burnishing of the metal and a subsequent fracture. Long span fixed partial dentures must have connectors that are large enough to resist the flexing that could cause the porcelain to fracture.

The thickness of the substructure and porcelain is important. The metal may be reduced to a minimum of 0.2 mm., and the porcelain should not exceed 2 mm. in thickness but it may be increased to as much as 2.5 mm. in nonstressed areas.

Laboratory procedures are of critical importance. During casting procedures the technician must make sure that the alloys are not overheated, that the crucibles are not contaminated, that investment contaminated gold is not remelted, and that differing alloys are not mixed.

When the metal is being treated care must be taken not to use contaminated stones to reduce metal. Prepared metal surfaces must be decontaminated. After degassing it is important not to touch the metal with fingers.

The porcelain technique must use adequate condensation and avoid any contamination from air or manipulation. The porcelain and water or medium must be carefully and properly mixed.

During soldering, the joint must have an adequate size and location. The surfaces must be free of contamination to ensure a porosity-free joint.

The last major cause of porcelain-fused-to-metal restoration failures is occlusion. Occlusal disharmony with prematurities and cuspal interferences can and does cause many failures.

REFERENCES

1. Shillingburg H.T., Hobo S., Fisher D.W.: Preparation design and margin distortion in porcelain-fused-to-metal restorations. *J. Prosthet. Dent.* 29:276, 1973.
2. Riley E.J.: Ceramo-metal restoration state of the science. *Dent. Clin. North Am.* 21:669, 1977.
3. Shell J.S., Nielsen J.P.: Study of the bond between gold alloys and porcelain. *J. Dent. Res.* 41:1424, 1962.
4. Miller L.L.: Framework design in ceramo-metal restorations. *Dent. Clin. North Am.* 21:699, 1977.

BIBLIOGRAPHY

Baker C.R.: A porcelain-fused crown. *J. Prosthet. Dent.* 18:1, 1967.

Brecker S.C.: Porcelain baked to gold—a new medium in prosthodontics. *J. Prosthet. Dent.* 6:801, 1956.

Brecker S.C.: Improved porcelain fused to gold bridge. *Dent. Clin. North Am.*, 163, March, 1959.

Cowger G.T., Woycheshin, F.F.: Gold plating to enhance the appearance of porcelain-faced crowns. *J. Prosthet. Dent.* 11:925, 1961.

Custer F., Asgar K., Payton F.A.: The effect of certain variables in the bond strength of porcelain fused to gold. *(Abst.) Int. Assoc. Dent. Res.* 40:94, 1962.

Dahl B.L.: Some biological considerations in crown and bridge prosthetics. *J. Oral Rehabil.* 1:245, 1974.

Dykema R.W., Johnston J.F., Cunningham, D.M.: The veneered gold crown. *Dent. Clin. North Am.* 653, Nov., 1958.

Ewing J.E., Bentman D.: Porcelain-veneered full-crown restorations made with cadmium patterns. *J. Prosthet. Dent.* 18:140, 1967.

Farah J.W., Craig R.G.: Distribution of stresses in porcelain-fused-to-metal and porcelain jacket crowns. *J. Dent. Res.* 54:255, 1975.

Gage J.P.: Anterior porcelain crowns in general practice. *Br. Dent. J.* 138:256, 1975.

Gettleman L., et al.: Studies on a new dental casting gold alloy. *J. Dent. Res.* 45:595, 1967.

Hagan W.H.B.: Combination gold and porcelain crown. *J. Prosthet. Dent.* 10:325, 1960.

Hoffman E.J.: How to utilize porcelain-fused-to-gold as a crown and bridge material. *Dent. Clin. North Am.*, 57, March, 1965.

Howard W.W.: Porcelain-fused-to-gold for Class IV inlays. *J. Prosthet. Dent.* 13:761, 1963.

Howell R.A.: Gold/porcelain anterior crowns. *Br. Dent. J.* 11:118, 1961.

Howell R.A.: Gold/porcelain bridge work, *Br. Dent. J.* 116:80, 1964.

Johnston J.F., et al.: Construction and assembly of porcelain veneer gold crowns and pontics. *J. Prosthet. Dent.* 12:1125, 1962.

Knap F.J., Ryge G.: Study of bond strength of dental porcelain-fused-to-metal. *J. Dent. Res.* 45:1047, 1966.

Lavine M.H., Custer F.: Variables affecting the strength of bond between porcelain and gold. *J. Dent. Res.* 45:32, 1966.

Leinfelder K.F.: Heat treatment of alloys to be used for the fused porcelain technique. *J. Dent. Res.* 43:927, 1964.

Leinfelder K.F., et al.: Hardening of high fusing gold alloys. *J. Dent. Res.* 45:392, 1966.

Leinfelder K.F., Servais, W.J., O'Brien, W.J.: Mechanical properties of high fusing gold alloys. *J. Prosthet. Dent.* 21:523, 1969.

Leone E.F., Fairhurst C.W.: Bond strength and mechanical properties of dental porcelain enamels. *J. Prosthet. Dent.* 18:155, 1967.

Lyons D.M., et al.: Porcelain-fused-to-gold—evaluation and esthetics. *J. Prosthet. Dent.* 10:319, 1960.

Meadows T.R.: Clinical comparison of cast gold crowns with acrylic and fused porcelain veneer facings. *J. Am. Dent. Assoc.* 66:772, 1963.

Medwedeff F.M.: Porcelain-fused-to-gold: Fixed partial dentures. *J. Prosthet. Dent.* 18:46, 1967.

Mintz V.W., Caputo A.A., Belting C.M.: Inherent structural defects of porcelain-fused-to-gold restorations. *J. Prosthet. Dent.* 32:544, 1974.

Moffa J.P., Jenkins W.A.: Status report on base-metal crown and bridge alloys. *J. Am. Dent. Assoc.* 89:652, 1974.

Morrison K.N., Warnick M.E.: Investment compounded specifically for ceramic procedures. *J. Dent. Res.* 38:762, 1959.

Mumford G.: The porcelain-fused-to-metal restorations, *Dent. Clin. North Am.* 241, March, 1965.

Mumford G., Ridge A.: Dental porcelain. *Dent. Clin. North Am.* 15:33, 1971.

O'Brien W.J., Kring J.E., Ryge G.: Heat treatment of alloys to be used for the fused porcelain technique. *J. Prosthet. Dent.* 14:955, 1964.

Pruden H.H.: Solder connections with porcelain-fused-to-gold. *J. Prosthet. Dent.* 22:679, 1967.

Ryge G.: Current American research on porcelain-fused-to-metal restorations. *Int. Dent. J.* 15:385, 1965.

Schiffer R.: Soldering technique for high fusing gold in porcelain. *J. Prosthet. Dent.* 22:4, 1969.

Schnell R.J., Mumford G., Phillips R.W.: An evaluation of phosphate bonded investments used with a high fusing gold alloy. *J. Prosthet. Dent.* 13:324, 1963.

Shelby D.S.: Practical considerations and designs of porcelain-fused-to-metal. *J. Prosthet. Dent.* 15:542, 1966.

Shell J.S., Nielson J.P.: Study of the bond between gold alloys and porcelain. *J. Dent. Res.* 41:1424, 1962.

Silver M., Klein G.: Precision attachments in conjunction with cast platinum-porcelain restorations. *Dent. Dig.* 62:296, 1956.

Silver M., Klein G., Howard M.C.: Platinum porcelain restorations. *J. Prosthet. Dent.* 6:695, 1956.

Silver M., Howard M.C., Klein G.: Porcelain bonded to cast metal understructure. *J. Prosthet. Dent.* 11:132, 1961.

Silver M., Klein G., Howard M.C.: An evaluation and comparison of porcelain fused to cast metals. *J. Prosthet. Dent.* 10:1055, 1960.

Straussberg G., Katz G., Kuwata M.: Design of gold supporting structures for fused porcelain restorations. *J. Prosthet. Dent.* 16:928, 1966.

Swartz M.C., Phillips R.W.: A study of adaptation of veneers to cast gold crowns. *J. Prosthet. Dent.* 7:817, 1957.

Tuccillo J.J., Nielson J.P.: Creep and sag properties of porcelain-gold. *J. Dent. Res.* 46:597, 1967.

Weinberg L.A.: A new design for porcelain-fused-to-metal prosthesis. *J. Prosthet. Dent.* 17:178, 1967.

CHAPTER 7

Pin Retained Restorations

PETER M. JACKIN, D.D.S.

MANY METHODS of restoring function and esthetics to lost tooth structure are available to the dentist. Unfortunately, some of these restorative procedures, especially those that involve the use of porcelain, are expensive for the patient and necessitate a radical removal of tooth structure, a task that is far too easy with high speed rotary instruments.[1] The patient may demand an esthetically pleasing result, but an excessive amount of tooth structure may be needlessly wasted to achieve such a result with complete tooth coverage (Fig 7–1). Despite many claims to the contrary, acid-etch composite restorative material can only be considered a temporary restoration. Their esthetic appearance is impaired in the mouth by food, drink, and tobacco. There is no doubt that gold restorations have proved longevity but they demand an exacting restorative technique to be successful.

Black's original classification[2] of the principles of cavity preparation apply only to compound cavities for gold foil, although these were revised to provide bulk for amalgam. More recently Rosensteil[3] considered the problem of inlay and crown retention as a function of cavity form and concluded that a preparation was retentive if the restoration had a single path of insertion. In addition, it has been shown that retention depends on the length of the path of insertion.[4] Opposition to displacement in the direction of withdrawal is a result of the keying action of the cement, which in turn depends on the shear strength of the cement, the surface area of the bond, the microscopic irregularities, the pitch of the restoration, and the thickness of the cement film.[5] Eccentrically acting forces, however, tend to produce a torque on the restoration, so that if the restoration is retentive, displacement cannot occur unless the tooth fractures or the restoration distorts.[6] In relatively sound teeth, therefore, good retention form may be achieved by preparing opposed axial walls of adequate length. In teeth with less sound tooth structure, a single path of insertion of adequate length can be achieved by careful preparation of the remaining tooth substance[7] aided by the use of multiple miniature parallel pins to confer a single path of insertion for the restoration.

The use of pins to aid inlay retention has been advocated for a number of decades.[8–17] Their use to aid retention of Class IV, V, and VI gold foil[18] and porcelain inlays[19] has also been advocated. The construction of a core of amalgam or composite followed by a full crown restoration may be simpler to perform than partial coverage aided by pin retention, but it is not always necessary to produce a full crown when only parts of a tooth are destroyed. There is often insufficient primary retention for even a core unless this is pin retained also. Accidental termination of a gold margin on amalgam that is in contact with oral fluids may produce undesir-

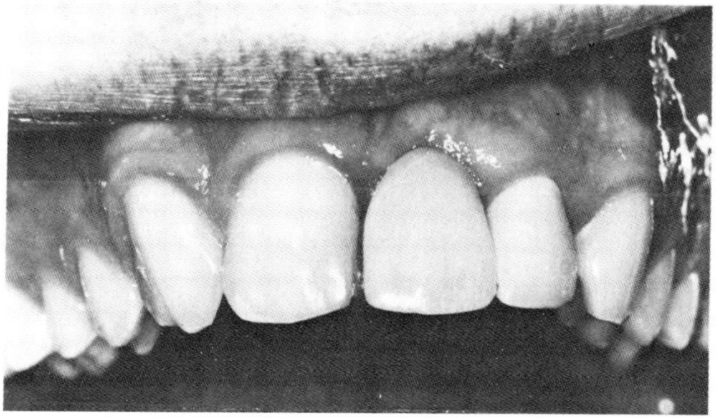

Fig 7–1.—A three-unit restoration replacing the maxillary left central with a pinledge on the right central incisor and a porcelain-fused-to-metal crown on the left lateral incisor. Conservation of the tooth structure has been achieved on the central along with an acceptable esthetic result.

able metal corrosion. When composite cores are not completely covered they are exposed to the oral fluids and potential deterioration.

The modern composite materials rarely offer a long-term esthetic appearance because of surface staining. They are more susceptible to wear than gold or porcelain. But composite restorative materials are advantageous because of their reduced cost and because they require little operative technique relative to cavity preparation. They certainly offer no challenge to the operator to maintain high standards of skill. There is, as yet, no evidence that composite restorative materials enjoy the long-term durability of cast gold.

Resistance form may be defined as protection of the remaining tooth substance against fracture caused by forces of mastication. The resistance depends on cavity preparations being designed to distribute loads over a large area of tooth substance. In extensive cast restorations cavities must be designed to produce:

1. A single path of insertion;
2. A close mechanical coupling between tooth and restoration;
3. An effective spread of loads; and
4. An outline form that satisfies the requirements of extention for prevention, conservation, and esthetic appearance.

These objectives may be achieved through a variety of techniques. Preparations should be well defined, although sharp internal line angles should be avoided as they produce high local stress concentrations in both tooth and restoration.[20] Axial walls should converge slightly (5°) in an occlusal direction, with pulpal and gingival walls flat and at 90° to the axial walls. Such a design will result in axial loads being resisted without horizontal force components developing to displace the restoration.[21] Reverse bevelling should be used to oppose displacement of obliquely acting forces by spreading the load to other cusps.[22] This is limited by the effectiveness of the angle of the bevel, which must allow the gold margin to be easily burnished. Grooving the incisal edge of capped cusps further improves the resistance to rotational failure by increasing the purchase of the casting on the cusp.[23] Increased proximal coverage spreads the load over a greater area of tooth substance. A three-quarter crown type of restoration enables weakened cusps to be "locked into the casting," thereby improving the resistance force by opposing rotational forces. To effectively use the remaining tooth substance, linings should be kept minimal to allow the closest mechanical coupling between restoration and tooth substance.

USE OF PINS

Whereas the retentive qualities of pin retainers result from the single path of insertion provided by the pins, the actual retention is dependent on the length, diameter, number, and surface texture of the pins.[24, 25] Tapered pins are less retentive than parallel sided ones. Pins can enhance resistance form by allowing the casting to act more effectively as a "tie-bar" between weak cusps. The use of pins, however, is limited by the risk of pulp exposure and the problem of parallelism.

The efficient use of pins in teeth requires a knowledge of the anatomy of the cervical third of both crown and root, and a knowledge of the thickness of dentin at various levels within the tooth. There is a limited amount of data, however, available about dentin thickness.[26, 27] More recently, Gourley[28] studied 100 sound caries-free molars using casts, radiographs, and sections. This study showed that the favorable locations to place pinholes in molars are the line angles or corners. To establish the proper direction of the pinhole, the drill is placed in the sulcus parallel to the root surface and moved to the desired location without changing the angulation before drilling the hole.[29] Alternatively, a small instrument may be placed in the sulcus parallel to the root surface as a guide in establishing the desired angulation for the drill. Two locations where there is an adequate amount of dentin, but where this method of determining angulation of the hole is contraindicated, are the lingual aspect of the maxillary molars and the distal aspect of the mandibular molars. The difficulty in finding the proper direction of the pinhole in these locations comes from the abrupt angulation of the roots just apical to the cementoenamel junction. Placing a pinhole parallel to the crown outline in these areas tends to direct the pinhole into the pulp. Furthermore, the middle of tooth surfaces is not a good location for pins because of internal anatomy. Placing pins in these areas can easily involve root furcations of the maxillary molars or flutings on the roots of the mandibular molars. The high incidence of furcations extending to within 3 mm of the cementoenamel junction greatly increases the danger of perforating the surface of the tooth if pins are placed in the middle of the facial, mesial, or distal surfaces of maxillary molars. The location of the bifurcation of the roots of mandibular molars also contraindicates the placing of pins in the middle of the facial and lingual surfaces of these teeth. Of particular importance is that large teeth tend to have furcations nearer to the cementoenamel junction and deeper fluting on the roots.

The recommended minimum thickness of dentin for a pinhole is three times the diameter of the pinhole. Thus, a pinhole of 0.5 mm diameter requires at least 1.5 mm of dentin, allowing 0.5 mm of dentin between the hole and the pulp, and between the hole and the tooth surface. If the holes are not completely surrounded by dentin, the incidence of pulp involvement, root perforation, or enamel fracture will be greatly increased.

LINGUAL PIN VENEER

Most patients are opposed to any visible gold on their anterior teeth. A type of restoration is possible, however, that enables the dentist to provide the patient with a good esthetic appearance without losing the strength and durability characteristics of cast gold restorations. This type of restoration is called the lingual pin veneer.

The cavity preparation for lingual pin veneer differs from that for the conventional three-quarter crown in two respects. First, the three-quarter crown is inserted in a direction parallel to the incisal two thirds of the labial surface, whereas the lingual pin veneer is inserted perpendicularly to the lingual surface. Secondly, the classic three-quarter crown relies on axial grooves for retention, whereas the lingual pin veneer depends entirely on miniature cast gold pins.

The crowns of anterior teeth have contours that do not readily lend themselves to conventional three-quarter crown preparations, particularly the mandibular incisors. In all anterior teeth the greatest mesiodistal width of a tooth is found to lie well toward the labial surface. When the incisors or the cuspids are viewed from the lingual aspect, the lingual surface and the major part of the mesial and distal surfaces can be seen. The contact points are generally near the incisal edge. As a result, castings are more suited for anterior restorations when they are inserted from the lingual rather than the incisal aspect.

Ideally, the path of insertion should be directly perpendicular to the lingual surface of the tooth. The following questions should be considered before beginning the preparation: Will the proximal margins of the restoration include any carious or potentially overlapped teeth and will the overlapped teeth prevent the seating of the finished restoration because of obstruction from adjacent teeth?

Restorations made using this technic do not have to be inserted from the lingual aspect. Large span fixed partial dentures and periodontal splints may require insertion from the incisal or occlusal aspect. In this instance, the parallelometer may be aligned with ease. A casting prepared from the occlusal or incisal aspect forms an excellent type of retainer for posterior fixed partial dentures when the anterior abutment tooth is a canine with no previous carious involvement.

It is difficult to gain retention where previous carious lesions, chips, and fractures or abrasions have caused a considerable loss of tooth structure. There is general agreement that pins are superior to axial grooves in such situations. Pins, however, have not been popular for two basic reasons. First, such preparations are not easy to make, and second, it is difficult to reproduce pins in wax patterns. The latter reason may be overcome by accurate reproduction of pinholes using sized nylon bristles.

There are many indications for this type of cavity preparation. It has been successfully used as a substitute for most anterior three-quarter crowns, for restorations of fractured angles of young anterior teeth, abraded maxillary incisors, mandibular incisors, anterior fixed partial dentures, and for splinting anterior teeth (Fig 7–2).

The initial step in cavity preparation is the reduction of the lingual surface and incisal edge to provide for adequate gold thickness when the teeth are in centric and eccentric occlusal relations. Next, a finish line is established at the gingival border. After this, a tapered diamond stone of the desired size is used to extend and carry the finish line interproximally. The proximal extension may be carried as far toward the labial aspect as is judged advisable, or this finish line may end along the lingual ridge or line angle. Lingual insertion of a casting eliminates undercuts and the potential fracture of a fragile corner of labioincisal enamel.

After the gross reduction and establishment of the finish line, the tooth is surveyed for pinholes. A good roentgenogram should be studied to avoid penetrating

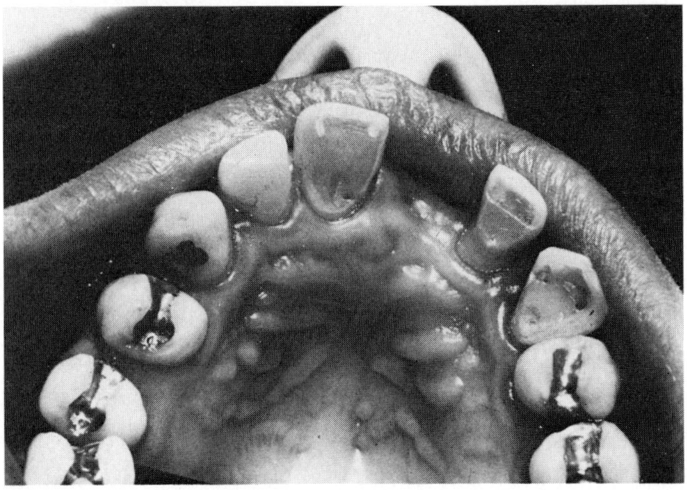

Fig 7–2.—Multiple pinledge preparations on the central and lateral incisor, and canine. The central incisor and canine are of the unilateral design, whereas the lateral, for soldering purposes, is of the bilateral design.

the pulp chamber or perforating the side of the tooth. An exposure will seldom occur if reasonable care and judgment are used. Pinholes that will fall mesial or distal to the pulp chamber may be drilled to their maximum depth (2.5 mm), whereas those that are aimed directly toward the pulp should not be longer than 1 mm. As many as five pinholes can be placed in even the smallest tooth although three or four are usually adequate.

The next step is the marking of the drill sites. After the locations are marked and centered, the parallelometer is positioned and attached to the teeth with compound. The pinholes are drilled to their desired depth at slow speed.

After the pinholes have been prepared, the parallelometer is removed and the cavity preparation is complete (Fig 7–3). Obtaining an impression of the cavity preparation is not difficult. The lingual angulation of the cavity preparation requires that the impression must be removed lingually, not incisally. To eliminate tearing or distortion during withdrawal, the operator must prevent the impression material from flowing through the gingival embrasures and locking on the labial surface. The labial gingival openings, therefore, are sealed with a soft compound. A thick layer of utility wax placed over the compound and the labial portion of the tooth eliminates distortion caused by material that might otherwise flow over the incisal to the labial surface.

For purposes of reproducing the miniature pinholes in the impression, special nylon bristles of .022 in. in diameter are used. The bristle is inserted in the pinhole so that the knob protrudes 2 or 3 mm, thereby engaging the impression material. Customary technics are used to mix the impression material, which is then placed in a syringe and injected around the bristles. To prevent them from floating out of the holes, a finger or instrument may be held over the bristles while the material is being injected. A small amount of material is placed on the impression tray and carried to place. After it has set, the impression is removed in a lingual direction.

The impression is poured into any one of the improved dental stones and care is

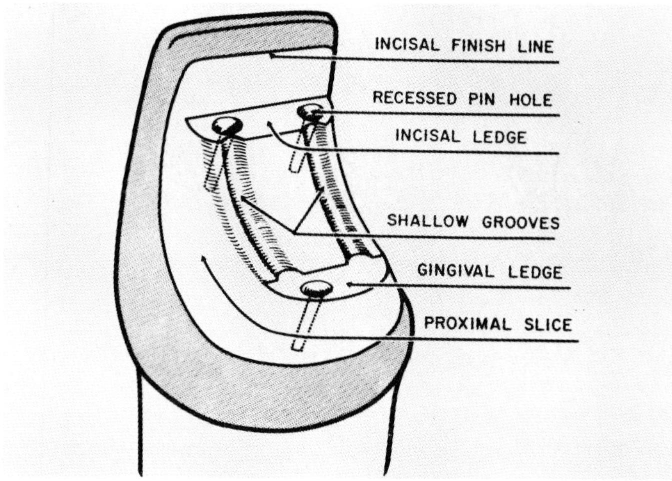

Fig 7–3.—This schematic diagram identifies the salient features of the pinledge preparation.

taken to eliminate all air bubbles. As the impression is separated from the stone model, the bristles may pull out of the impression material and be retained in the stone die. If this occurs, they may be removed easily with a small pliers. After the die has been separated, trimmed, and lubricated, it is ready for the pattern. To obtain a reproduction of the pins in the wax pattern and to permit free withdrawal of the pattern, nylon bristles that are smaller than .022 in. diameter must be used. The end of the bristle that is inserted into the die hole should be cut clean with a sharp razor blade while the outer end is melted to a head with a hot instrument so that it projects about 0.5 mm from the stone die. Molten wax is added to engage the bristles and provide bulk for the pattern. Distortion of the wax pattern is avoided if it is removed from the stone die in a direction parallel to the bristles.

Conventional methods of investing and casting will yield good results. The nylon bristles will burn out of the mold as readily as the wax and no difficulty should be encountered in reproducing the pins in the gold. A hard inlay or fixed partial denture type of gold is used if maximum rigidity and strength are desired.

Before the casting is seated, a no. 4 round bur should be used to chamfer or bevel the sharp edges around the pin holes in the tooth. The slight funnel-shaped opening that is formed will guide the pins to place and will provide a slight relief area around the base of the pins, thereby permitting the casting to assume a better adaptation. After the casting has been adjusted for occlusion and polished, it is cemented in a conventional manner. Care must be taken that the cement covers the pins and the inside of the casting completely. As an added precaution, some cement may also be placed over the preparation and worked into the holes with a dull explorer or round periodontal probe. A lentulo spiral* in a contra-angle handpiece is effective for spinning cement into pinholes.

While the casting is being fabricated, temporary protection must be provided for the exposed dentin. Plastic crown forms filled with zinc oxide and eugenol cement are satisfactory if the contact points are opened. Temporaries may also be fabricated

*Union Broach Corp., 36–40 37th St., Long Island City, NY 11101.

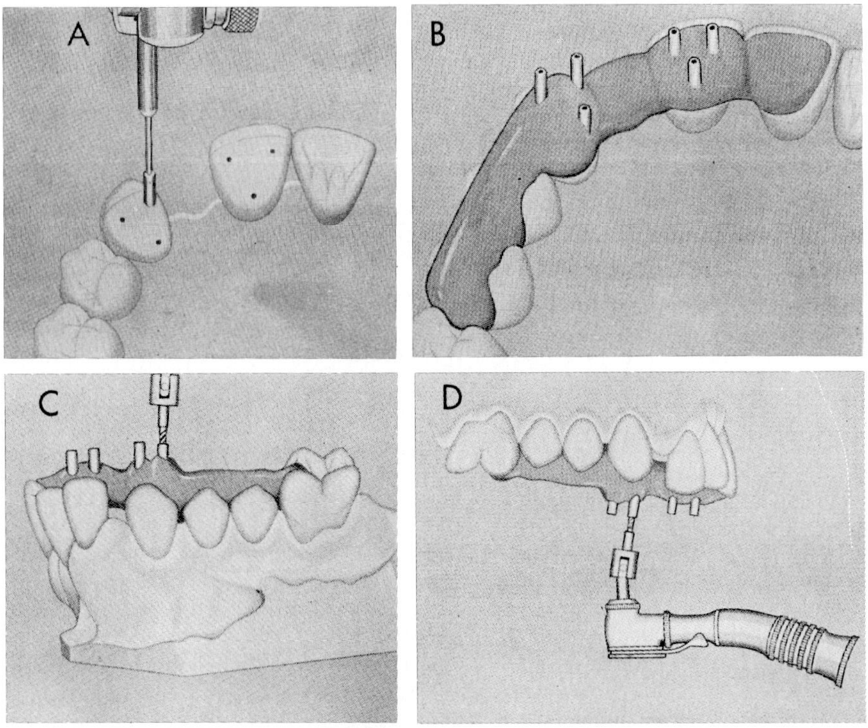

Fig 7–4.—A, an impression is made and cast poured of the pin veneer preparations before pin holes are drilled in the teeth. With the aid of the cast and radiographs, the location and direction of the pin holes are determined by the dentist. In the laboratory the bushings are located parallel to each other over the areas where the pin holes are to be drilled and paralleled with the aid of a surveyor. **B,** an acrylic index is made over the cast, including one or two adjacent teeth on either side, and supporting the bushings. **C,** using a self-limiting twist drill, holes are drilled in the stone master cast in the laboratory using finger pressure to rotate the drill. The index is then removed, serrated pins inserted in the pin holes, and the pattern for the restoration fabricated. The pattern is invested and the casting made, incorporating the serrated pins. The restoration is then completed. **D,** the completed restoration and the index with the bushings are returned to the dentist. The index is placed in the mouth and the pinholes are drilled in the teeth using the handpiece with the same length and diameter of the twist drill that was used in the laboratory. The restoration may be seated, fitted, and cemented immediately.

using nylon bristles that have been cut to clear the occlusion and then covered and incorporated in autopolymerizing resin. A tiny pledget of cotton in each pin hole will help to completely remove the temporary cement.

Initially, the operator should attempt to restore single teeth, after which smaller fixed partial dentures and periodontal splints may be attempted. With experience, these restorations can be made more rapidly than conventional three-quarter crowns with less stress on the operator and more conservative tooth preparation for the patient.

In addition to the system described for preparing and fabricating the lingual pin veneer, an interesting variation is the Ney Parallel Pin Technic.** The technique,

**The J. M. Ney Co., Hartford, CT. 06100.

which is described in detail with the kit, minimizes the problems of achieving parallelism of the pin channels. Pin holes are drilled in the teeth with the aid of an index that is developed in the laboratory and subsequently transferred for intraoral application (Fig 7–4, A–D).

PINLEDGES AND PINLAYS

The pin ledge casting is one in which the operator prepares a modified onlay or three-quarter crown. To enhance the retention of the casting, supplementary pins are placed into the dentin within strategically located areas. Ledges, or seats, for the pinholes are usually accompanied by a groove or a box in at least one proximal surface.

The pinlay differs from the pinledge in that is has no grooves, boxes, or flanges. It has only a chamfered finish line that surrounds a flat area of missing tooth structure. When this type of restoration is indicated, the cavity preparation is nothing more than a reduction for occlusal clearance followed by placement of small pinholes for retention. This preparation is extremely flexible in design, in that it does not have to include the contact. In the pinlay, pins are not auxiliary devices used to aid in securing the casting in position; they are the primary means of retention.

A primary use for the pinlay casting is for restoring those areas of a tooth that are destroyed by abrasion and wear. The abnormally worn incisor, maxillary or mandibular, and the cusp tips of canines are classic examples.

It should be pointed out that the dislodgement of any casting is a real possibility when it is subjected to heavy masticatory forces that induce tipping or bending. Pinlays are more susceptible to these forces than pinledges. The operator should select patients for pinlays carefully. Where masticatory forces might contraindicate their use, a different design should be selected.

The pinledge veneer is applicable in the case of an individual tooth and for a successful anterior fixed partial denture retainer. The technique permits conservative tooth reduction. Pulp damage is minimized by the use of small retention pins that are easily duplicated with nylon bristles and indirect impression techniques. Pinledges are contraindicated for grossly carious teeth, teeth too small or too thin for accurate positioning of the pins, patients with a high caries index, and long span fixed partial dentures without intermittent abutments.

To achieve satisfactory esthetic results with adequate retention and stability, pinledge preparations must be designed with an accurate study cast and radiographs to determine the size and location of the pulp. Sufficient tooth reduction is necessary to provide adequate metal bulk. The outline form, finishing lines, bracing grooves, resistance ledges, and retention holes require careful planning.

The retention pinholes are started in the center of each ledge with a no. 1/2 round bur. They are then made parallel to the proximal groove, when proximal grooves are used, and parallel to each other with a twist drill of 0.024 or 0.028 in. diameter. The drill must be driven slowly and intermittently withdrawn for chip clearance and to ensure against jamming or breaking. The drill selected should be the largest diameter that is safe, and the hole should be from 2 to 3 mm deep.

Reproduction of the pinholes is ensured by accurately sized nylon bristles placed in the drilled holes and checked to ensure against binding. A 0.022 in. diameter bristle is used in conjunction with the 0.024 in. drill, while a 0.027 in. bristle is fitted in the hole made by the 0.028 in. drill. A size differential of 0.001 to 0.002 in. between drill and bristle is recommended. Bristles are knobbed and extend 1 to 2 mm from the prepared tooth surface. No bristle should touch the impression tray as it could be bent to the side and be left undetected as the impression material is setting. When the tray is removed from the mouth, the bristle, securely held by the material, will straighten, leaving its terminal end in a completely misplaced position.

Reversible hydrocolloid or any of the elastomeric impression materials are excellent for duplicating pin preparations after thorough cavity lavage.[30, 31] After the gingival tissues have been deflected from the marginal areas, the teeth are carefully washed and dried, and the knobbed nylon bristles are inserted into the pinholes. If these bristles fit too loosely, they will float out during the impression procedure. A coating of vaseline will ensure placement and will not interfere with removal. If they fit too tightly, the bristles may tear out of the material when the impression is removed.

When set, the impression is removed, poured into die stone, and allowed to harden. The cast is removed from the impression and sectioned into dies. Any knobbed bristles that remain in the stone model are removed. The stone is lubricated, and new bristles of the smaller diameter are introduced into the pinholes. These will be incorporated into the pattern and must be 0.002 in. smaller than the bristles used for the impression. To engage the wax, these bristles are also knobbed. Wax is added and the pattern is carved, sprued, and removed in the usual manner. The resulting pinledge or pinlay should be made of type C or fixed partial denture gold for toughness and strength. After the casting has been made, it is fitted, polished, and cemented.

INDICATIONS, CONTRAINDICATIONS, AND USES

Experience gained through the use of pins has led to certain conclusions regarding their indications, contraindications, and uses. Some of these factors are discussed below.

Overlapped Teeth

Overlapped teeth are generally contraindicated for pinlays, especially if the casting involves proximal contacts. The problems encountered between proper pin alignment and contact points of adjacent teeth are often insurmountable. In some instances, the enamel of adjacent contacts may be reduced and contact rebuilt in the gold casting.

Incisors in Labioversion

Maxillary anterior teeth in labioversion are good candidates for cast pin splints, whereas those teeth whose long axis tips inward at the incisal are contraindicated.

Pin Location

The location of the pins is important. Placing pins close together in the area of the cingulum and leaving the incisal half of the restoration without retention invites failure. The tendency for the gold to flex fractures the cement bond along the incisal edge of the casting, and results in leakage or recurrent caries in this region. Teeth should, therefore, be prepared with pins near the incisal edge.

Pins can be used to good advantage in two surface onlays for posterior teeth. Rather than include the contact point of a sound proximal surface for retentive purposes, pins can be used and the margin terminated on the downward slope of the crest of the marginal ridge. Pins placed closer to the pulp than 0.85 mm promote cracks and pulpal stress.[32]

Pin Angulation

A diagonally directed or horizontally directed pin is much more subject to dislodgement than the vertical type.

Drill Breakage

The bibevel twist drill is different from the conventional dental bur. Because it cuts a clean channel and will not tolerate lateral thrust, as a dental bur will, it is subject to occasional breakage. The removal of a broken drill is virtually impossible. If this occurs, the operator should abandon the drill and select a new pin site alongside the broken drill. The broken drill is covered during cementation and remains entombed within the dentin.

Pulp Exposure

Pulp exposures are often thought of as a large clinical problem, but experience has shown that pulp exposed by a drill does not necessarily need endodontic therapy.[33, 34] It is of the greatest importance, however, to recognize a pulp exposure. Often, the drill touches the pulp without actually entering it and rupturing blood vessels. A fine smooth broach instead of a dental explorer, is used to probe pinholes that are potentially in a pulpal area. This unrecognized pulp exposure is the most dangerous, not because it is an exposure, but because the operator fails to treat it as an exposure.

Blocking Out of Embrasures for Impressions

Occasionally, an impression must be made of contacting surfaces from which it would be extremely difficult to withdraw the material because the interproximal spaces are narrow and constricted. To prevent this difficulty, it is wise to occlude or block out the labial embrasure with a bit of wax or compound.

Temporary Protection of Pinholes

Temporization of conventional crown preparations to protect exposed dentin is standard operating procedure. When pinholes are placed in dentin, especially permeable dentin, temporaries become a matter of utmost importance because such pinholes must be sealed against saliva and debris. As an additional safeguard against the blind channels of the pinholes becoming contaminated by bacteria and their toxins, it is wise to insert the finished casting as soon as possible. Protection does not require that the pinhole be filled; a simple sealing of the orifice is adequate. Regardless of the material or method selected, temporary protection should be easily placed and removed.

Cementation

The cementation of inlays has been subjected to much investigation.[35–39] Before fitting the casting to the tooth, each pinhole is chamfered with a no. 4 round bur to form a funnel-like guide for sliding the pin into its hole. This also removes the sharp edge of dentin around the orifice that could prevent the complete seating of the casting.

The drying and medicating of the pinholes before cementation can be enhanced by the use of the rubber dam. Some operators prefer the use of a paper point or a wisp of cotton on a barbed broach for application of Copalite varnish.

Cementation of the pin casting is best done by mixing an ample volume of slow-setting cement, spinning cement into the pinholes using a shortened lentulo spiral paste filler in a handpiece, and generously coating both the tooth and the casting with cement. There are little data to confirm the accusation[40] that it is difficult for cement to be adapted around pins. This problem was stated as the reason that these restorations are associated with relatively low retentive strength.

PROBLEM SOLVING WITH PINS

There are many reasons for gold inlay failures, including recurrent caries, periodontal breakdown, sensitive teeth, tooth fracture, poor esthetic appearance, and loss of retention. When retention of a restoration proves troublesome, pins are often an excellent solution.[41] In addition, grooves on the cavity floor may aid retention by allowing a thicker layer of cement between inlay and tooth surface.[42]

Where there is a loss of lingual cusps in premolars and molars, the restoration of choice is the pin retained three-quarter crown. It demands little loss of tooth substance and is esthetically acceptable. In a conventional three-quarter crown, the grooves are placed as near the buccal aspect of the tooth as possible, thereby providing the greatest resistance to lateral displacing forces. When the lingual cusps have been lost with undermining of the buccal cusps, resistance form may depend on capping the buccal cusps by a reverse bevel. Simply reducing the vertical heights of the buccal cusps does not produce the resistance to restoration displacement by lateral loads. In this situation, pins placed in the buccal cusps will resist lateral forces. Pins placed at the gingival floor increase retention form, whereas those placed at the cusp tips increase the resistance form by tying the weakened cusps together. The effects of lateral loads in the pins may be further countered by the provision of a groove at the mesial edge of the capped cusps to allow better frictional retention for the casting without showing any more gold. When there is total loss of all cusps, unless the pulp is involved, effective retention can only be achieved by the use of pins. In most situations these would retain a foundation to be covered by a full crown restoration.

REFERENCES

1. Tucker R.V.: Variation of inlay cavity design. *J. Am. Dent. Assoc.* 84:616, 1972.
2. Black G.V.: A restatement of the principles of extension for prevention and some correlated subjects. *Br. J. Dent. Sci.* 45:732, 1902.
3. Rosensteil E.: Retention of inlays and crowns as a function of geometrical form. *Br. Dent. J.* 103:388, 1957.
4. Kaufman E.G., Coelho D.H., Laurence C.: Factors influencing the retention of cemented gold castings. *J. Prosthet. Dent.* 11:487, 1961.

5. Smyd E.S.: Factors which influence casting accuracy: A universal casting technic. *J. Am. Dent. Assoc.* 36:160, 1948.
6. Lewis R.M., Owen M.M.: Mathematical solution of a problem in full crown construction. *J. Am. Dent. Assoc.* 59:943, 1959.
7. Tanner A.N.: Pin paralleling techniques. *Israel J. Dent. Med.* 19:13, 1970.
8. Reynolds C.B.: Pin-locked cast gold inlays in abutment teeth. *Dent. Items of Int.* 31:814, 1909.
9. Burgess J.K.: Consideration of some of the problems and details of the operative side of bridgework. *Pacific Dent. Gaz.* 25:498, 1917.
10. Wesserman H.: Pinledge bridge attachment for anterior teeth. *Dent. Cosmos.* 65:1310, 1923.
11. Trigger T.C.: Principles of cavity preparation as applied to gold and porcelain inlays. *Dominion Dent. J.* 45:53, 1933.
12. Iwansson R.: The pinledge attachment and its use for fixed bridges. *Dent. Items of Int.* 56:202, 1936.
13. Shooshan E.D.: Pin-ledge casting technique—its application in periodontal splinting. *Dent. Clin. North Am.* 189, March, 1960.
14. Schnepper H.E., Baum L.: Miniature parallel pins for retention of cast restorations. *J. Prosthet. Dent.* 11:772, 1961.
15. Auth V.C.: The large gold inlay with pin retention. *Dent. Dig.* 72:104, 1966.
16. Lorey R.E., Embrell K.A., Myers G.E.: Retentive factors in pin-retained castings, *J. Prosthet. Dent.* 17:271, 1967.
17. Caputo A.A., Standlee J.P.: Pins and posts—why, when, and how. *Dent. Clin. North Am.* 20:2, 1976.
18. Going R.E.: Pin-retained gold foil. *J. Am. Dent. Assoc.* 78:323, 1969.
19. Kinzer R.L.: Porcelain inlays using retentive pins. *J. Indiana State Dent. Assoc.* 53:8, 1974.
20. Douglass G.D.: Principles of preparation design in fixed prosthodontics. *J. Acad. Gen. Dent.* 21:25, 1973.
21. Farah J.W., Dennison J.B., Powers J.M.: Effects of design on stress distribution of intracoronal gold restorations. *J. Am. Dent. Assoc.* 94:1151, 1977.
22. Holland C.S.: Cast gold restorations for teeth with large carious lesions. *Br. Dent. J.* 131:16, 1971.
23. Mondelli J., Steagall L., Ishikiriama A.: Fracture strength of human teeth with cavity preparations. *J. Prosthet. Dent.* 43: 419, 1980.
24. Moffa J.P., Phillips R.W.: Retentive properties of parallel pin restorations. *J. Prosthet. Dent.* 17:387, 1967.
25. Lorey R.E.: Abutment considerations. *Dent. Clin. North Am.* 24:63, 1980.
26. Arnim S.S.: Conservation of the dental pulp—cavity preparation. *J. Prosthet. Dent.* 9:1017, 1959.
27. Dilts W.E., Mullaney T.P.: Relationship of pinhole location and tooth morphology in pin-retained silver amalgam restorations. *J. Am. Dent. Assoc.* 76:1011, 1968.
28. Gourley J.V.: Favourable locations for pins in molars. *Oper. Dent.* 5:2, 1980.
29. Markley M.R.: Pin reinforcement and retention of amalgam formations and restorations. *J. Am. Dent. Assoc.* 56:675, 1958.
30. Brannstrom M., Nyborg H.: Pulpal reaction to polycarboxylate and zinc phosphate cements used with inlays in deep cavity preparations. *J. Am. Dent. Assoc.* 94:308, 1977.
31. Leidal T.I., Eriksen H.M.: Microleakage along composite restorations in human premolars after treatment with different cleansing agents. *Scand. J. Dent. Res.* 87:470, 1979.
32. Trabert R.C., Caputo A.A., Collard E.W.: Stress transfer to the dental pulp by retentive pins. *J. Prosthet. Dent.* 30:808, 1973.
33. Dolph R.W.: Intentional implanting of pins into dental pulp. *Dent. Clin. North Am.* 14:73, 1970.
34. Suzuki M., Goto G., Jordan R.E.: Pulpal response to pin placement. *J. Am. Dent. Assoc.* 87:636, 1973.
35. Silness J.: Distribution of artificial crowns and fixed partial dentures. *J. Prosthet. Dent.* 23:641, 1970.

36. Jorgenson K.D.: Relationship between retention and convergence angle in cemented veneer crowns. *Acta Odontol. Scand.* 13:35, 1955.
37. McLean J.W.: Restoration of anterior teeth. *Ann. R. Coll. Surg. Engl.* 48:35, 1971.
38. Hembree J.H., George T.A., Hembree M.E.: Film thickness of cements beneath complete crowns. *J. Prosthet. Dent.* 39:533, 1978.
39. Hoard R.J., Caputo A.A., Contino R.M.: Intracoronal pressure during crown cementation. *J. Prosthet. Dent.* 40:520, 1978.
40. Burns B.B.: Pin retention of cast gold restorations. *J. Prosthet. Dent.* 15:1101, 1965.
41. Fayle H.E.: Gold inlay failures and some causes. *J. Prosthet. Dent.* 29:439, 1973.
42. Chan K.C., Boyer D.B., Reinhardt J.W.: Comparison of the retentive strength of two cast gold pin techniques. *J. Prosthet. Dent.* 42:527, 1979.

CHAPTER 8

Gingival Retraction and Tissue Management

KEITH E. THAYER, D.D.S.

GINGIVAL RETRACTION and tissue management are critical phases of fixed prosthodontics. Any preparation with a subgingival margin cannot be successfully and accurately recorded without proper and adequate tissue retraction. The retraction procedures used must not permanently alter or damage the gingiva. Consequently, tissue management becomes as important as tissue retraction.

The epinephrine-impregnated cord is most commonly used for gingival retraction. In a recent survey[1] epinephrine cord was the choice of more than 73% of the respondents. Nonepinephrine cord was the choice of only about 23%. There is considerable concern about the possible systemic effects of the epinephrine. Numerous studies, in both animals and humans, have been conducted during the past 20 years[2–8] that have reported varying and conflicting results. Some studies in dogs showed no significant increase in blood pressure[2] or heart rate,[4] whereas another study with monkeys disclosed a moderate elevation in pressure of 4% to 18%.[5] A later dog study[6] indicated that physical procedures, such as tooth preparation and tissue abrasion along with mechanical placement of the cord, affected pressure and rate. This suggests endogenous adrenalin production and supports an earlier speculation.[2] Another study on monkeys[8] reported an increase in blood pressure from electrosurgical retraction procedures.

One human study[3] reported a minimal variation in rate or pressure. Another human study[7] reported that an increased pulse rate depends more on anxiety and stress than blood level of epinephrine and that blood pressure is elevated by placement of epinephrine cords on an exposed vascular bed or lacerated tissue. Four percent racemic epinephrine cords produced less elevation than 8% cords.

It is generally accepted that the use of epinephrine retraction cords on patients with cardiovascular disease history of any kind is highly contraindicated. It is also contraindicated in patients with diabetes and those using antidepressant drugs that potentiate the effect of epinephrine.[9] Because epinephrine cords are so effective and so widely used it should be well understood that any cardiovascular system response to them will most likely be increased with use of a high concentration of epinephrine, increased number of teeth retracted, and increased area of exposed vascular bed including abrasion and trauma. An apprehensive or fatigued patient is more apt to respond negatively to the drug. If a large number of teeth are to be prepared in one arch it is advisable to schedule separate appointments for preparation and impression to allow abraded tissue surfaces to recover. The additional appointment may also result in a less fatigued and less apprehensive patient.

In cases of severe adverse reaction to epinephrine retraction cords the appropriate treatment is to place the patient in a prone position and give oxygen.

GINGIVAL RETRACTION MODES

Gingival retraction modes may be classified in three categories:[10] mechanical, chemical or mechanico-chemical, and surgical or electrical.

Mechanical

The typical mechanical retraction is done with a copper tube or band (Fig 8–1) where the tube mechanically displaces the tissue as the tube is seated to make a modeling compound impression. Copper tubes, which provide mechanical retraction, may also be used with the elastomeric impression materials.

Another mechanical retraction technique uses leather rings that are placed in the sulcus apically to the prepared margin while the impression is made. A modified and flared copper band[11] may also be placed around the prepared tooth and incorporated into an elastomeric impression in a full arch tray while mechanically displacing the gingival tissue away from prepared margins. The key to successful mechanical retraction is to carefully fit and festoon the copper tube or band.

Delayed mechanical retraction may be done with an overextended temporary protection, usually of aluminum, filled with temporary stopping, gutta percha, or another thermoplastic material. The temporary crown is placed on the prepared tooth and allowed to remain for 24 or more hours. This usually results in nonreversible tissue displacement and possible gingival attachment relocation. It is never indicated except when such changes are acceptable to the treatment plan.

Chemical

Chemical retraction is done with the aid of some sort of chemical agent (Fig 8–2 A,B). The agent is applied with the aid of a cotton cord, string, or pellet. The placement of this material adds a mechanical component to the procedure and thus the term mechanico-chemical is applied by some dentists.

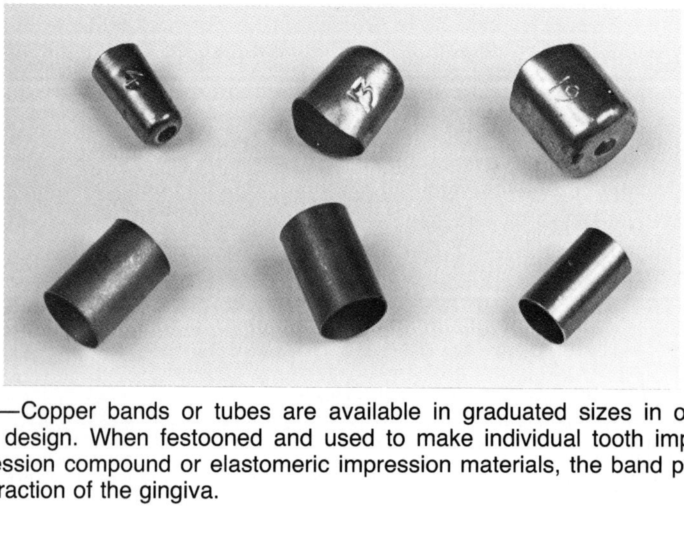

Fig 8–1.—Copper bands or tubes are available in graduated sizes in open end or closed end design. When festooned and used to make individual tooth impressions in either impression compound or elastomeric impression materials, the band provides mechanical retraction of the gingiva.

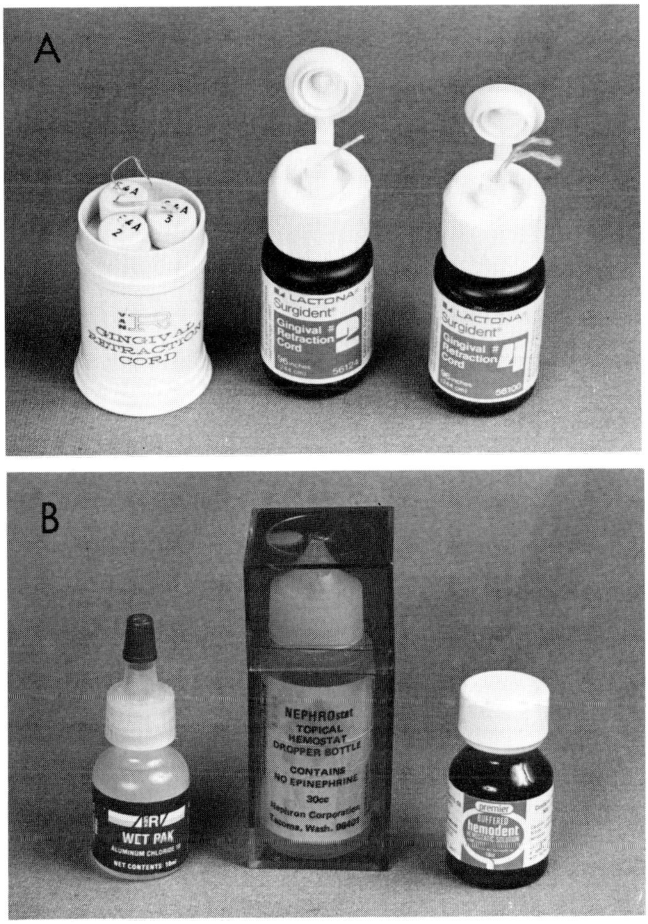

Fig 8–2.—A, epinephrine impregnated gingival retraction cord is available from numerous manufacturers. It is available in varying diameters and numbers of strands, and the weave or hardness of the cord also varies. There is also a choice of epinephrine concentration. **B,** aluminum chloride is the second most popular chemical agent. In liquid form it may be applied to an untreated cotton cord and is recommended for patients with a medical history that would contraindicate the use of epinephrine. Aluminum chloride solution may also be added to epinephrine cords for additional hemostatic effect. Aluminum chloride solution may be added to the cord before or after placement in the gingival sulcus.

The chemicals that are most commonly used for this method are epinephrine or adrenaline chloride, aluminum chloride, alum, or zinc chloride. As previously mentioned, epinephrine is the most popular and widely used. When the health history contraindicates epinephrine, aluminum chloride is the usual choice. Another common technique is the use of an epinephrine impregnated cord with an aluminum chloride liquid solution added to the cord either before or after it is placed in the gingival sulcus. Either drug can be used alone effectively, but they work well in combination. Epinephrine cords are available in 4% and 8% concentrations. The 4% is normally recommended and is more popular as it produces adequate retraction with fewer side effects. A .033% solution of aluminum chloride is recom-

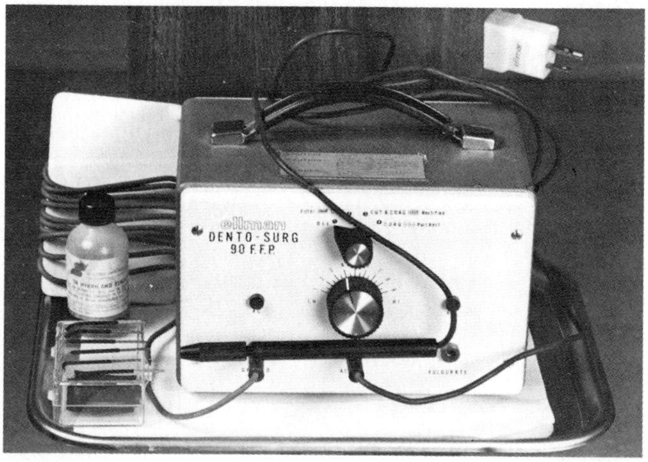

Fig 8–3.—The electrosurgery unit provides effective gingival retraction and hemorrhage control. It is also effective in removing excess tissue in problem areas such as deep subgingival margins and irregular edentulous ridge contours.

mended. Concentrated aluminum chloride solution is not recommended, as it will produce an inflammatory reaction followed by ulceration and exudate.[12]

Alum impregnated cords are available for gingival retraction. Alum is a styptic and uses a different chemistry to provide retraction. It is probably less effective than the other agents for hemorrhage control on freshly abraded tissue. It is quite effective on intact healthy gingiva. It has no contraindication for use with the patient with cardiovascular disease history. Like aluminum chloride, alum may also be used in combination with epinephrine. One study[13] reports this combination to be the most effective for reduction of gingival exudate for impression making. Alum is recommended for use in a 100% concentration.[14]

Zinc chloride is now seldom recommended and little used as a gingival retraction agent. It is available in 8% and 40% impregnated cords. Chemically, it is escheratic and can produce permanent soft tissue and bone damage if used in high concentrations or left in contact with tissue for extended periods. At best, the tissue recovery time is more than twice that of any other retraction mode.[14]

Surgical

Electrosurgery (Fig 8–3) is an effective and safe mode of gingival retraction. Used properly, it is effective in hemorrhage control as well as for providing a trough for introduction of the impression material into the sulcus.[15–17] Electrosurgery is also recommended for use in conjunction with the chemically acting gingival retraction cords.[14]

Technical skill and dexterity are important in electrosurgical retraction. The adjustment of the surgical unit is also important. Once learned and mastered it becomes routine. Without proper use and care it is possible to cause serious or permanent tissue damage.

CLINICAL TECHNIQUES

Copper bands or tubes are available in open or closed end design. The open end allows better vision for fitting and festooning the band. The closed end, which usually has a small perforation to allow for the escape of excess impression material, provides more rigidity and resists metal deformation and distortion at the time of removal of the tube impression.

The band should be plainly and consistently marked on the facial surface so that it may be repeatedly replaced accurately on the prepared tooth. The band should be heat softened so that it can be easily and accurately adapted to the circumferential tooth contours. To prevent trapping of tissue between the band and the tooth it should be the smallest diameter that will fit over the prepared margin. It is accurately festooned to correspond to the festoon of the prepared margin on the tooth. After trimming with a scissors the margin must be crimped and smoothed to provide close adaptation to the tooth and prevent trapping or traumatizing of gingival tissue.

The technique of placement of gingival retraction cord can have a profound effect on the success and quality of elastomeric impressions. The word retraction may be a misnomer as it might imply a vertical change in the tissue level. This is not done with any cord placement technique nor is it desired. The desired effect is the lateral displacement of the tissue away from the prepared tooth margin. The displacement is done mechanically with the cord but it is the chemical in the cord that maintains that displacement long enough to make the impression. The tissue gradually returns to its previous position over a period of up to 12 minutes.[10]

There are variations in the technique of cord placement but generally a dry cord and a dry sulcus are best. A dry field can usually be established easily with cotton rolls and gentle drying of the tooth with air. If the sulcus is filled with saliva or other fluid, the view is impaired and the cord becomes saturated making it more difficult to manipulate. In addition, any oral fluids absorbed by the cord dilutes the effective action of the drug in the cord. When a second retraction agent is desired, such as a combination of epinephrine and aluminum chloride, the cord is usually impregnated with epinephrine and the aluminum chloride added in solution. If this is done before cord placement, the cord should be blotted dry with a gauze sponge. A preferred method is to apply the aluminum chloride to the epinephrine cord with a cotton pellet after the cord is in place in the sulcus.

The selection of a cord with the proper diameter is important. The cord should be small enough to be completely placed in the most shallow sulcus of the prepared tooth. The sulcus depth will usually vary around the circumference of the prepared tooth. If the cord cannot be completely placed in the sulcus it is difficult to be certain that the cord is in the proper position to gain adequate tissue displacement for the impression. After one cord is accurately placed in the sulcus additional cords are placed to fill the sulcus to the level of the crest of the free gingiva. The only gingival retraction cord that effectively displaces tissue is between the tooth and the tissue. Any cord incisal or occlusal to the free gingival margin only serves to obscure vision in observing if the cord is in proper position in the sulcus (Fig 8–4,A,B).

The placement of the cord in the sulcus is best done with the aid of a double-ended instrument with opposite blade orientation on the two ends (Fig 8–5). This allows instrument access to all surfaces of the tooth. In the extremely narrow or shallow sulcus a flat periodontal probe may be helpful. The instrument end should be smooth, rounded, and thin. Most double-ended plastic instruments need some thinning and recontouring for optimum use. The instrument is used to press the cord against the hard tooth structure and to carry it subgingivally with a rolling

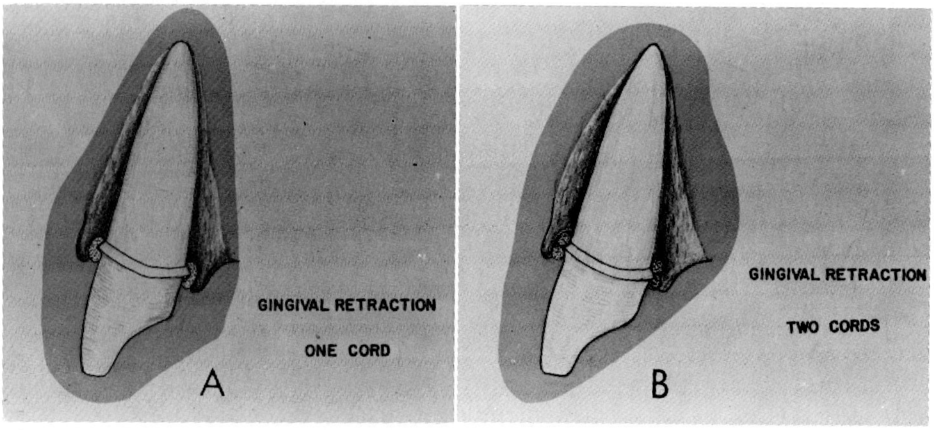

Fig 8–4.—**A,** the gingival retraction cord should fill the sulcus to the crest of the free gingiva. Any cord incisal to the free gingiva obscures vision of the cord in the sulcus. Only the cord in the sulcus displaces tissue laterally away from the prepared tooth margin that results in the desired retraction and tissue management. **B,** when the sulcus is so deep or the cord so small in diameter that it disappears in the sulcus, additional strands of cord are placed until the sulcus is filled. Because the sulcus depth varies around the circumference of most preparations, a single cord that is twice the length of the tooth circumference is recommended. This allows the first strand to be accurately placed and, where necessary, a second strand placed in one operation.

action.[18] Without the rolling action the cord is merely pressed against the elastic and compressible gingiva that springs back immediately on release. A firm but gentle pressure should be used with the instrument. Jabbing or poking with the instrument is ineffective and only serves to traumatize or irritate the gingiva and the periodontal attachment. Cases of foreign-body reaction after crown cementation have been reported.[19] The care in placing the cord and the instrument selected are important. This is especially true when the band of attached gingiva is narrow.

The cord placement is always examined and checked from the incisal or occlusal

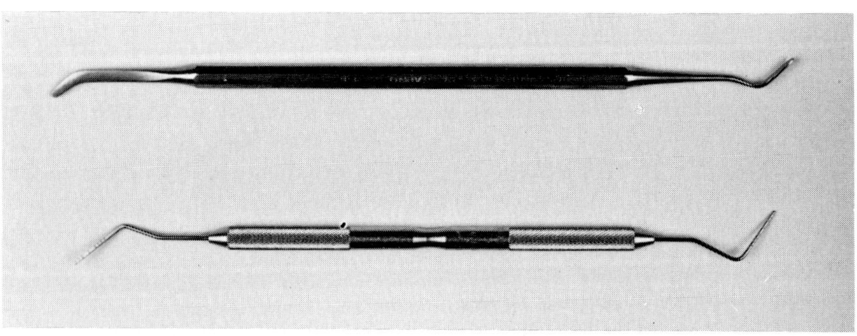

Fig 8–5.—Gingival retraction cord is most effectively placed with a thin, smooth, and rounded end instrument of a double-end design with opposite blade orientation on the two ends. This allows easy access to the entire circumference of the tooth. A flat blade periodontal probe may be helpful if a smaller instrument is required for a narrow and shallow sulcus.

aspect of the prepared tooth. The cord should be between the gingiva and the prepared tooth and should fill the sulcus to the crest of the free gingiva. If the cord is so small or the sulcus so deep that the cord disappears in the sulcus, additional strands are placed to fill the sulcus (Fig 8–4,B).

Dentists develop their own preferences in selecting materials and techniques. If medical history does not contraindicate, an effective retraction procedure is to establish a dry field, place a dry epinephrine impregnated cord, apply aluminum chloride solution to the cord in the sulcus with a cotton pellet, and allow it to remain for approximately five minutes. The moisture of the aluminum chloride solution may help to prevent any surface clot from attaching to the dry cord and resulting in the reopening of the vascular bed on removal. This defeats part of the purpose of retraction in that hemorrhage may reoccur in the sulcus before the impression can be made.

Placement of an eprinephrine gingival retraction cord before subgingival tooth preparation is a technique preferred by some operators.[20] This technique is not used in chronic disease patients where epinephrine is contraindicated. Although the technique involves the placement of three cords, the benefits of better visibility and reduced tissue hemorrhage may save time during the preparation and impression appointment.

REFERENCES

1. Shillingburg H.T., Jr. et al.: Impression materials and techniques used for cast restorations in eight states. *J. Am. Dent. Assoc.* 100:696, 1980.
2. Thayer K.E., Sawyer J.D.: Gingival retraction agents: Retraction in dogs. *Iowa Dent. J.* 49:382, 1963.
3. Houston J.B., et. al.: Effect of R-epinephrine-impregnated retraction cords on the cardiovascular system. *J. Prosthet. Dent.* 24:373, 1970.
4. Goldberg A.T., Yoder J.L., Thayer K.E.: Analysis of heart rate in dogs during retraction in impression procedures. *J. Dent. Res.* 50:645, 1971.
5. Forsyth R.P., et al.: Blood pressure responses to epinephrine-treated gingival retraction strings in rhesus monkeys. *J. Am. Dent. Assoc.* 78:1315, 1969.
6. Houston J.B., Mettler L., Shapiro N.: Epinephrine absorption from retraction cord: A study in dogs. *Pharmacol. Ther. Dent.* 3:17, 1978.
7. Pelzner R.D., et al.: Human blood pressure and pulse rate response to racemic epinephrine retraction cord. *J. Prosthet. Dent.* 39:287, 1978.
8. Stark M.M., et al.: The effect of retraction cords and electrosurgery upon blood pressure and tissue regeneration in rhesus monkeys. *J. Dent. Res.* 56:881, 1977.
9. Shaw D.H., Krejci R.F.: Epinephrine containing gingival retraction cords—how safe are they? *J. Nebr. Dent. Assoc.* 52:7, 1976.
10. Harrison J.D.: Prevention of failures in making impressions and dies. *Dent. Clin. North Am.* 23:13, 1979.
11. Holmes H.M.: Gingival displacement, not retraction. *Dent. Surv.* 44:35, 1968.
12. Shaw D.H., Krejci R.F., Cohen D.M.: Retraction cords with aluminum chloride: Effect on the gingiva. *Oper. Dent.* 5:138, 1980.
13. Wilson C.A., Tay W.M.: Alum solution as an adjunct to gingival retraction: A clinical evaluation. *Br. Dent. J.* 142:155, 1977.
14. Fisher D.W.: Conservative management of the gingival tissue for crowns. *Dent. Clin. North Am.* 20:273, 1976.
15. Flocken J.E.: Electrosurgical management of soft tissues in restorative dentistry. *Dent. Clin. North Am.* 24:247, 1980.
16. Scrivner E.I., Jr.: Gingival tissue management during fixed prosthodontic procedures. *Dent. Clin. North Am.* 15:587, 1971.
17. Oringer M.J.: Reason and remedy for conflicting reports on comparative effects of steel

scalpel and electrosurgical cutting on gingival tissues and alveolar bone. *J. Am. Dent. Assoc.* 92:850, 1976.
18. Nemetz H.: Tissue management in fixed prosthodontics. *J. Prosthet. Dent.* 31:628, 1974.
19. Fine L., et al.: Foreign body-type reaction following crown cementation. *J. Periodontol.* 48:294, 1977.
20. Reiman, M.B.: Exposure of subgingival margins by nonsurgical gingival displacement. *J. Prosthet. Dent.* 36:649, 1976.

CHAPTER 9

Impression Materials and Techniques

SATISH C. KHERA, D.D.S.

THE GLOSSARY OF PROSTHODONTIC TERMS[1] defines an impression as: "1) An imprint or negative likeness. 2) The negative form of the teeth and/or other tissues of the oral cavity, *made* in a plastic material which becomes hard or set while in contact with these tissues. An impression is *made* in order to reproduce a positive form or cast of the recorded tissues."

In this definition, the word "made" has been underlined to emphasize that impressions in dentistry are "made" rather than "taken."[2] In fixed prosthodontics before the actual seating of the impression tray in the mouth, the clinician retracts the soft tissue surrounding the prepared tooth on all subgingival margins. The preparation is cleaned of any debris and completely isolated from saliva and blood. When the impression tray is seated, it must be properly positioned in the buccolingual and anteroposterior aspects, and stabilized with gentle pressure. The position must be maintained constantly throughout the polymerization or setting of the impression material. Heavy pressure could slightly displace teeth or compress soft tissue. The resulting impression would not accurately record the true relationship of the soft tissue and the teeth adjacent to the prepared tooth. If the impression tray is not stabilized during the setting of the material, it could be displaced by gravity, hydraulic effect, or by movement of the patient's tongue, lips, or cheeks. This would likewise result in an inaccurate impression. The entire procedure must be carefully managed to obtain an accurate, detailed negative imprint of the area that will facilitate the fabrication of the restoration. Clearly, with proper management of oral structures, the clinician is *making* rather than taking an impression of the area to satisfy the requirements.

PREREQUISITES FOR GOOD IMPRESSIONS

The quality of the impression will reflect the efforts of the dentist. The materials available for making impressions are accurate, workable, and can produce excellent results if the conditions in which they are used are ideal. The materials must be properly manipulated.

The minimum conditions required to make good impressions are:

1. A tooth preparation that is free from debris and saliva, blood, or plaque films;
2. An adjacent free marginal gingiva that is properly retracted from the tooth preparation thereby exposing the finish line, and an area approximately 1 mm apically, to ensure the accurate recording of this most critical area in the preparation.

The space made available in the gingival sulcular area must allow sufficient thickness of the impression material to ensure against a thin film of the set material tearing and destroying the recorded detail when it is removed from the mouth. Any thin subgingival extensions of the impression material may also be distorted or displaced by the die material when the impression is poured; and

3. The quadrant or area of the tooth preparation must be completely isolated and must remain dry while the impression is made. If the operating area is contaminated with saliva, blood, or other debris, an accurate impression is virtually impossible.

Cleaning the Preparation

Many methods and agents have been used to clean the tooth preparation and the surrounding area before impression making. The use of a water spray is among the most common and effective methods. A solution of 3% hydrogen peroxide can also be used for this purpose. Some clinicians[3] have advocated the use of commercially prepared products such as Acriphen* to both cleanse and disinfect the cavity preparation. A mild citric acid, Epoxylite 9060 cavity cleaner,** may be used to clean the tooth preparation and the surrounding tissue. Some of these products may have potential damaging effects on the pulp and also the adjacent soft tissue if not properly and carefully used. This is especially true if the tooth preparation is deep or if the soft tissue is badly lacerated and not adequately protected. The use of this type of cleanser should be limited to selected and ideal conditions and every effort should be made to be sure that the tooth preparation and the surrounding soft tissue is thoroughly and completely washed and rinsed with water to eliminate any possible irritation from residual agents.

Tissue Management

Subgingival margins must be exposed by lateral displacement of the tissue for impression making. Retraction agents and materials must be compatible with the patient's general health. They must provide effective hemorrhage control and sufficient tissue displacement to allow for adequate marginal bulk of impression material for an accurate impression.

Isolation of the Preparation

After the preparation has been thoroughly cleaned and any hemorrhage from the soft tissue controlled, it is gently air dried. Blowing that is too vigorous could lead to a dessicated preparation and to hypersensitivity of the pulp. Severe dessication leads to pulpal emphysema that results in hypersensitivity and possibly, eventual death of the pulp.

Cotton rolls, gauze, and suction are aids in maintaining a dry and isolated field. Saliva, tongue, cheeks, and lips should not come in contact with the preparation area. The area should remain isolated throughout gingival retraction procedures, injection of syringe material, and seating of the impression tray. The cotton rolls, gauze, and gingival retraction materials should be removed just before injecting the syringe impression material into the sulcular area.

---

*Obergfeb Bros., Los Angeles, CA

**Lee Pharmaceuticals, South El Monte, CA

IMPRESSION MATERIALS FOR FIXED PROSTHODONTICS

Impression Compound

Many impression materials have been used for making impressions of prepared teeth. One of the very earliest commonly used materials was impression compound. It is used in a festooned copper tube or band for making impressions of individual tooth preparations.[4] With the advent of newer and better impression materials including reversible hydrocolloids, polysulfides, silicone rubbers, polyethers, and vinyl polysiloxanes the use of impression compound is becoming obsolete. The techniques using this material for making impressions will not be discussed here.

Hydrocolloids

Reversible hydrocolloids (Fig 9–1) have enjoyed popularity in the profession ever since the technique of using the material was described in 1937.[5] It has proved to be a good impression material for many clinicians. It is relatively inexpensive and is not as unpleasing in color, odor, or taste as are some of the newer final impression materials. Hydrocolloids are slightly hydrophilic and will tolerate the presence of small amounts of moisture in the sulcular area.

Hydrocolloid is not as immediately available for use for impression making as the elastomeric materials as it has to be specially prepared before use. This requires the use of a hydrocolloid conditioning unit. The operation and maintenance of the unit itself requires attention for accuracy of temperature. Inaccurate or improper temperature of water in the units will directly affect the viscosity, handling characteristics, and accuracy of the material as well as patient comfort. Special water cooled rim-lock trays with water tubes are also required. The cost of the conditioning unit and special trays partially negates the cost saving of the material itself.

Some dentists find the finish lines as recorded in the impression difficult to read. The material has weak edge strength and may tear in deep sulcus areas and thin interproximal spaces common in partial coverage preparations. Hydrocolloid distorts rapidly in a normal atmospheric environment. Therefore, the impression must be poured with die material immediately after removal from the mouth. The impression cannot be stored or sent to a commercial laboratory for pouring without running a great risk of dimensional distortion in the process. Hydrocolloid impres-

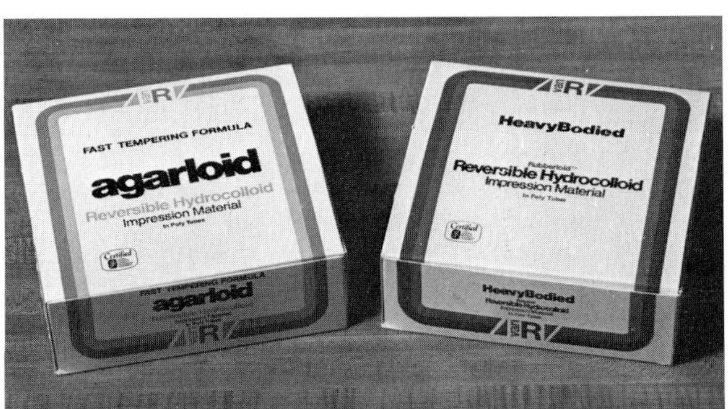

Fig 9–1.—A representative example of reversible hydrocolloid impression material for tray and syringe use. (Courtesy of Patterson Dental Supply Co., Cedar Rapids, Iowa.)

sions are not recommended to be electroplated for making dies because of the physical instability of the material before and during electrodeposition.[6] From the standpoint of the patient, the material could be uncomfortably warm if the tempering bath of the conditioning unit is not functioning properly.

It is quite possible that some of the above factors have led to the decrease in popularity of the use of hydrocolloid. A recent survey[7] showed that the newer elastomeric impression materials were almost four times as popular as the hydrocolloids. The availability of even newer materials, like vinyl polysiloxanes which have high dimensional stability even after several days, will probably further affect the clinical use of hydrocolloids. Hydrocolloids remain popular in many areas of the world. The use of these materials has been well described and documented in the literature,[6] so detailed description of manipulative techniques of hydrocolloids will not be undertaken here.

Polysulfides

Polysulfide impression materials were the first in a long line of elastomeric impression materials. The rapid and general acceptance of the elastomeric materials that were introduced to the profession in the early 1950s[8] are attributed to some clinically important factors. These materials do not require any special equipment for their use, as do hydrocolloids. The pouring of the dies immediately after removal of the impression from the mouth is less critical than for hydrocolloids. The pouring of the die material may be safely delayed for up to a half hour for polysulfide impressions if the clinical schedule demands. The dimensional stability shown by these materials is superior to that of the hydrocolloids.

Polysulfide rubber base material (Fig 9–2), also referred to as mercaptan rubber impression material, is probably the most popular of the elastomeric impression materials. Shillingburg's survey[7] showed that this material was used by about 45% of the clinicians responding. This popularity may be attributed to several factors. It was the first elastomeric impression material introduced to the profession and has

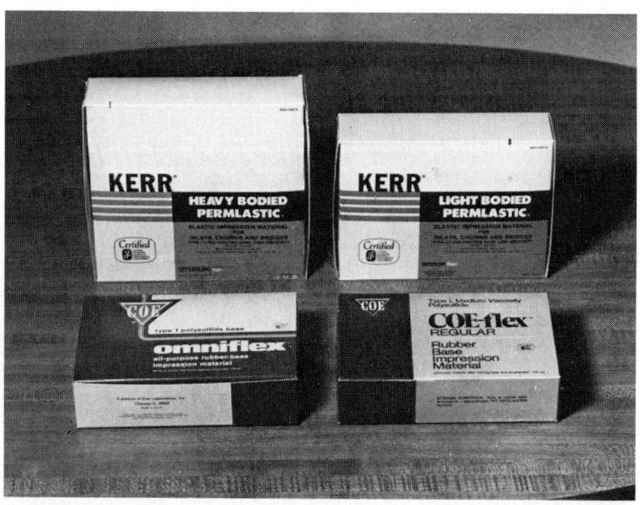

Fig 9–2.—Two brands of varying consistency of polysulfide rubber base impression materials. (Courtesy of Patterson Dental Supply Co., Cedar Rapids, Iowa.)

been taught quite widely in dental schools. Another important factor may be the cost. Compared with other elastomeric materials, polysulfides are the least expensive and produce equally good results. The material has good body and edge strength for recording the deep gingival sulcus areas. Multiple casts and dies can be obtained from a single impression. If first pour dies are defective, a second pour, made immediately, will be accurate if the impression has not been physically damaged during the separation of the first die. Polysulfide impressions can be silver plated if desired.

Because dimensional changes in the form of shrinkage[9] may start to occur in this material after 30 minutes, sending rubber base impressions to a commercial laboratory unpoured will most likely result in dimensional changes leading to less accurate castings. A custom resin tray will help to minimize the dimensional change discrepancies. A custom tray allows a uniformly thick layer of impression material,[10–13] whereas a stock tray will produce an impression that may be thick in certain areas and thin in others. This variation in thickness of impression material will increase the likelihood of a distorted impression. Polymerized polysulfide rubber is elastic but quite firm. Therefore, any severe anatomical undercuts in the mouth should be blocked out before the impression is made. Soft utility wax may be used to block out undercuts around pontics or open gingival embrasures. Rubber base is hydrophobic in nature and does not tolerate the presence of moisture in the gingival sulcus. A completely dry field, devoid of any saliva or blood, is required for accurately recording preparation margins.

The color and odor of this material are quite objectionable to some. If the unpolymerized material is allowed to come in contact with clothing, it cannot be removed from the garment.

Silicones

Early silicone base elastomeric impression materials of the condensation type were introduced in the late 1950s.[14] These early products had many defects. The material produced gases during continuing polymerization that lead to porosities on the surface of the cast. They had a short shelf life and critical working time. Their accuracy was inconsistent and erratic. Time and persistent research produced the silicone base impression materials that are now consistently accurate and widely accepted for clinical use.

These silicones (Fig 9–3) polymerize by a condensation type chemical reaction. The catalyst for the reaction is either stannous octate or dibutyl tin dilaurate, which promotes cross linkage of the silicone polymer molecule by alkyl silicates.[9] This is accomplished by a condensation reaction between the hydroxyl group of the silicone polymer and the ethoxy group of the alkyl silicate. This results in the splitting out of methanol or ethyl alcohol molecules. These molecules evaporate in a gaseous form leading to subsequent contraction of the impression material and pitting of the dies if the die material is poured into the impression immediately after removal from the mouth. Some manufacturers suggest that the impression should be poured approximately 1 hour after it is removed from the mouth. These alkyl silicates are highly unstable, particularly if mixed with the organo-tin component to form a single catalyst liquid. A limited shelf life may result because of oxidation of the tin component within the catalyst. Two catalysts are sometimes supplied to keep the alkyl silicate and organo-tin compounds separate until the time of mixing. This

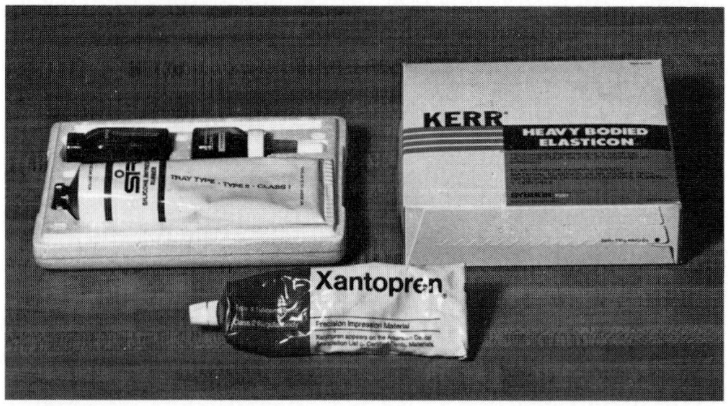

Fig 9–3.—Representative brands and consistencies of condensation type silicone base impression materials. (Courtesy of Patterson Dental Supply Co., Cedar Rapids, Iowa.)

prolongs the shelf life of the catalyst system. Shelf life may also be affected as a result of degradation or cross-linkage of the base during storage.

The contemporary silicone base materials have some distinct advantages over polysulfide rubber base impression material. The color and the odor of silicone is much more pleasant. Some of the undesirable sticky or messy properties encountered during manipulation of polysulfides have been eliminated. The silicone base materials possess excellent properties in terms of edge strength and discrimination of finish lines. They do not require any special equipment for handling and manipulation. The shelf life is still somewhat shorter than that of the polysulfides. Like polysulfides, the impressions made with these silicone base elastomers need to be made in custom trays.

The original condensation type silicone base elastomers were supplied in a two-paste system using a double mix technique. They are now also available in a putty-wash system that does not require the use of a custom tray (Fig 9–4). The technique for use of the two different systems will be discussed later. Although putty-wash impressions can be used to produce multiple dies from a single impression,

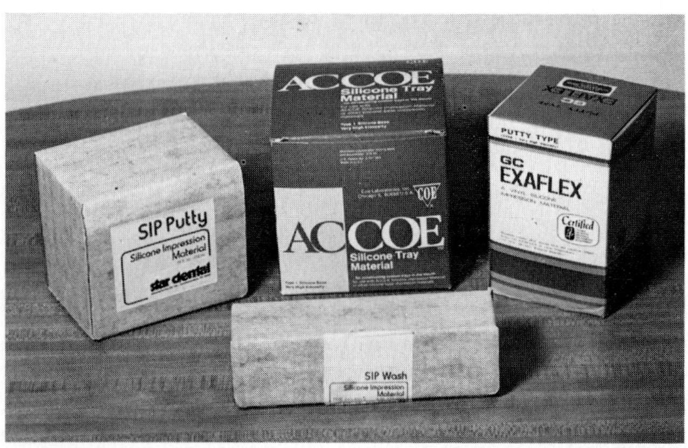

Fig 9–4.—Examples of both condensation and addition reaction silicone base impression materials for use with the putty-wash impression technique. (Courtesy of Patterson Dental Supply Co., Cedar Rapids, Iowa.)

dimensional changes are more likely to become apparent in successive pour dies. Different putty-wash systems can vary. A recent study reports that the putty-wash system of condensation type materials was not consistently reliable.[15]

Silicone base elastomers also are hydrophobic and as such do not tolerate the presence of moisture around the tooth preparation. These impressions require special care in pouring. As silicones have low wettability, this may cause bubbles or voids when the die and cast materials are poured.

Silicone base materials have reasonably good tear strength, better than the hydrocolloids but not as good as the polysulfides. Impressions made with silicone base materials are compatible with most die-making materials and techniques including silver plating. Copper plating the condensation type silicone base impressions is not recommended because of increased inaccuracies in the electroformed dies.[16] A recent study has found nickel-plating to be compatible with this material.[17]

Polyethers

Introduced in 1969,[18] the polyether type impression materials are gradually increasing in popularity (Fig 9–5). One of the advantages of this type of material is that it is faster setting and saves valuable chair time. Another advantage is that the pouring of the impression can be delayed for more prolonged periods. The impressions made with this material are easily read and there is no need to have any special equipment for handling or manipulating. The superior dimensional stability[19, 20] also allows the die material to be poured more than once to obtain multiple dies and still maintain good accuracy.[21]

In a series of research projects,[22–25] it was shown that polyethers have the highest modulus of elasticity and greatest ultimate strength 10 minutes after mixing of all the materials tested. The polyethers, along with silicones, demonstrated the least effect on setting time because of temperature rise. This material showed excellent properties during spatulation and syringing. It is resistant to displacement in the subgingival areas. These properties, along with good edge strength, make this material effective in clinical applications.[26] Polymerized polyether absorbs water. Impressions must be rinsed, dried, and stored dry until they are poured to avoid deformation.

Like the polysulfide and early silicone base impression materials, polyethers require custom trays. They require more than the usual spacing between the teeth

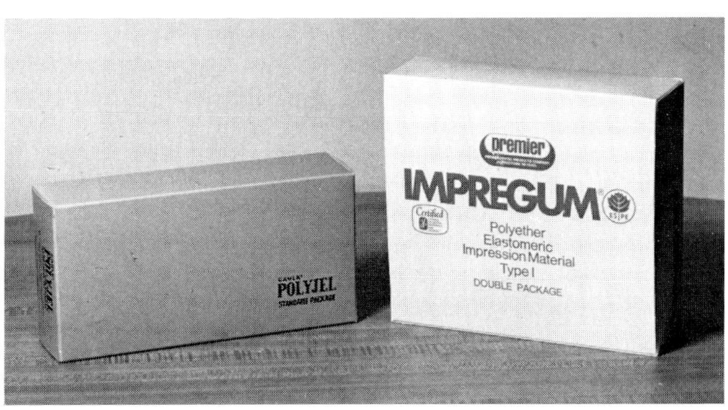

Fig 9–5.—Two popular brands of polyether impression materials. (Courtesy of Patterson Dental Supply Co., Cedar Rapids, Iowa.)

and the tray to compensate for the high rigidity of the set material. The blocking out of undercuts is important. If undercuts are not blocked out, not only is the removal of the tray from the mouth difficult, but the removal of the working cast and dies from the impression often results in fracture of dies and adjacent teeth. Manufacturers[27] and researchers,[28] suggest a spacer of 3 to 4 mm between the teeth and tray to counter this extreme rigidity. As with other elastomers, polyethers do not tolerate the presence of fluids in the gingival sulcus so preparations must be dry and well isolated before and during the impression-making procedure.[29]

Vinyl Polysiloxanes

The most recently developed elastomeric impression materials are the vinyl polysiloxanes (Fig 9–6). These are silicone materials with a different setting chemistry from the earlier condensation reaction-type silicones. They are classified as addition reaction materials. The base of both of these materials is compounded in a similar manner. It is essentially the catalyst that is different. In the addition material, the catalyst is a platinum salt and the reaction is an addition reaction.[9] The polymer is terminated with vinyl groups and is cross-linked with silane groups. This type of reaction does not leave any by-products, such as methanol in condensation silicone. This leads to excellent dimensional stability even for prolonged periods.

The setting time for the addition material is an improvement over other types of elastomeric impression materials. Comparatively, these materials offer a slightly longer working time than the condensation silicone base and polyether impression materials but much shorter than that of the polysulfides. The working time for these materials is approximately four minutes.

The addition type silicone base impression materials have better recovery properties after deformation than any other elastomeric impression materials and show the least amount of permanent deformation after set. The tear resistance of addition silicone materials is greater than the condensation materials and the polyether impression materials but less than the polysulfides.[9]

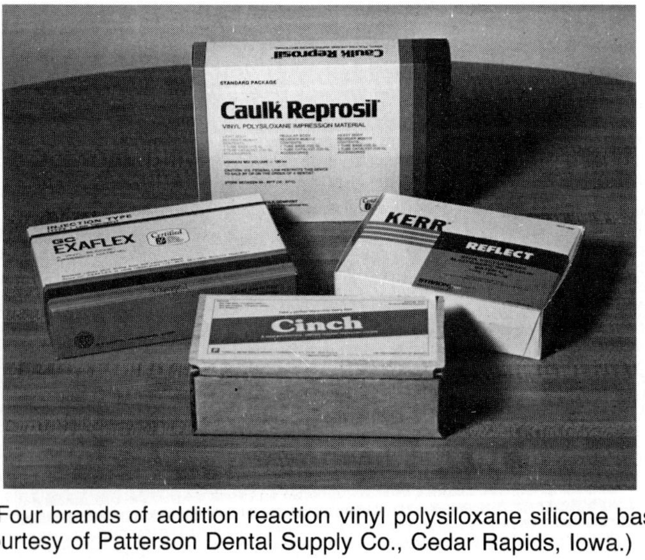

Fig 9–6.—Four brands of addition reaction vinyl polysiloxane silicone base impression materials. (Courtesy of Patterson Dental Supply Co., Cedar Rapids, Iowa.)

The most important improvement shown by the addition type vinyl polysiloxane impression materials is the dimensional stability. In a recent study,[30] this material showed the least dimension change of all the elastomeric impression materials. This quality could have far-reaching clinical implications in that the pouring of the impression could be delayed for a prolonged period and repeated highly accurate pours could be made for multiple or replacement dies. The use of a custom tray for making impressions is recommended. Undercut areas of the arch must be properly blocked out before the impression is made. Additional relief space for the impression material of up to 4 mm is recommended when the custom tray is being fabricated.[14, 31]

Addition silicone base impression materials are the most expensive elastomeric materials available. In general, the cost increases in the order the materials have been developed, polysulfides being the least expensive followed by silicones, polyethers, and vinyl polysiloxanes.

MANIPULATION OF IMPRESSION MATERIALS

Fabrication of Custom Trays

Most of the elastomeric impression materials require the use of a custom tray for best results. The only exception is the putty-wash system silicones. The tray should be fabricated at least 24 hours before the impression is made. It has been shown repeatedly [10–13, 32] that custom trays allow uniform thickness of impression material and provide greater accuracy. For polysulfides, it is recommended that the space allowed for impression material in the impression tray should be 2 to 3 mm. Other elastomeric impression materials need 3 to 4 mm of uniform space. A custom tray can be easily fabricated using autopolymerizing acrylic resin as the tray material. The following steps are recommended for the fabrication of the custom tray:

1. A preliminary cast in dental stone is made from an alginate impression of the patient (Fig 9–7);

2. The soft tissue area on the cast is marked with a pencil to the desired margin of the tray (Fig 9–8). The tray should extend at least 3-4 mm beyond the free

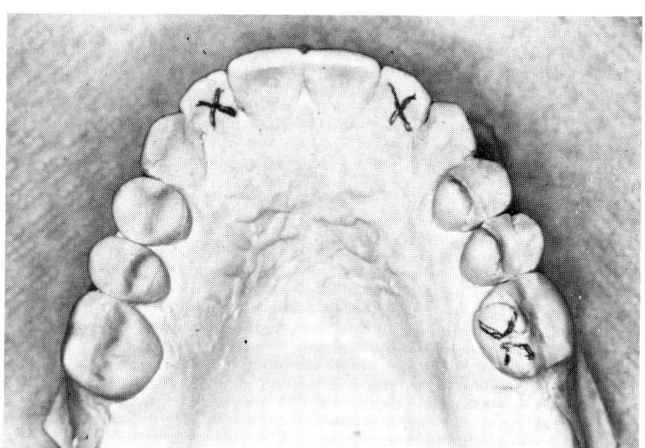

Fig 9–7.—Study cast with teeth to be prepared marked.

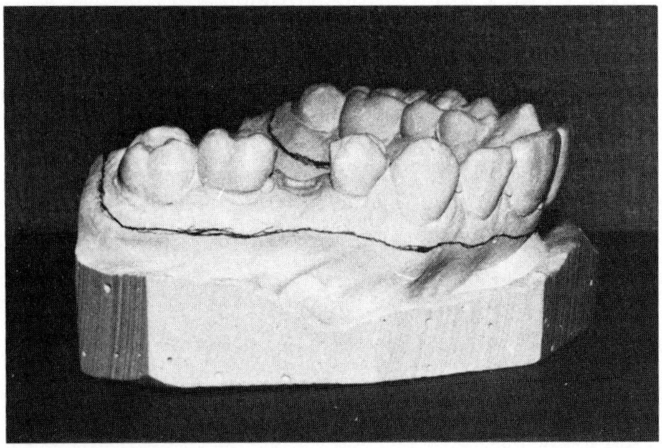

Fig 9–8.—The desired extension of the tray outlined on the study cast.

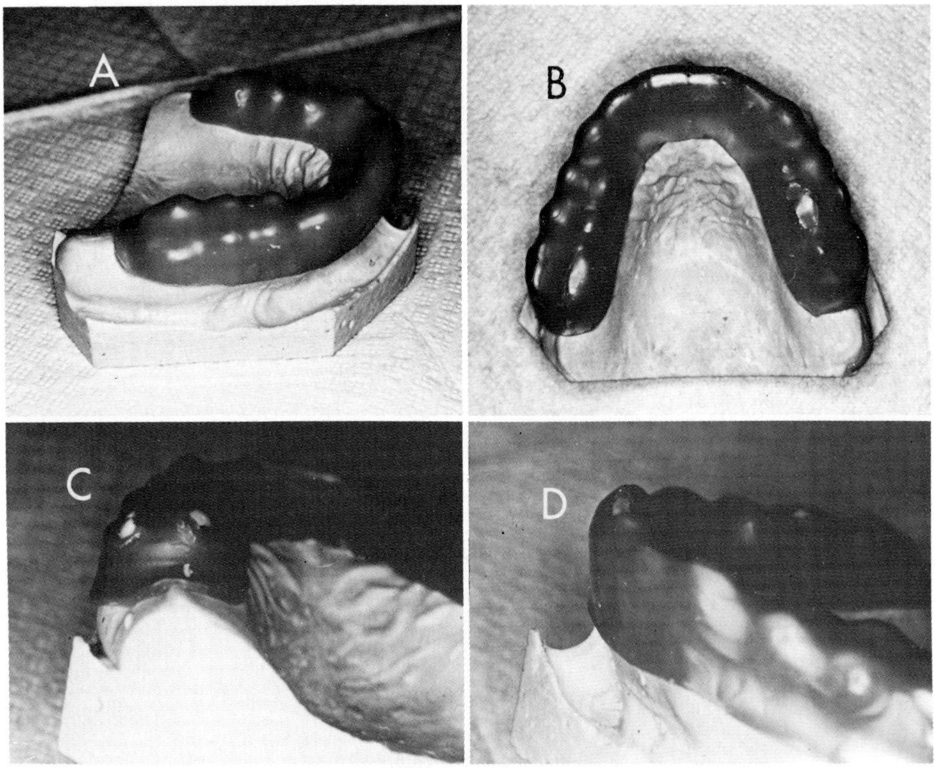

Fig 9–9.—**A,** study cast with two layers of softened base plate wax adapted on the area of the arch to be incorporated in the impression. **B,** occlusal stops established in the base plate wax so that they make a triangle. Note stops are developed to the facial and lingual aspects on both anterior and posterior teeth not involved with preparations. **C,** the flat surface of wax exposing cast to the buccal and lingual aspects, forms a flat guiding plane on the inner surface of the tray, which acts as a lateral centering guide when seating the impression. **D,** the same flat surface is developed to the labial and lingual aspects of the central incisal edges. These inclines in the tray center the impression anteroposteriorly.

gingival margin. It should include the distal surface of the most distal tooth in the arch;

3. The cast is dipped or soaked in water and 2–4 mm of softened baseplate wax is adapted on the cast (Fig 9–9,A). The baseplate wax should be trimmed to the pencil mark on the cast. Relief may also be accomplished by dipping the wet cast in melted baseplate wax or adapting wet asbestos to the cast;

4. Stops are developed on three or more widely separated teeth. Two of these stops should be placed on teeth adjacent to the teeth to be prepared. Additional stops should be placed on the opposite side of the arch or as far away from the preparation site as possible for a tripoding effect (Fig 9–9,B). If no tooth is available posterior to the most posterior preparation, a stop may be developed in an area of firm and stable soft tissue away from any proposed pontic contact area. Stops are developed at a 45° angle to the occlusal plane. Wax is removed in a flat surface down to contact with buccal inclines of buccal cusps and lingual inclines of lingual cusps (Fig 9–9,C) and labioincisal and linguoincisal angles of anterior teeth (Fig 9–9,D). These stops provide an automatic centering effect both laterally and anteroposteriorly as the tray is seated and engages buccal and lingual cusps and incisal edges. They also prevent overseating or underseating of the tray that can occur if stops are developed on cusp tips or in the sulcus;

5. Autopolymerizing acrylic tray resin is mixed in a wax paper cup. When it is still pliable but nonsticky to fingers, the material is formed into a roll that is approximately the length of the dental arch. This roll is placed over the wax shim and adapted and thinned with finger pressure to about 3 mm in thickness (Fig 9–10). All of the wax should be covered with the tray material. If care is taken to press the resin only to the margin of the wax shim, little or no excess will remain to be trimmed with a knife while the tray material is still soft. After the material is set, any necessary trimming is done with an arbor band on a lathe. This tray should not be more than 3 mm thick or the insertion and the seating of the tray in the oral cavity will be cumbersome. A 3 mm thickness of the tray is required for rigidity. A short handle in the anterior may be desired to facilitate the handling of the tray (Fig 9–11);

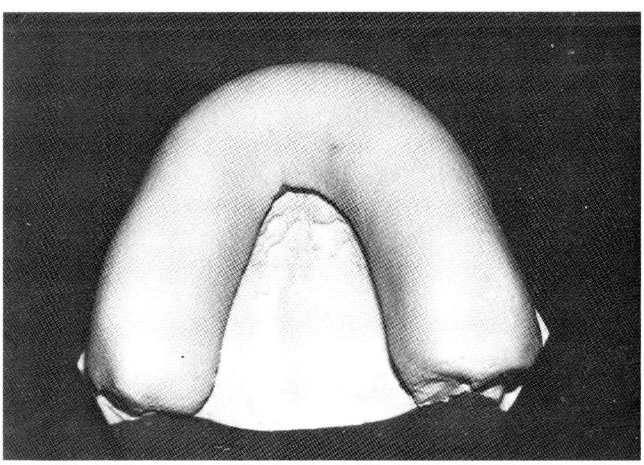

Fig 9–10.—Autopolymerizing acrylic tray resin adapted to completely cover the base plate wax.

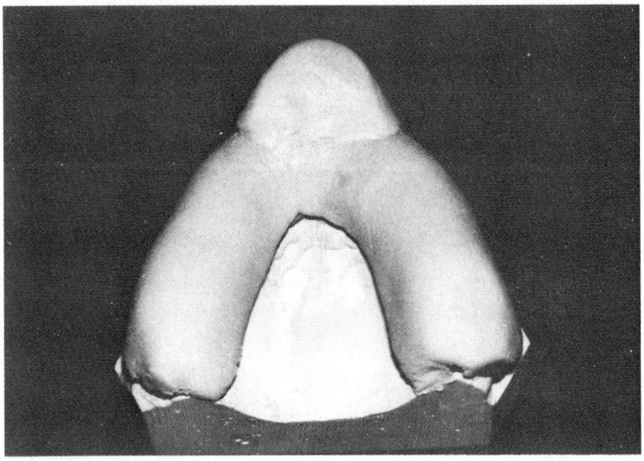

Fig 9–11.—A handle adapted in the anterior segment of the tray may help to facilitate the handling of the tray.

6. When the exothermic heat of curing occurs the cast and tray may be submerged in cold water to prevent the wax shim from melting and sticking to the tray. If preferred, when exothermic heat begins the tray may be carefully removed, the wax shim discarded, and the tray returned to the cast to finish polymerizing with the stops in contact with the cast teeth. Any wax adhering to the tray after complete polymerization must be removed;

7. Any tray extending apically to the wax shim is trimmed and rounded so that no tray comes in contact with the buccal or lingual mucosa. Any rough areas of the tray may be pumiced (Fig 9–12); and

8. A thin layer of the tray adhesive is applied on the inner surface and the periphery of the clean, dry tray (Fig 9–13). It is important to use the adhesive supplied by the manufacturer for each different impression material. Thick layers of

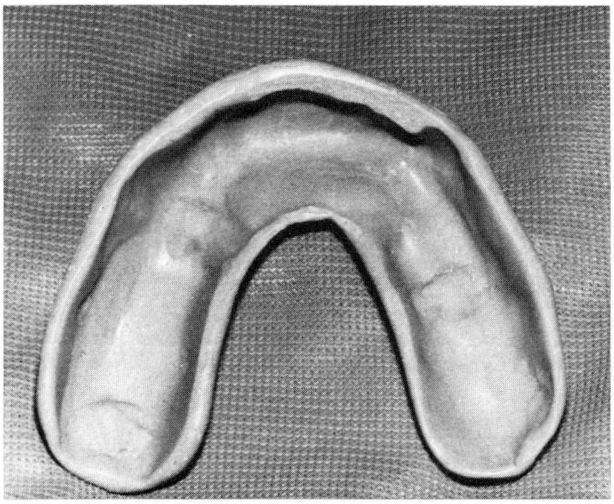

Fig 9–12.—The properly trimmed and cleaned tray ready for the application of tray adhesive.

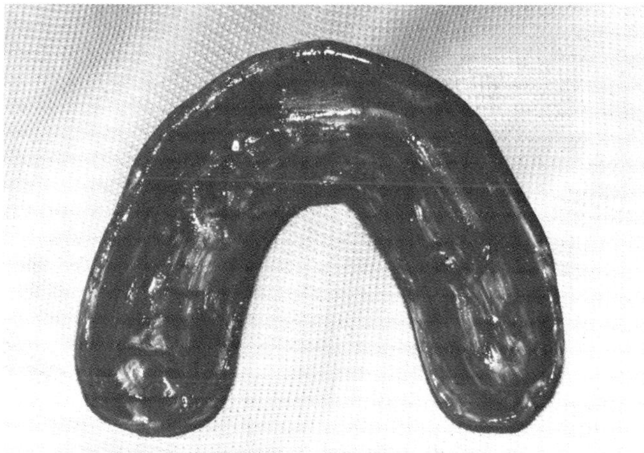

Fig 9–13.—A thin coating of tray adhesive applied on the inside of the tray and on the peripheral areas.

adhesive should be avoided. If any pools of adhesive occur in the tray, they can dry on the surface and leave a fluid interface. This renders the adhesive totally ineffective for securing the impression material to the tray. The adhesive should also be completely dry before the impression material is loaded into the tray. Wet adhesive could produce a distorted impression from nonattachment to the custom tray. The tray is now ready for use in the impression-making procedures.

DISPENSING AND MIXING THE IMPRESSION MATERIALS

Two Paste Systems

Proper dispensing is an important factor in the manipulation of the impression materials. Manufacturer's diretions should be strictly adhered to for best results. Most of the two paste systems are supplied in tubes containing base in one tube and catalyst in the other. Some techniques use the same consistency material for both syringe and tray whereas others use light bodied material for the syringe and heavy bodied for the tray. The latter is commonly referred to as a double mix technique. The following steps are recommended in the making of impressions:

1. Equal lengths of both the base and the catalyst are exuded on a paper pad usually supplied with the impression material. The base and catalyst should be placed as closely together as possible without allowing them to come in contact (Fig 9–14). If premature contact occurs before spatulation begins, polymerization will start and affect the working and physical properties of the mix. The paper pad is stabilized with one hand and the catalyst and base mixed with a firm metal spatula using a stirring action. Only the tip of the spatula should be used (Fig 9–15). If the base and the catalyst have been properly dispensed on the paper pad, the mixing will be effortless and quick. If the base and the catalyst have been dispensed too far apart or if the entire length of the blade of the spatula is used to mix and spatulate the base and the catalyst, the mixing will become messy and cumbersome. It will also take more time and will require a greater physical effort to obtain

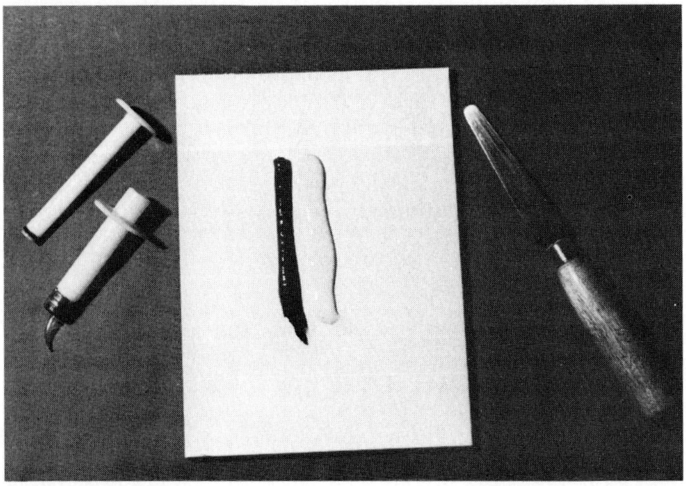

Fig 9–14.—Properly dispensed impression material. Notice that the catalyst and the base are dispensed in the middle of the pad but not touching each other. Properly cleaned and prepared syringe is placed close to the pad.

properly mixed material. The stirring of the base and the catalyst should continue until a homogenous streak-free mix is obtained. Then the blade of the spatula may be used to obtain the final homogeneity in the impression material and to remove any air bubbles that may have been trapped during stirring (Fig 9–16). The material is now ready for loading into the injection syringe;

2. The injection material is loaded into a syringe that will assure the free flow of the impression material. The inside of the syringe and the plunger should be clean and free of any remnants of impression material from previous use. The plunger of the syringe may be lightly lubricated to facilitate its free movement in the syringe

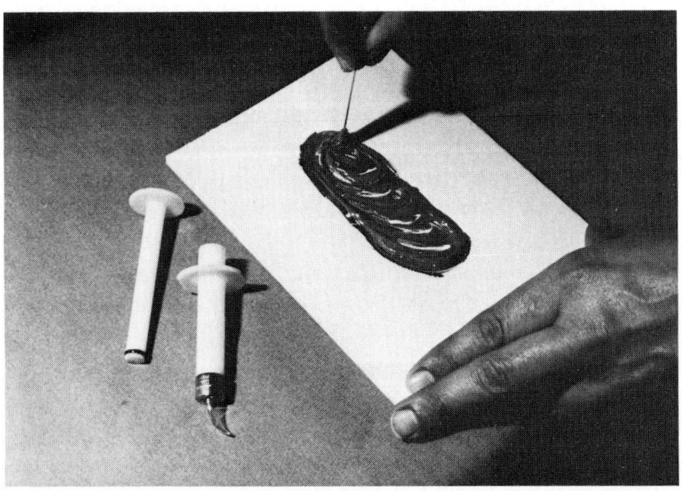

Fig 9–15.—Proper mixing of the material using only the tip of the spatula. Note the circular movement of the tip as evidenced by the pattern in the impression material.

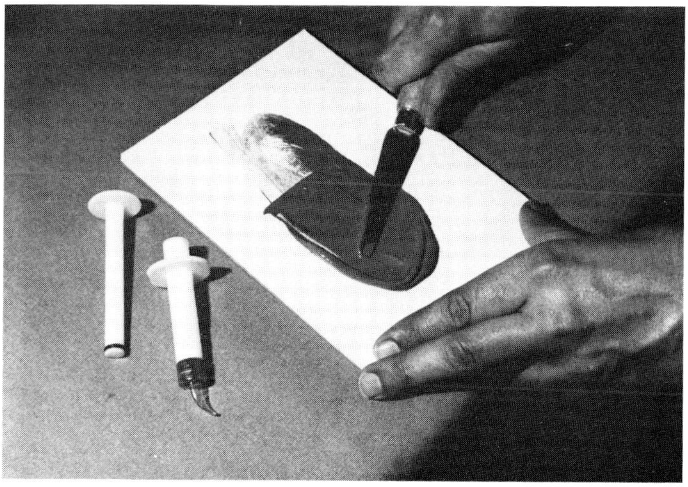

Fig 9–16.—Final homogeneity is obtained by using the flat portion of the spatula.

barrel. The tip of the syringe should also be clean and clog-free. The hole in the tip should not be too small because it should not block the free flow of the impression material. Frequently, it is advisable to enlarge the hole of the disposable tip by cutting a short section from the end with a pair of scissors. Many techniques are described in the literature on loading the syringe. All are equally good. The Kerr's* Free-Flo syringe has been chosen as a representative example (Fig 9–17). The prepared plastic tip and its retainer hub are assembled on the barrel. To load the syringe, the end of the barrel is scraped through the impression material at approximately a 45° angle from the surface of the mixing pad (Fig 9–18). When the desired amount of material is in the barrel, the outside is wiped with gauze and the plunger inserted into the barrel. The syringe is now ready for use (Fig 9–19);

3. Dispensing and mixing the heavy body impression material for use in the custom tray is similar to the technique described above. While loading the tray, it is critical to avoid the incorporation of subsurface air bubbles in the impression material. The base and catalyst must be thoroughly and homogeneously mixed. There should be no streaks in the mix. All the impression material is scraped on to the blade of the mixing spatula (Fig 9–20). To load the tray the part of the spatula closest to the handle is positioned along the lingual flange of one end of the tray (Fig 9–21). The tray is loaded by gradually moving the spatula downward at the same time it is moved around the lingual border (Fig 9–22). This technique allows for an easy and clean loading of the tray, and more importantly avoids the incorporation of air bubbles. Once the tray is properly loaded it is ready to place in the mouth;

4. Injecting the light body impression material is very critical. The field of operation must be well isolated and free and clean from blood, saliva, and any other debris. The gingival tissue must have been properly manipulated to expose the finish line of the preparation. All retracting agents must be carefully removed from

*Sybron-Kerr Manufacturing Co., Romulus, MI

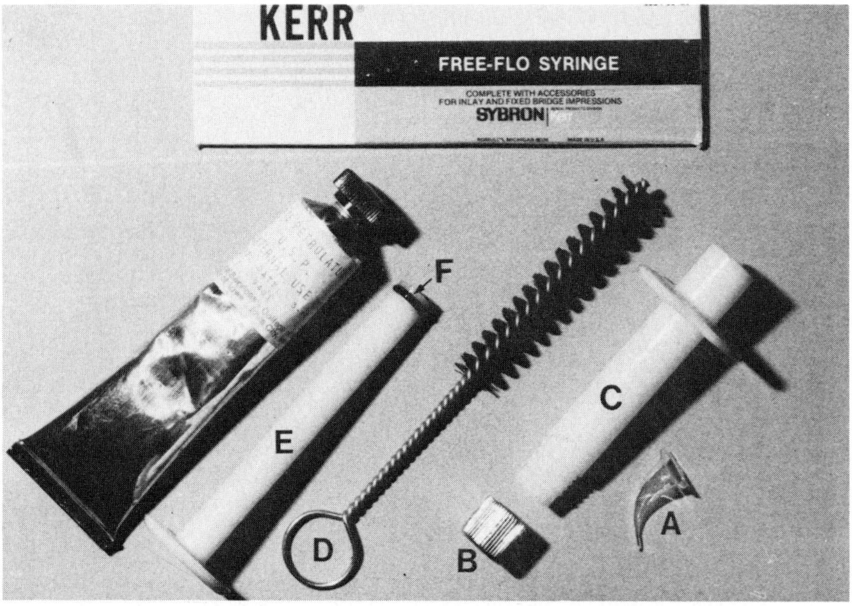

Fig 9–17.—Armamentarium display for proper use of injection syringe. A clean, clog-free plastic tip *(A)* is inserted into the retainer *(B)* and properly seated. The barrel of the syringe *(C)* should be thoroughly cleaned with the cylindrical brush *(D)* to remove any remnants of material from previous use. The retainer is screwed tightly on the barrel. The plunger *(E)* should also be cleaned and the ring washer *(F)* on the plunger should be lightly lubricated with petroleum jelly to facilitate easy action of the plunger in the barrel.

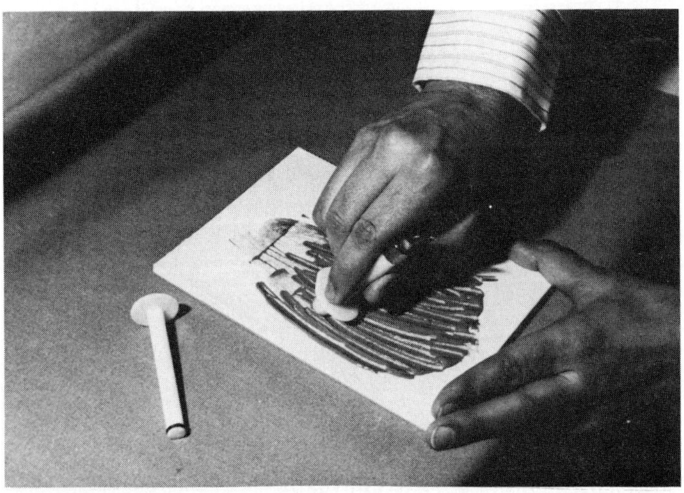

Fig 9–18.—After the material has been properly mixed, it is scraped with the spatula to one area on the pad. Holding the barrel at a 45° angle from the surface of the pad, the end is scraped through the material for filling.

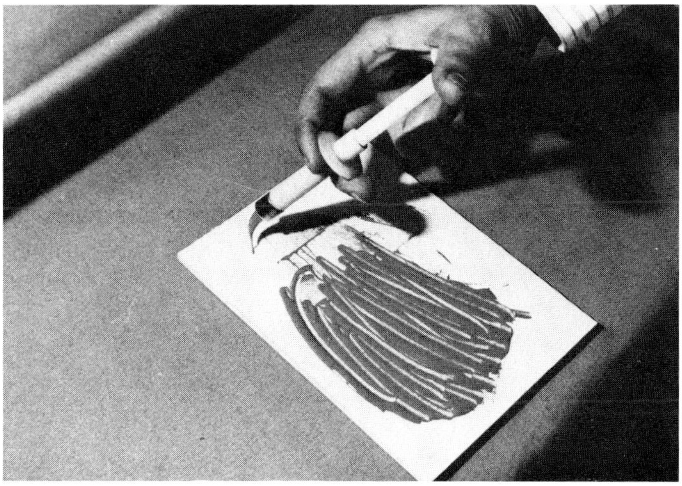

Fig 9–19.—After the desired amount of material is collected in the barrel, the plunger is inserted. The syringe is now ready for use.

the gingival sulcus. The light body impression material in the syringe is injected into the sulcus around the prepared tooth starting in the area where access is most difficult (Fig 9–23). The sulcus is filled while pushing the impression material ahead of the tip to minimize bubbles and voids in the margin areas;

5. After the light body impression material has been injected into the gingival sulcus and around the preparation, the loaded custom tray is seated. The tray stops will guide the seating of the tray buccolingually and anteroposteriorly. If the tray touches any prepared tooth surface it will result in a defective impression. If the tray touches any soft tissue surrounding prepared teeth the impression will probably fail. When the tray is fully and accurately seated, gentle continuous pressure

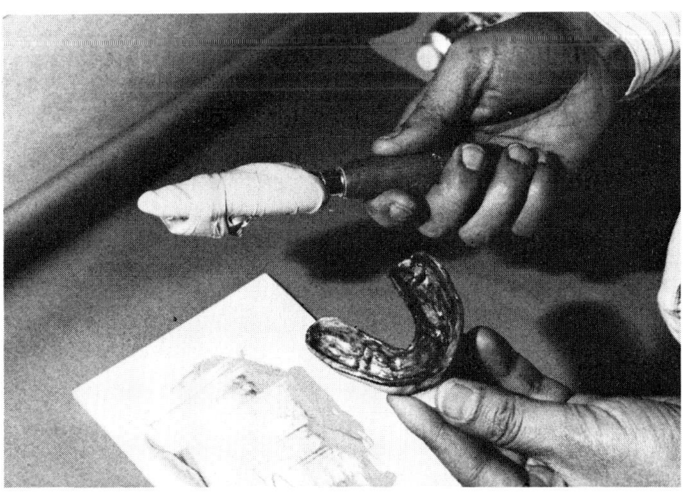

Fig 9–20.—To load the tray with heavy bodied impression material, the entire mass of mixed material is picked up on the blade of the spatula. The tray is held in the other hand as shown.

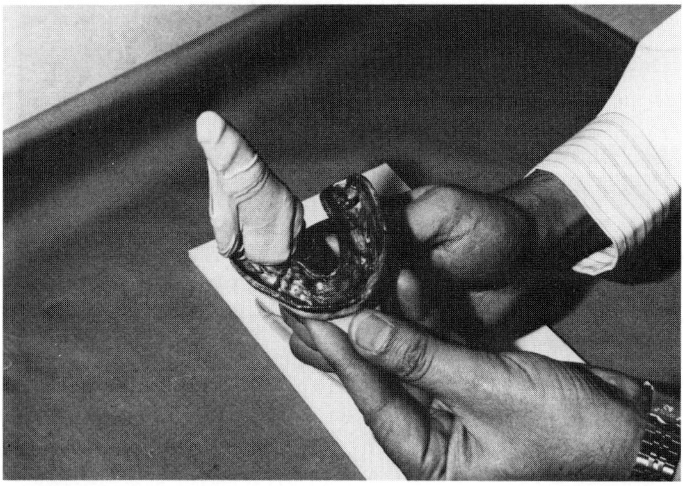

Fig 9–21.—Start loading the tray at the heel on one side and move the spatula both anteriorly and downward.

should be maintained to stabilize the impression tray until the material is set. The impression should remain in the mouth until a dull instrument will not permanently deform the set material when pressed into it; and

6. After the impression material is set, the tray is carefully removed from the mouth. The clinician must re-examine the mouth, particularly the gingival sulcular area, for any tags of the impression material that may have torn and remained. It is crucial that this be done carefully before the temporary restoration is placed. If any impression material tags are allowed to remain, ensuing complications could include continuous and constant irritation of the soft tissue and sensitivity possibly leading to periodontal abscess and cellulitis.[33–37] After removal from the mouth the

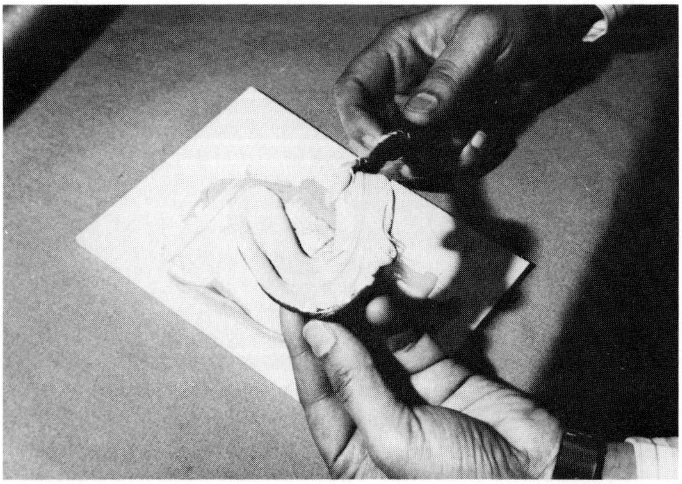

Fig 9–22.—Keep the spatula moving along the lingual flange of the tray until the opposite heel of the tray is reached and the tray is fully loaded.

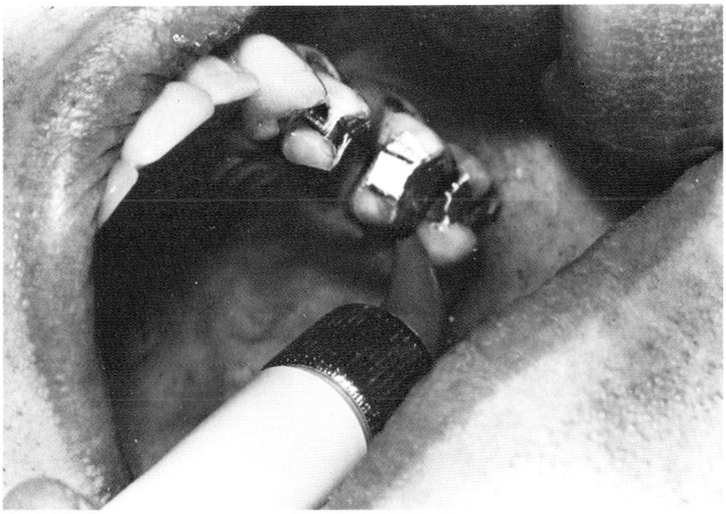

Fig 9–23.—Syringe material is injected first in the area of most difficult access. The tip of the syringe should be placed on top of the gingival sulcus and not in it. During injection, the impression material should always be pushed ahead of the tip to help prevent voids or the incorporation of air bubbles in the sulcus.

impression is rinsed with water and cleaned of any saliva or blood. After drying with an air syringe, the impression is examined carefully for the detailed negative replication of the prepared tooth and its surrounding tissue (Fig 9–24). An accurate and acceptable impression will show the following characteristics.

A. A complete and accurate impression of the prepared teeth, particularly of the finish line. It should also record, in detail, any retention grooves or boxes in the preparation.

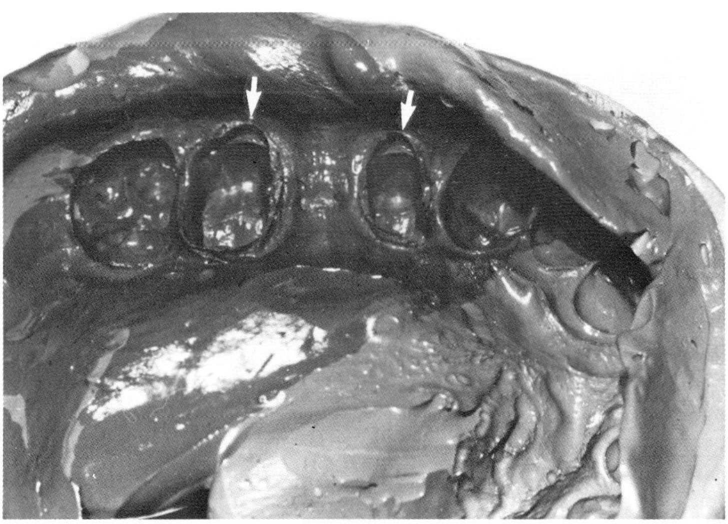

Fig 9–24.—A good final impression will show a thin flash *(arrows)* of impression material beyond the finish line. No air bubbles should be present on the impression surface.

B. True and accurate relationship between the prepared teeth and the adjacent teeth.

C. Complete and accurate record of the soft tissue detail, particularly of the soft tissue immediately adjoining the prepared teeth and ridge tissue in pontic areas.

D. No air bubbles on either the prepared teeth or adjacent teeth.

E. No tears in the impression material, particularly in narrow interproximal areas and the gingival sulcus.

F. Equal thickness of the impression material on all sides of the prepared and nonprepared teeth. The tray should not show through the impression except in the area of the tray stops.

G. An impression that is firmly attached to the tray.

H. An impression that is clean and is easily readable.

If the impression does not have all of the above mentioned characteristics, it is not acceptable and should be remade.

Putty-wash Systems

The condensation silicone materials were the first to be available in a putty-wash system as well as a two-paste system. More recently some manufacturers have marketed polysulfides in a putty-wash system. Vinyl polysiloxanes are also available in the putty-wash system, leaving polyethers as the only material not available in the putty-wash system.

The main difference of this system over the two-paste system is that the putty-wash system does not require a custom tray. An initial impression is made using the putty material in a stock tray. This initial impression serves as the custom tray for the wash impression material that is light bodied. The following technique steps are recommended for this system of impression making:

1. Before tooth reduction and preparation for cast restorations, a stock tray that fits the arch and allows at least 3 mm of space on either side of the teeth is selected.

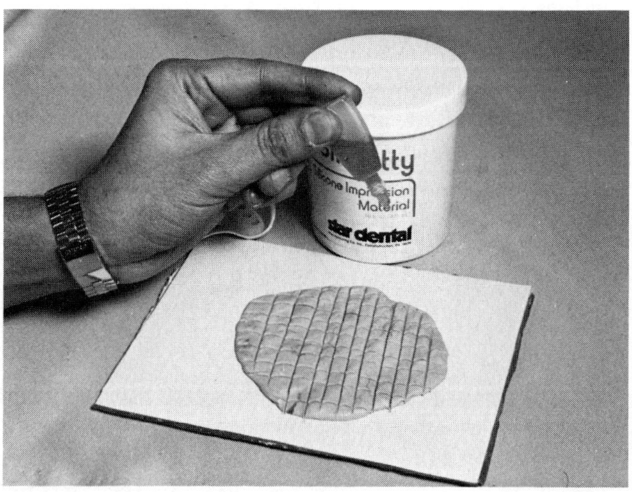

Fig 9–25.—The putty-base material is flattened on a pad in a disc shape and then cross scored with the spatula. This pattern helps to hold and incorporate the catalyst into the putty.

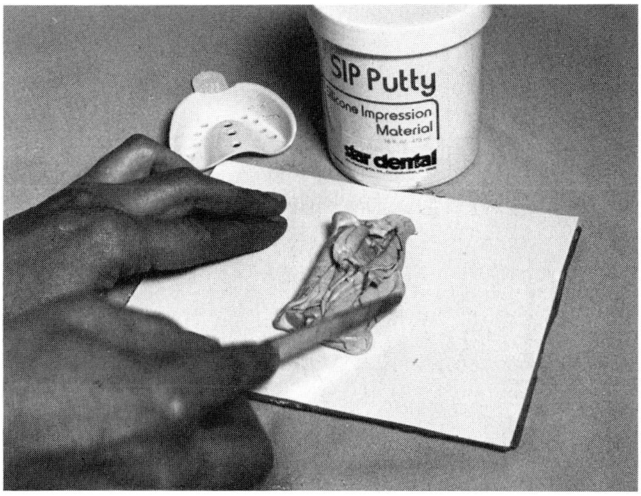

Fig 9–26.—After adding the catalyst, the material is folded on itself with the spatula.

The tray is lightly and evenly painted with the tray adhesive provided and allowed to dry;

2. An adequate amount of putty material to fill the stock tray is dispensed on a pad and spread in the shape of a thin disc. A spatula is used to cut shallow, cross-hatched grooves into the putty. This prevents the accelerator liquid from running on application and aids in its incorporation into the putty (Fig 9–25). Drops of accelerator are added according to the manufacturer's directions. The accelerator is incorporated into the putty by carefully folding with the spatula until the accelerator is completely enveloped (Fig 9–26). The material is then transferred into the palm of the hand and kneaded with the fingers for another 30 seconds (Fig 9–27). If any of the accelerator liquid remains on the pad, it may be blotted into the putty

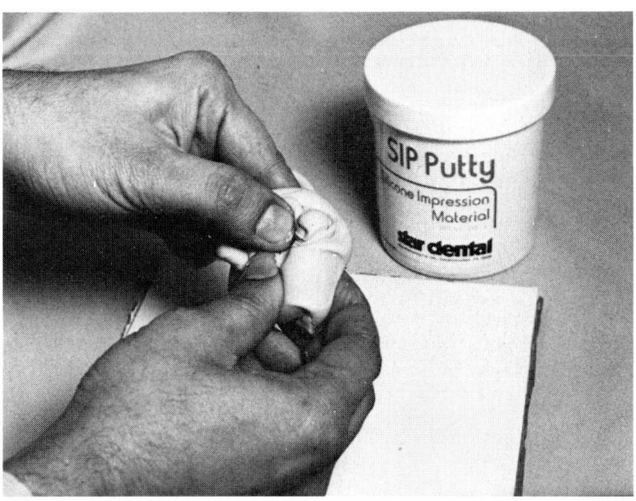

Fig 9–27.—The material is picked up and kneaded with fingers according to manufacturer's instructions.

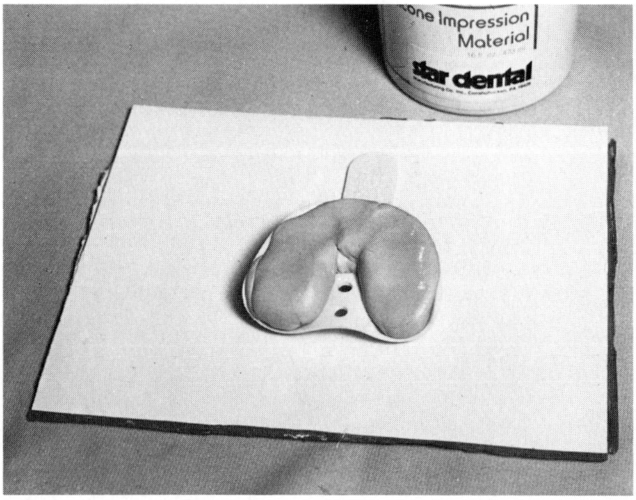

Fig 9–28.—When proper mixing is finished, the putty material is loaded in the stock tray and placed in the mouth for an impression.

as kneading is completed. The material is formed into a roll and pressed into the tray (Fig 9–28). If a polyethylene sheet spacer is provided with the putty material, it may be placed over the putty in the tray before seating in the mouth;

3. The tray is removed from the mouth after the initial polymerization of the material has taken place. If a spacer was used it is removed. Any excess material from the periphery of the tray is removed using a sharp knife. If a spacer was not used, any material that flowed into any embrasures is removed (Fig 9–29). This will allow easier seating of the tray in the mouth when the final wash impression is made. The tray is set aside for use after the tooth preparation has been completed;

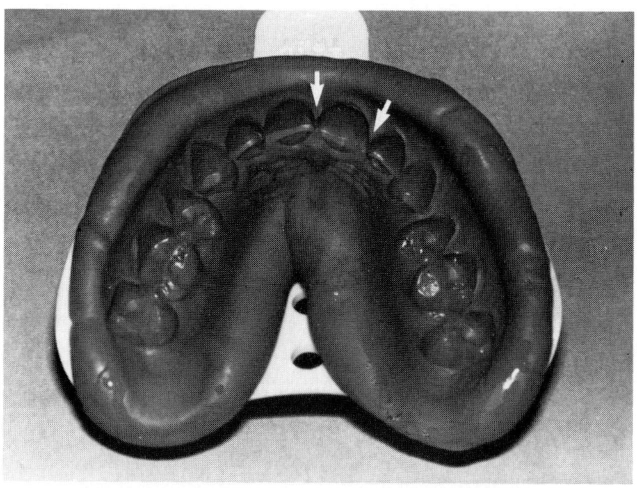

Fig 9–29.—If a spacer is not used, the interproximal embrasure material *(arrows)* should be trimmed out with a sharp knife to facilitate replacement of the impression in the mouth. This is most important adjacent to teeth to be prepared, but should be done throughout the arch.

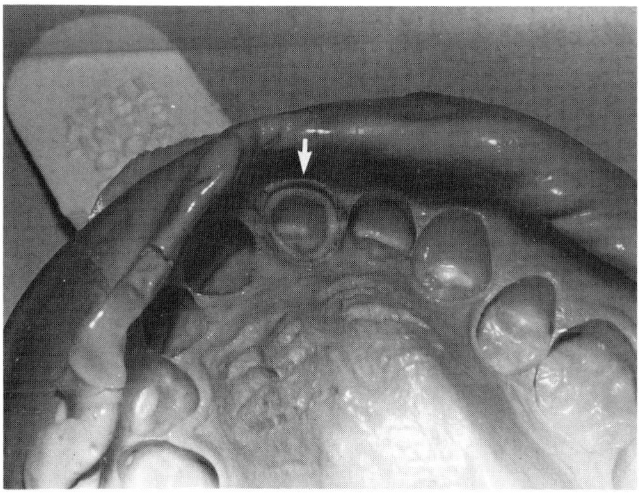

Fig 9–30.—A good final impression will show the preparation, the finish line, and tissue contour in detail. It will also show a flash *(arrow)* of impression material cervicle to the finish line and will be devoid of any air bubbles.

4. Light bodied wash material is used to make the final impression after the preparations have been completed. With the prepared tooth or teeth isolated and the tissue properly retracted, attention is given to dispensing and mixing the wash material. About four inches of material is placed on a paper pad for a full arch impression. Accelerator is added according to the manufacturer's directions. The material is spatulated for 30 seconds to a streak-free mix. The injection syringe is loaded as previously described and the remainder of the mixed material loaded into the putty impression. After removing any cotton rolls and retraction cord from the gingival sulcus, the material is injected as described earlier. When the preparation has been completely covered with the light body material, the tray is slowly and carefully seated in the mouth until firmly in place. At this point, the tray should only be stabilized, with no pressure. Any pressure exerted, while the light body wash material is polymerizing, will produce stresses in the already set yet compressible putty. When it is removed from the mouth, the putty will rebound to distort and deform the final impression. The impression tray should be held in place until the wash material is completely set; and
5. When the material is set the impression is carefully removed. The mouth is checked for any remaining tags of impression material in the sulcus or gingival embrasures. The impression is washed, dried, and examined (Fig 9–30). It must satisfy the previously listed requirements of an acceptable impression.

REFERENCES

1. Glossary of Prosthodontic Terms (pamphlet): *J. Prosthet. Dent.* 20:447, 1968.
2. Nagle R.J., Sears V.H.: *Denture Prosthetics: Complete Dentures.* St. Louis, C.V. Mosby Co., 1962.
3. Baum L.: *Advanced Restorative Dentistry: Modern Materials and Techniques.* Philadelphia, W.B. Saunders Co., 1973.
4. Kapin S.H.: Compound copper band impressions: How and why. *Quint. Int.* 12:23, 1979.

5. Sears A.W.: Hydrocolloid technique for inlays and fixed bridges. *Dent. Digest* 43:230, 1937.
6. Charbeneau G.T., et al.: *Principles and Practice of Operative Dentistry.* Philadelphia, Lea & Febiger, 1975.
7. Shillingburg H.T., et al.: Impression materials and techniques used for cast restoration in eight states. *J. Am. Dent. Assoc.* 100:696, 1980.
8. Myer G.E., et al.: The thiokol rubber base impression materials. *J. Prosthet. Dent.* 8:330, 1958.
9. Phillips R.W.: *Skinner's Science of Dental Materials.* Philadelphia, W.B. Saunders Co., 1982.
10. Bailey L.R.: Acrylic resin tray for rubber base impression materials. *J. Prosthet. Dent.* 5:658, 1955.
11. Myers G.E., Stockman D.B.: Factors that affect the accuracy and stability of mercaptan rubber base impression materials. *J. Prosthet. Dent.* 10:525, 1960.
12. Shippee R.W.: *An Evaluation of Reproduction of Partially Edentulous Mouth with Elastic Impression Materials* (master's thesis). Ann Arbor, University of Michigan, 1958.
13. Shippee R.W.: Accuracy of impressions made with elastic impression materials *J. Prosthet. Dent.* 10:381, 1960.
14. Asgar K.: Elastic impression materials. *Dent. Clin. North Am.* 15:81, 1971.
15. Lacy A.M., et al.: Time-dependent accuracy of elastomer impression materials. Part I: Condensation silicones. *J. Prosthet. Dent.* 45:209, 1981.
16. Stackhouse J.A.: Linear dimensions of electrodeposits and impression materials substrates. *J. Dent. Res.*, I.A.D.R. Program and Abstract #195, 1979.
17. Stackhouse J.A.: Impression materials and electrodeposits. Part I: Impression materials. *J. Prosthet. Dent.* 45:44, 1981; Part II: Electrodeposits. *J. Prosthet. Dent.* 45:146, 1981.
18. Yeh C.L., Powers J.M., Craig R.G.: Properties of addition-type silicone impression materials. *J. Am. Dent. Assoc.* 101:482, 1980.
19. Christensen R., Christensen G.J.: Dimensional stability and working characteristics of polyethers and polysiloxanes. *J. Dent. Res.*, I.A.D.R. Program and Abstract, #34, 1978.
20. Wallace S.W., Suway N.B., Eames W.B.: A comparison of the dimensional accuracy and stability of elastomeric impression materials. *J. Dent. Res.*, I.A.D.R. Program and Abstract, #22, 1978.
21. Luebke R.J.: *The Effect of Delayed and Second Pours on Elastomeric Impression Materials* (master's thesis). Iowa City, University of Iowa, 1976.
22. Kaloyannides T.M.: Elasticity of elastomer impression materials. I. Measurement of Young's modulus of elasticity and the coefficient of elasticity. *J. Dent. Res.* 52:439, 1973.
23. Kaloyannides T.M.: Elasticity of elastomer impression materials. II. Permanent deformation. *J. Dent. Res.* 52:719, 1973.
24. Kaloyannides T.M.: Elasticity of elastomer impression materials: Breaking limit and ultimate strength. *J. Dent. Res.* 53:630, 1974.
25. Kaloyannides T.M., Kapari D.J.: Setting time and consistency of elastomer impression materials. *J. Dent. Res.* 53:653, 1974.
26. Herfort W., et al.: Viscosity of elastomeric impression materials. *J. Prosthet. Dent.* 38:396, 1977.
27. Premier Espe—Instruction for Use of PREMIER ESPE Impregum Polyether Elastomeric Impression Material.
28. Doukoudakis A.: *The Effect of Bulk on Accuracy of Polyether Impression Materials* (master's thesis). Iowa City, University of Iowa, 1979.
29. Hembree J.H., Jr., Nunez L.J.: Effect of moisture on polyether impression materials. *J. Am. Dent. Assoc.* 89:1134, 1974.
30. Ciesco J.H., et al.: Comparison of elastomeric impression materials used in fixed prosthodontics. *J. Prosthet. Dent.* 45:89, 1981.
31. McLean J.W.: Silicone impression materials. *Dent. Pract.* 9:56, 1958.
32. Schmitt N., et al.: Elastomers from polyethers and ethylene amine derivatives. U.S. Patent, 3,453,242; July 1, 1969.
33. Miller T.H., et al.: A tissue locked impression: Report of a case. *Iowa Dent. J.* 26, April, 1969.

34. Clark S.M.: Rubber base foreign body. *J. Prosthet. Dent.* 31:439, 1974.
35. Garey R.C., Narang R.: An unusual foreign body in the buccal vestibule. *Oral Surg.* 42:314, 1976.
36. Gullett C.E., Caulder S.L.: Residual fragment of rubber base material. *Oper. Dent.* 3:131, 1978.
37. Eliasson, S.T., Holte, N.O.: Rubber base impression material as a foreign body. *Oral Surg.* 48:379, 1979.

CHAPTER 10

The Provisional Restoration

DANIEL L. HALL, D.D.S.

THE MANAGEMENT OF teeth that have been prepared for fixed prostheses presents a challenge to the restorative dentist. The term "provisional" restoration was chosen over the more common term, "temporary" restoration, for a particular purpose. The use of the term temporary restoration may place this phase of care in a less important position in the mind of the dentist and most certainly demises its value in the mind of the patient. This should be avoided, as the provisional restoration is an important phase of treatment. This phase must not be compromised.[1-4]

The results of an inadequate provisional restoration haunt the dentist daily. A gingival margin that has receded from the time of final impression to delivery of the maxillary incisor crown serves as an example of frustration and disappointment for both the dentist and the patient. Care in construction of the provisional restoration is important to the maintenance of tissue levels. There are many requirements placed on the protection used for a tooth between preparation and the final restoration. When any or all of these requirements are not met the result may well be economically undesirable for the dentist, painful and disappointing for the patient, and time consuming for both. The success or failure of a treatment may rest with the properly constructed provisional restoration. This phase of care increases in importance with the increase in complexity of the treatment.

REQUIREMENTS FOR THE PROVISIONAL RESTORATION

The requirements for the provisional restoration are the mechanical, physiologic, and esthetic requirements.

Mechanical Requirements

There are many mechanical requirements for the intermediate restoration. First, the tooth must be maintained in the same relationship as before the preparation. This relationship is between both adjacent and opposing teeth. To maintain the proper relationship between adjacent teeth the provisional must have intimate contact with any teeth that previously contacted. It is also important to have a stable occlusal contact with the opposing tooth or teeth. A second mechanical requirement is that the protection be strong enough to withstand the stress placed on it for the time required. Thirdly, the restoration must be retentive, having enough contact with the prepared tooth for adequate retention for the duration of its use. A fourth requirement is that the material be smooth and contoured well enough to allow normal hygiene care. A fifth requirement is that the restoration must be able to be relined or repaired if more extensive restoration or changes are anticipated or become necessary. The appliance should also be able to be removed with relative ease without destroying it, thus enabling it to be reused as necessary, and it must be dimentionally stable. Lastly, the appliance must be within the skill level of the average dentist and must be practical from both time and cost factors.

Physiologic Requirements

There are many physiologic requirements for the provisional restoration. Pulpal protection is important in vital teeth, so the material used must be tolerated by the pulp so as not to cause an irreversible pulpal irritation. The maintenance of the pulpal health by the provisional restoration is aided by the luting medium used. No luting medium, however, will overcome the problems of an inadequate provisional restoration. Secondly, the protection must maintain good gingival health. The requirements include: good marginal fit and correct contour of the restoration in the marginal area. The contour that is anatomically correct has been shown to cause less tissue recession than alternate contours.[5] Correct contour of the embrasure spaces is also important for gingival health.[2, 6] Thirdly, the protection must not cause tissue irritation mechanically or chemically. When these three requirements are met the appliance will be physiologically accepted. Furthermore, a nonconductive material is most desirable. This is a property shared by the currently popular provisional restoration products.

Esthetic Requirements

Esthetic requirements are important when the restoration is in the anterior portion of the mouth and sometimes the premolars. The tooth-colored provisional restoration can be preformed or constructed in the mouth. The esthetic considerations for the provisional restoration are the same as those for the final restoration. To have an acceptable esthetic result, there must be a proper contour, a reasonably close shade match, and polished surfaces.

A good esthetic restoration helps to gain the confidence of the patient. The anterior provisional restoration made in conjunction with diagnostic wax-ups aids in developing proper esthetics, when necessary.[7] The flexibility of the provisional restoration should not be overlooked whenever the development of esthetics is needed for the finished restoration.

TYPES OF PROVISIONAL RESTORATIONS

There are many types of provisional restorations in use. Each has its own advantages and disadvantages, ranging from the expensive and time-consuming, such as the cast metal, to the least customized aluminum shell. The provisional restoration can be divided into the preformed metal or aluminum shell crowns that are used for posterior tooth protection and the preformed or custom-made resin crowns and fixed partial dentures used in the anterior and posterior segments. Polycarbonate crowns may be used for anterior and premolar teeth. The provisional restoration may also be categorized into the single unit and multiple unit appliance, the multiple unit being either a fixed partial denture or a group of single units. The metal preformed shell is only recommended for the single unit. This method of protection frequently falls short of the mechanical and physiologic requirements.

The Single Posterior Provisional Restoration

Materials used for the single unit include the custom constructed acrylic crown and the preformed metal shell crown. The acrylic crowns are made with an alginate impression, wax impression, or vacuum-pressed template. Posterior intermediate restorations are necessary for any prepared tooth, vital or nonvital, since the tooth must also be protected against position change.

The Single Preformed Shell Crown

The single aluminum shell provisional restoration is the single unit whereby a temporary can be festooned using crown shears and contouring pliers to meet the physiologic requirements of the gingiva. Caution should be used with this crown. Meeting all of the requirements of the provisional restoration is difficult with this technique. The single preformed shell crown may involve the selection of a crown that is too narrow mesiodistally to have it fit the tooth well enough to be retained. The solution is to select a crown with mesial and distal contact, and to reline it with an acrylic resin for an adaptation that will ensure retention. This will give a proximal and occlusal contact, and suitable retention.

Various brands of preformed metal shell crowns offer different contours, such as bell-shaped or flat occlusogingival contours. Both have their advantages and disadvantages and may be customized to meet both mechanical and physiologic requirements. When using the less bell shaped variety the following technique can be used:

1. Select a crown that fits securely at the proximals. Frequently, this crown does not offer the required gingival retention (Fig 10–1);

2. Festoon the margins to fall approximately 0.5 to 1 mm short of the prepared tooth margin when the occlusal contact is positive but not interferring with complete closure. It is frequently necessary to have the patient bite with force to actually bend the soft aluminum occlusal surface of the crown to allow proper func-

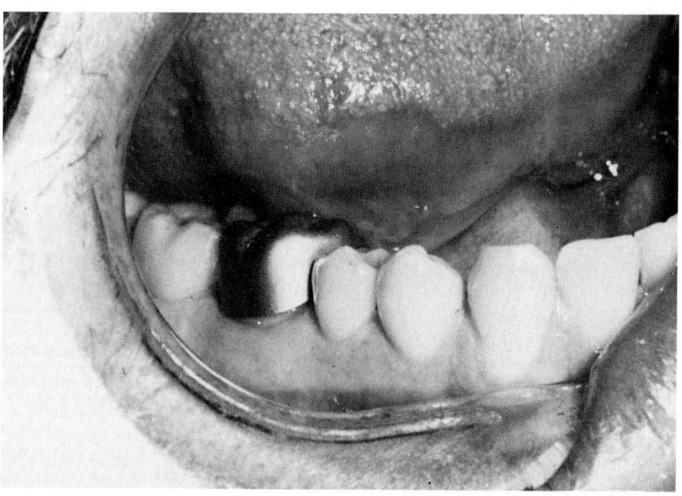

Fig 10–1.—Selected aluminum shell crown with correct mesiodistal width. Note loose gingival fit.

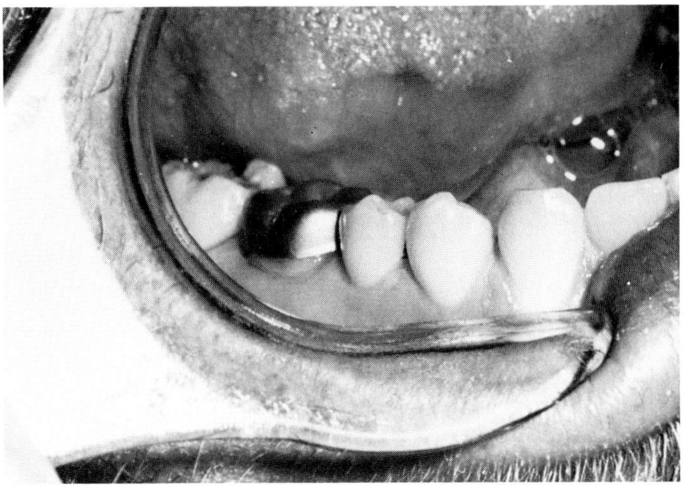

Fig 10–2.—Crown festooned short of preparation margin.

tion. This is not necessarily undesirable, as the action frequently creates a positive occlusal stop. It is undesirable to use a wooden stick or cotton roll between the teeth when forming the crown to the opposing occlusion. This will cause the provisional crown to be forced out of occlusion and will destroy the positive occlusal contact that prevents the extrusion of the prepared tooth or opposing teeth. Care must be used to maintain occlusal relationships;

3. After festooning and adjusting the occlusion, the contacts and the occlusion can be checked to be sure that they meet the physiologic and mechanical requirements. When this is accomplished, the operator may proceed with customizing the marginal fit and gaining adequate retention (Fig 10–2);

4. Then the crown is filled with a temporary acrylic resin (the types will be discussed under anterior provisional restorations), and placed on the tooth. Excess resin should flow from around the crown in all areas (Fig 10–3). Close attention

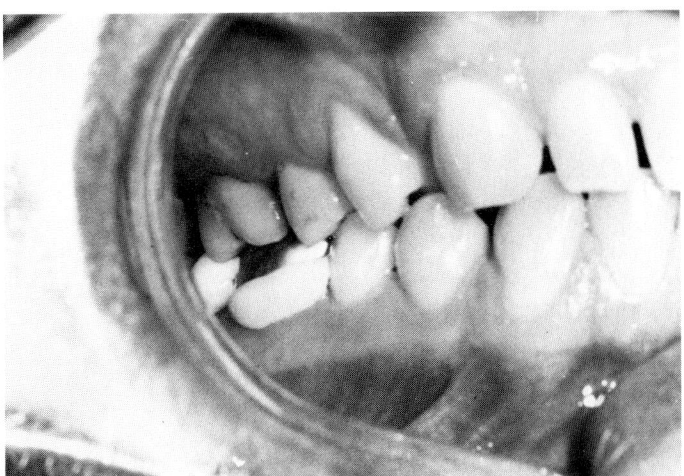

Fig 10–3.—Crown in place, teeth in occlusion, and excess acrylic at margins.

must be kept on the crown and as the acrylic reaches rebound stage, the crown is removed and replaced every few seconds until near the final set. Failure to do this will cause the crown to adhere to the tooth because of polymerization shrinkage. Excess interproximal material may also lock under adjacent tooth contours and make removal difficult;

5. This acrylic liner finishes polymerization out of the mouth. The operator will then be able to read the margin within the acrylic and, using acrylic burs, trim back the excess acrylic giving a narrow band of acrylic beyond the margin of the festooned metal provisional restoration. This can then be smoothed with pumice giving a fine, smooth, well-fitting margin; and
6. The protection is now ready for cementation (Fig 10–4).

Customized Acrylic Provisional

The customized acrylic provisional is the preferred treatment when the esthetic appearance of the restoration is a factor. The customized intermediate restoration is superior in mechanical, physiologic, and esthetic requirements, but requires more chair time than the preformed aluminum shell crown. Chair time must be weighed against the need for esthetics, the time the restoration will need to be worn, and patient comfort. The construction of the customized temporary crown can meet the necessary mechanical, physiologic and esthetic requirements.

The patient's unprepared teeth are the best models for reproducing an acceptable provisional restoration.[8]

The Wax Impression Technique[9]

This technique lends itself to the single unit provisional restoration. It may be used for posterior or anterior teeth. The impression material is base plate wax. The impression is made directly in the mouth before tooth preparation. This impression may be made at the initial examination or at the preparation appointment. The base plate wax is adequately stable to allow storage for an extended time. The technique is as follows:

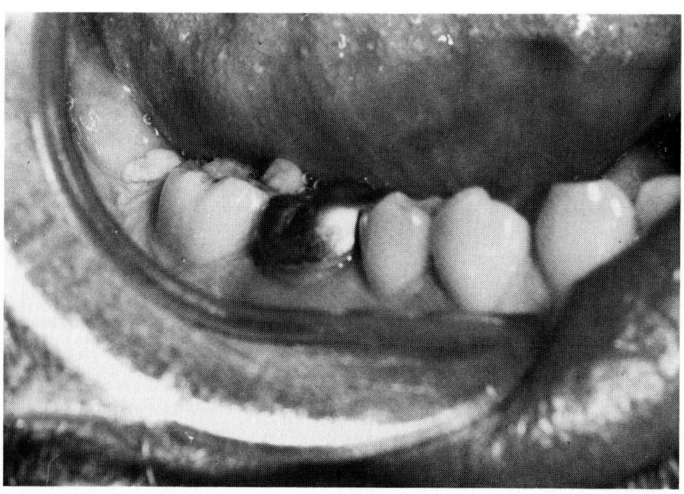

Fig 10–4.—Excess acrylic removed and finished to prepared tooth margin. Restoration smoothed and ready for cementation.

1. With the patient present, a base plate wax is heated and rolled into a half to three-quarter inch diameter of adequate length to extend over mesial and distal adjacent teeth;

2. The wax is molded over the teeth with finger pressure. The patient is instructed to close in centric occlusion and to mold the wax against the lingual of the teeth while the dentist uses finger pressure to mold the wax firmly on the facial;

3. The wax impression is then removed and set aside until the preparation has been done;

4. An additional wax impression may be made for use should the protection need to be remade in the future; and

5. After the tooth is prepared, the wax impression is filled with a temporary acrylic resin, placed over the preparation when the gloss disappears from the resin surface, and the patient is instructed to close in centric occlusion.

This technique does not differ from the manipulation of the resins when provisional fixed partial dentures are constructed using templates or alginate impressions. The use of the wax impression for any provisional restoration allows the patient to close in full occlusion while the resin is polymerizing.

The advantages of this technique over the performed shell crown are:

1. The shape is more nearly anatomic;
2. The occlusion is more stable and functional;
3. More ideal proximal contacts are established;
4. The wax stability allows long-term storage;
5. More esthetic requirements are met; and
6. The technique is inexpensive and time efficient.

The Anterior Single Unit Intermediate Restoration

The anterior provisional restorations are a challenge. They are indicated whenever a single unit or multiple units are to be placed and an interim restoration is necessary. Examples of materials that have acceptable tooth shading are the methyl methacrylates such as Jet (Lang),* ethyl methacrylates such as Trim II (Bosworth),** and the epimine plastic Scutan (Premier).† Currently, there is a controversy as to whether these materials should be placed directly on prepared tooth structure. The setting of both methyl and ethyl methacrylate produces an exothermic reaction. The generated heat must be prevented from causing pulpal damage when it is used directly. Removal and cooling under tap water or cooling of the material by air-water syringe while in the mouth is recommended. The exothermic reaction is increased as the volume of material is increased. A four abutment, six unit temporary fixed partial denture will create much more heat than the relining of a well adapted polycarbonate single crown. The setting of the epimine plastic creates only a slight exothermic reaction.[10]

The second concern is the free monomer in the autopolymerizing resins. These two concerns have not been researched individually so it is not possible to make a definite statement as to the free monomer effect alone. It is known that free monomer is not a long range problem.[11] The epimine does not have free monomer.[10] Studies have shown that using methyl methacrylate directly on the tooth can cause

*Lang Dental Mfg. Co., Inc., Chicago, IL 60607.
**Harry J. Bosworth Co., Skokie, IL 60076.
†Premier Dental Products Co., Norristown, PA 19401.

pulpal irritation,[12–14] but the reaction was reversible. Reparative dentine has been shown to be effective for walling off chemical assault.[14] It was also shown that with 1.5 mm remaining dentine there was a similar reaction to epimine, methyl methacrylate, and zinc oxide and eugenol cement.[15] Some authors recommend coating the teeth with petroleum jelly for protection.[16, 17] It is also prudent to use a cavity liner such as copalite and/or a thin layer of a calcium hydroxide material when the preparation could be near the pulp. There are many authors who advocate the direct technique,[2, 9, 16, 18–21] and many who support the indirect method.[4, 7, 22–24] Both will be presented.

The single anterior unit may be constructed with the materials mentioned. The more popular methods include the alginate impression, the wax impression, the clear plastic template, the celluloid crown form, or the polycarbonate crown form. The technique for the clear celluloid crown form (Caulk)* and the polycarbonate Ion crown form (3M)** are the same. The polycarbonate form is somewhat stronger than the all resin crown made with the celluloid form.[25] The polycarbonate crown does not have the shade selection capability offered by the resins. The flexibility of the celluloid forms give them an advantage over the polycarbonate forms in some situations.[19] Both products are supplied in varying sizes for premolar, canine, lateral, and central incisor teeth.

The direct technique with either type of form is as follows:

1. Tooth preparation is done;
2. Proper width crown form is selected (Figs 10–5 and 10–6);
3. Form is festooned to proper length and gingival contour (Figs 10–7 and 10–8);
4. The crown form is filled with the selected tooth colored material;
5. When the gloss disappears from the material, the crown is placed on the prepared tooth that has been appropriately protected as previously discussed;
6. When the excess material around the margins shows rebound, the crown is

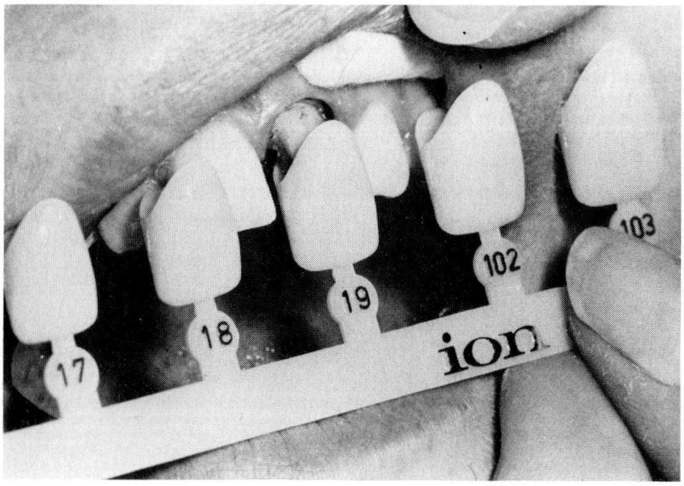

Fig 10–5.—Selection of mesiodistal width using polycarbonate crown form.

---

*Caulk Division of Dentsply International, Inc., Milford, DE 19963.
**3M Company, Costa Mesa, CA 92626.

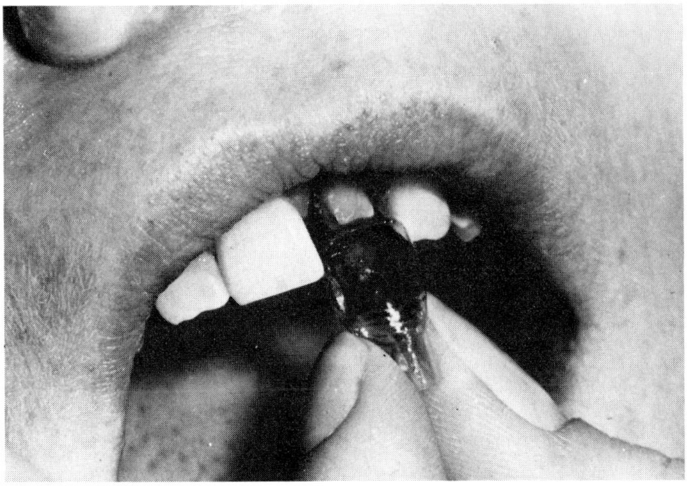

Fig 10–6.—Selection of mesiodistal width using celluloid crown form.

removed and replaced intermittently on the tooth (Fig 10–9) until the resin has hardened. The material must not be allowed to set completely while on the tooth. This will result in locking on the tooth, because of shrinkage and any excess material hardening in adjacent infrabulge areas;

7. When the material has gained final set out of the mouth, it should be trimmed to ideal contour and gingival fit (Fig 10–10). This step must be done accurately to ensure good tissue response between this phase and final restoration.[5] These margins deserve the same consideration as do the final restoration;[26]

8. The occlusion is adjusted with both eccentric and centric occlusion in mind (Fig 10–11); and

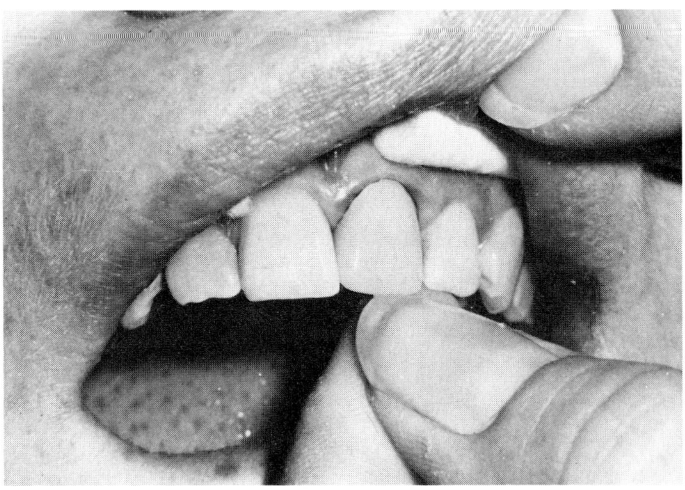

Fig 10–7.—Proper gingival festooning of polycarbonate form.

*Omnidental Corp., Harrisburg, PA 17105.

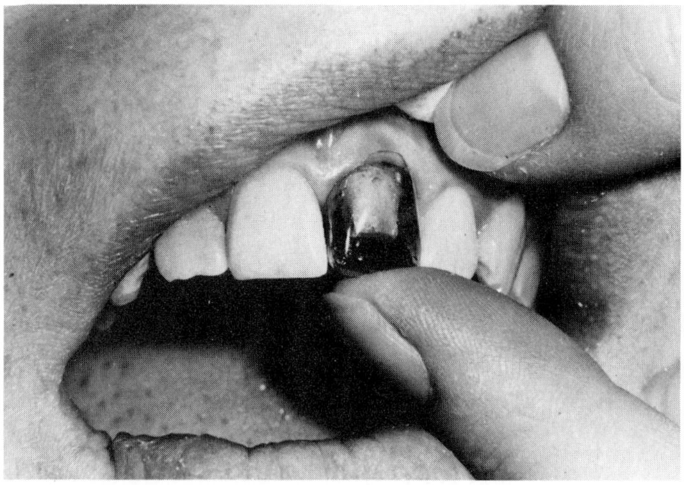

Fig 10–8.—Proper gingival festooning of celluloid form.

9. After polishing with pumice and a high luster acrylic polish, the provisional restoration is ready for cementation (Fig 10–12).

The clear shell should be removed before the temporary cementation of the intermediate restoration, as this shell does not bond with the acrylic and may cause an unesthetic and unhygienic situation.

Alginate impressions, wax impressions, and vacuum-formed templates (to be discussed next), may also be used for single unit provisionals.

PROVISIONAL FIXED PARTIAL DENTURE FOR MULTIPLE ADJACENT UNITS

The construction of a provisional appliance for the fixed partial denture and multiple adjacent units presents a greater challenge. Among the more popular techniques are the relined alginate impressions or wax impressions made from an altered study cast, and the relined clear acrylic template made on a study cast or a

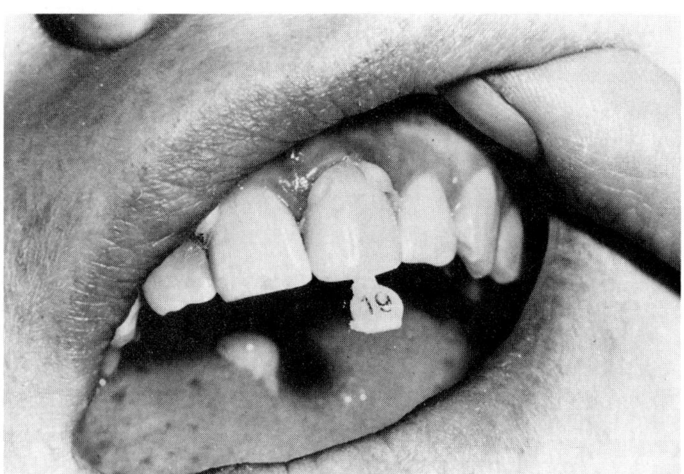

Fig 10–9.—Crown showing excess acrylic at rebound stage.

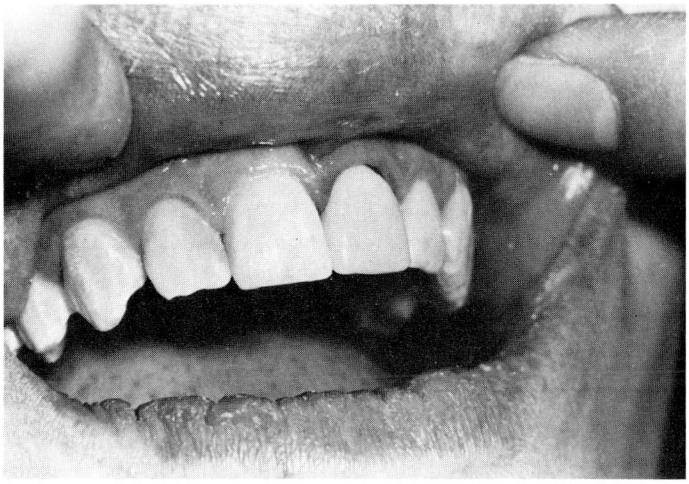

Fig 10–10.—Corrected gingival fit.

cast made from the impression of an altered study cast. All three techniques may be done directly[18] or indirectly.[4] There are also many variations of these basic techniques. The basic provisional restoration is meant to function for 2 to 3 weeks, but the periodontal splint, with longer projected usage, needs a different technique for a longer life.[27] This does not mean that the attention to form and function is less important for the short-term appliance. When a trial restoration is needed for diagnostic purposes a more involved technique than the one to be described will be necessary.[7] This technique may use the tooth-shaded materials previously discussed with the proper preparation protection.

Vacuum Formed Acrylic Template Technique

1. A study model must be obtained;
2. The study model should be altered if edentulous spaces need to be filled (Fig 10–13). A denture tooth can be used or spaces waxed in to provide an appropriate

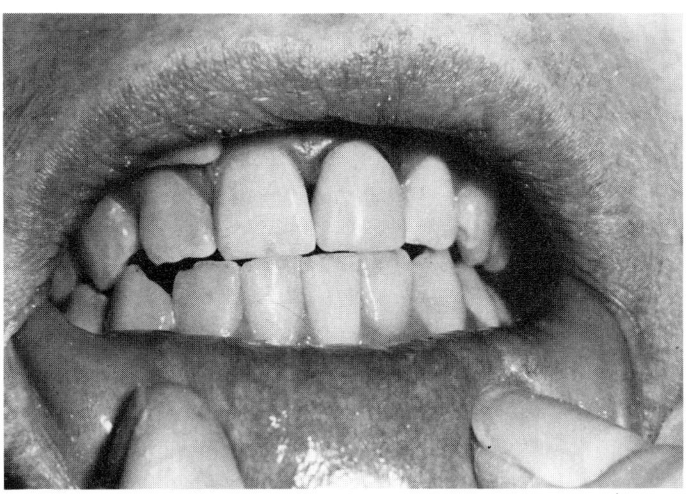

Fig 10–11.—Occlusion check in excursive positions.

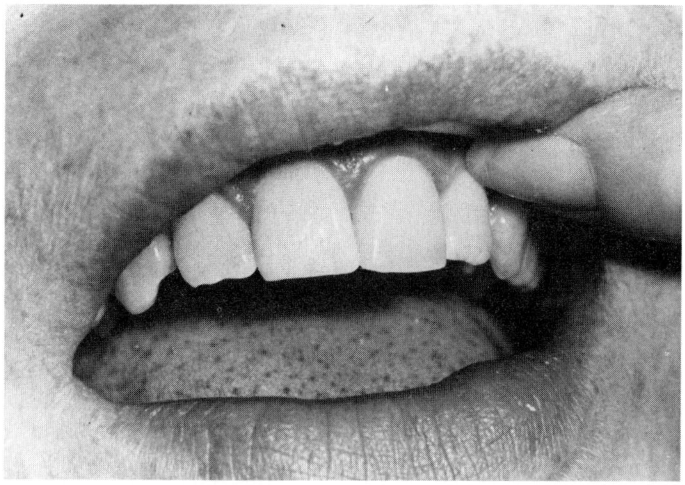

Fig 10–12.—Provisional restoration ready for cementation.

contour. Tooth shape and position may be altered with a diagnostic wax-up. When wax is used in any of these procedures an alginate impression should be made of the altered study cast, reproduced in dental stone and allowed to set with a moderately thin base of 2 to 4 mm (Fig 10–14). When the altered study cast is sufficiently set, it is placed in a vacuum-forming machine such as Omnivac (Omnidental)* and a clear acrylic sheet .02 mm in thickness is adapted as closely as possible to the altered study cast. A standard pencil eraser can be used to press the material into interproximals to help to closely adapt the template to the cast. This forms the matrix;

3. The clear acrylic matrix is cut away, maintaining full arch coverage (Fig 10–15). If the distal tooth is an abutment, some 2 to 5 mm of matrix must be allowed to extend posteriorly over the edentulous area to give an index to placement of the

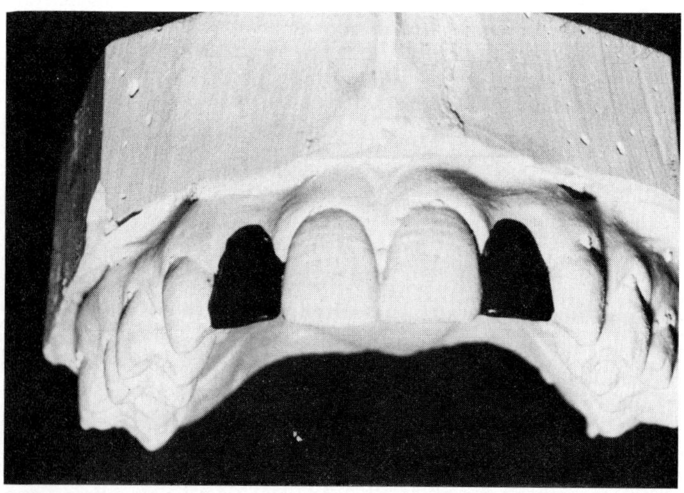

Fig 10–13.—Diagnostic wax-up of edentulous spaces using inlay wax.

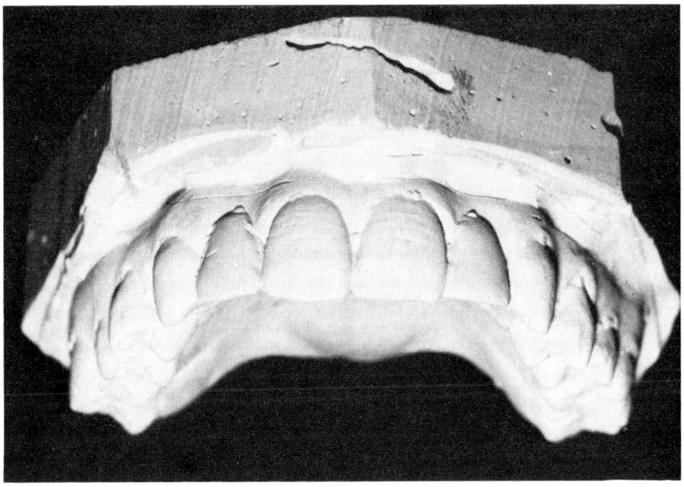

Fig 10–14.—Diagnostic wax-up reproduced in stone cast ready for vacuum-forming step.

matrix in the mouth. An accurate study cast, well-extended, is a must in this situation. The matrix should extend 2 to 3 mm past the tooth-gingiva margin;

4. After preparations have been done in all areas, the adapted and trimmed clear acrylic matrix is removed from the altered study cast and placed in the mouth to check for landmarks during placement and fit. Adequate tooth reduction may be verified at this point as the template is clear (Fig 10–16);

5. The form is filled rapidly, with a salt and pepper technique until the pontics and abutment teeth to be protected are completely filled with material. This eliminates bubbles in the material that can be a problem when the material is poured into the matrix;

6. With the prepared teeth appropriately protected, the matrix is quickly carried

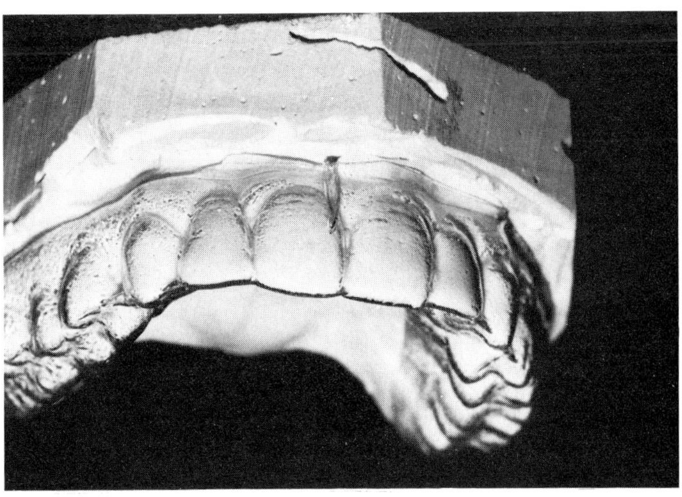

Fig 10–15.—Trimmed vacuformed matrix on cast showing proper extension and coverage.

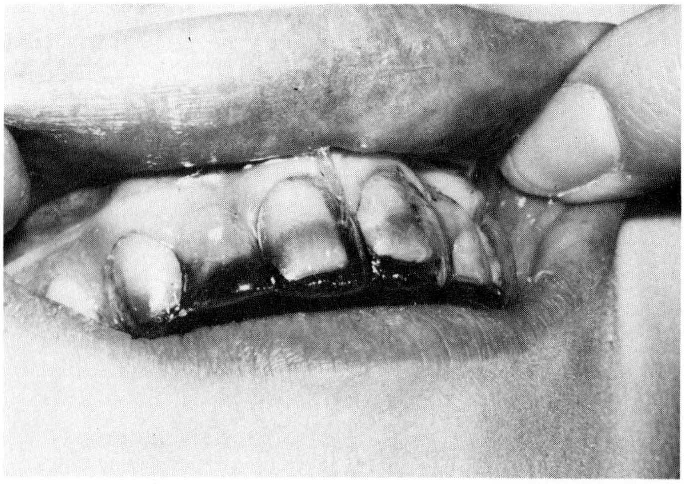

Fig 10–16.—Matrix in place, allowing for tooth reduction check and identifying landmarks to assure correct seating.

to the mouth and seated firmly. Flash will extend from the edge of the clear matrix. At this point, it should be confirmed that there are no voids in the provisional restoration. The excess material is available to test for the progress of the set;

7. Once the set has reached the dough stage, the acrylic should be removed and replaced. Should methyl or ethyl methacrylate be used some heat will be generated. If this is the case, cool it under tap water and replace, alternating every 15 to 30 seconds. The acrylic should not be allowed to gain its final set on the teeth. The material must be nearly set before removing for the last time (Fig 10–17). If not, the provisional will shrink and not fit after trimming;

8. Once the final set has taken place, the clear acrylic matrix is removed from the acrylic provisional. Shaping and finishing is done with acrylic burs and fine diamond wheels or discs. The finished restoration takes on its final shape (Fig 10–18);

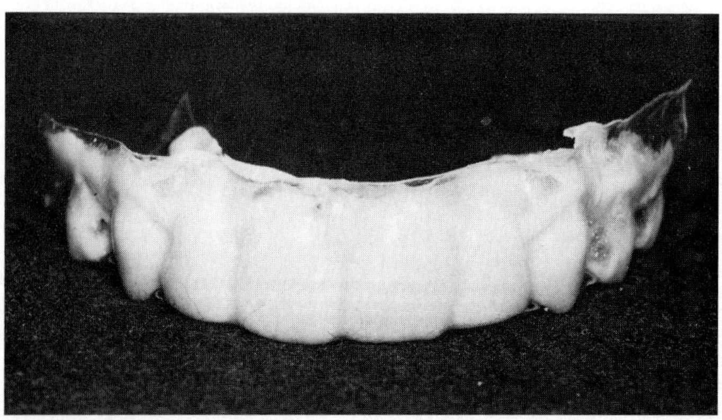

Fig 10–17.—Matrix removed showing expected flash of material.

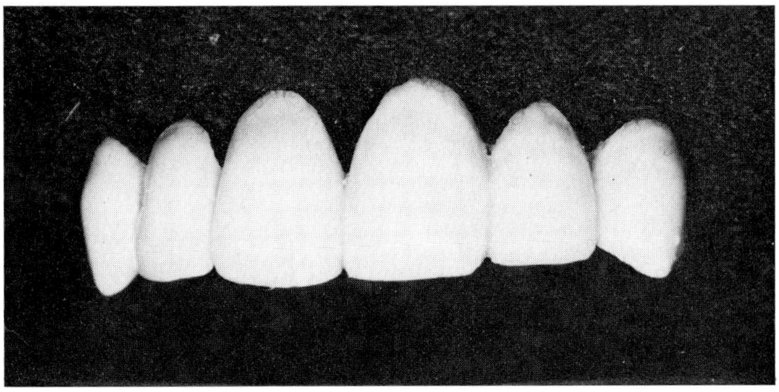

Fig 10–18.—Restoration finished to final shape and contours.

9. Once the final shape has been finished and the dentist and patient are satisfied with the esthetics and the occlusion, a final polish with pumice followed by a high luster polish will result in an acceptable provisional restoration; and

10. The restoration is ready for cementation (Fig 10–19).

This is the direct technique for the construction of a provisional fixed partial denture and can be used for multiple adjacent single units without alteration. When constructing multiple adjacent single units, it is suggested that they be left in one piece. The embrasure spaces should be opened sufficiently so as not to impinge on tissue but to allow for the passage of a floss threader to thoroughly remove all temporary cement.

Indirect Vacuum-Formed Acrylic Template Technique

A variation of this template technique is the indirect technique using the same materials. Steps one through four are done in the same manner. After the preparations are completed, an alginate impression is made of the prepared teeth and poured in quick-setting plaster. After separation, the template is fitted to the cast

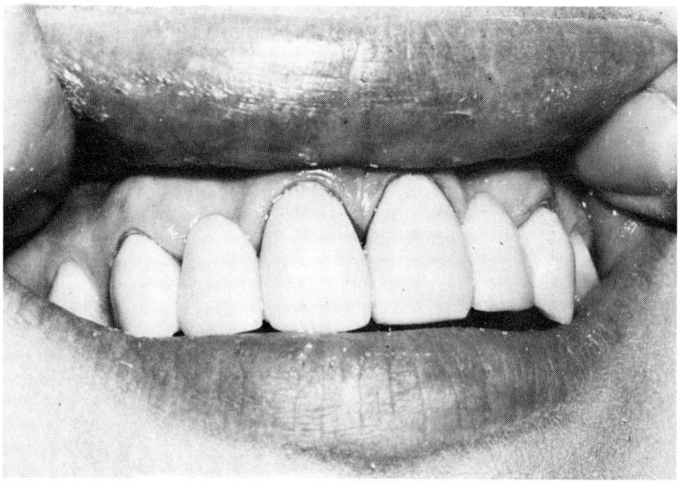

Fig 10–19.—Provisional restoration ready for cementation.

and the cast is covered with a foil substitute. The template is removed and filled with the selected resinous material, placed over the model of the prepared teeth, and held firmly in place. After complete setting the model is broken out and the restoration polished and fitted. In most instances, relining is not necessary, hence no exothermic heat or free monomer of acrylic materials is a problem.

The advantages of the clear template are:

1. The ability to evaluate tooth reduction;
2. The ability to visualize when the template is properly seated;[19]
3. The ability to assess the degree of set by testing the flash material;
4. The surfaces not requiring alteration are very smooth; and
5. The ability to have the template ready in advance.

The value of the diagnostic wax-up for the model for the provisional restoration cannot be over-emphasized. This allows:

1. The patient and the dentist to preview the esthetics of the final restoration and adjustments can be made until goals are met;
2. Desired occlusion may be developed;
3. Desired contours may be developed; and
4. Laboratory communications are made more precise as casts of the acceptable provisional appliance may be forwarded to the laboratory for duplication in the final restoration.

Alginate Impression or Wax Impression Technique

An alginate or wax impression may be used in a manner similar to the template. Either may be used with both the direct or indirect technique.

The major advantage of the alginate is the improved detail of the protection allowing for shorter finishing time. This may or may not be an advantage of the wax impression. It also eliminates the need for special equipment to fabricate the template.

A direct reline is possible with any of the above techniques, should gingival fit not be satisfactory initially. When relining, venting of the occlusal of the abutments will accomplish a better fit.[28]

One additional variation to this technique is to slightly underprepare the abutment teeth on an unaltered study cast and construct a provisional appliance as in the direct method. This would require a direct reline on the preparations at preparation time but could conserve some chair time.

The Protection for the Endodontically Treated Tooth

This is one of the more difficult of provisional restorations and can be time-consuming considering the brief time it is in use. The best solution to this problem is to plan the patient's appointment to extend over a single day. This allows the dentist to develop a pattern, invest, cast, and deliver the post and core. In this case, no protection will be required. If the patient is made aware of the plan in advance, in most circumstances they will accommodate the dentist. This can be done with approximately two hours between appointments. When the post is delivered, the preparation may be finalized and a provisional constructed that will be useful throughout the procedure.

If this is not an option, the dentist may use scored paper clip wire that extends to the depth of the prepared canal and 2 to 4 mm into the crown. The provisional is then made over the wire in the same manner as the single restoration. Caution must be used to avoid the introduction of temporary cement into the canal. Retrieval is difficult and can result in altering the shape of the canal. This renders the casting less satisfactory because of a compromised fit.

CEMENTATION OF THE PROVISIONAL RESTORATION

There are numerous cements currently being used. The mechanical requirement of a temporary luting agent is to retain the provisional restoration until the dentist wishes to remove it, and then to allow the removal without undue force or damage to the provisional restoration or the tooth or teeth being protected. Additional considerations include: pulpal protection, working time, easy cement removal from provisional and tooth, and compatibility with the material used to fabricate the provisional restoration. Cements are divided into soft, medium, and hard.[2] The soft is used most often as it will usually meet the requirements stated. An example of soft cement is Temp Bond (Kerr).* When more retention is needed or an extended period of use is required, IRM (Caulk)** is an acceptable choice. Should the mechanical requirements be even greater, one of the zinc oxide cements such as Fynal (Caulk)** may be used.

Zinc phosphate cement is not recommended because of its irritating effect on the pulpal tissue. Trial (Opotol)† is not recommended as a luting agent for provisional restorations as it lacks adequate retention. Trial is, however, an excellent product for temporary cementation of finished multiple unit fixed partial dentures.

When the provisional restoration is constructed with care and accuracy the soft cement will most often be the most satisfactory. When cementing a provisional restoration it is important to note that the restoration should not be forced completely to place with the finger or have the patient occlude with a cotton roll or other interposing material between the teeth. The reason is, if the provisional restoration is over-seated on the tooth, it will not be in contact with the opposing tooth and not meet the mechanical requirement of maintaining the occlusal relationship. This can be achieved by placing the provisional restoration on the tooth firmly, but leaving it 1 to 2 mm in hyperocclusion and then having the patient close gently on the provisional restoration. This completes its seating and maintains contact of all the teeth in centric occlusion while the cement sets. This will assure occlusal contact from the opposing teeth. Occlusal contact in itself is important; however, it also should be noted that the occlusal contact must be in a stable position so as not to create undue forces on opposing teeth or create a minor movement of the prepared tooth.

Extreme care must be exercised for the removal of the temporary cement from the margins. Thorough removal will prevent gingival irritation and periodontal injury.[29] If this step is neglected, receded and inflamed tissue will result with their accompanying problems. The coating of the exterior of the provisional restoration with petroleum jelly will facilitate removal of the temporary cementing material from the restoration.[8]

---

*Kerr Mfg., Romolus, MI 84174.
**Caulk Division of Dentsply International, Inc., Milford, DE 19963.
†Teledyne Dental Getz Opotol Division, Elk Grove Village, IL 60007.

REMOVAL OF THE INTERMEDIATE RESTORATION

There are many ways to remove the provisional restoration. A technique for removal of the aluminum shell crown is to use a towel clamp such as those used in surgery to drape the patient. The towel clamp is placed with the prongs on the buccal and lingual aspects and closed as a pair of scissors. By piercing a hole in the buccal and lingual aspects and gently rotating in all directions, the crown is usually dislodged easily, leaving only two perforations in the crown. This makes it possible to reuse the temporary if that is necessary. This technique can also be used for removing the acrylic temporary restorations but is less effective. The removal of the acrylic temporary restorations is usually done with the use of a light tapping from a back-action crown remover or the wedging of a spoon excavator. If the dentist uses the marginal ridge or cingulum of adjacent teeth as a fulcrum and the largest spoon excavator, enough force can be exerted to dislodge the restoration with minimum of stress to the abutment tooth. The key to removal of the temporary appliance is placing force in the path of withdrawal and using only the minimum force necessary. Damage to crown bases and margins is to be avoided.

SUMMARY

In conclusion, the importance of the provisional restoration must be reemphasized. The dentist must take care to meet the mechanical, physiologic, and esthetic requirements in all treatment. The provisional restoration may be neglected for a number of reasons. Often, the time required to construct an adequate restoration is underestimated, resulting in a hurried and unsatisfactory result. The dentist must be sure to save adequate time in the appointment for the construction of the provisional restoration. The construction may take place before the making of the final impression, thus assuring adequate time. This solution is also applicable in offsetting the problem of fatigue on both the dentist's and patient's part. Fatigue can play a role in poorly constructed provisional restorations. When construction is left until the last step, neither the patient nor the dentist has the stamina to persevere to an acceptable result. A final impression may be relegated to a subsequent visit whereas a provisional restoration must be fabricated before dismissal. The provisional restoration should be constructed to last for an adequate time. Frequently, this restoration is required to serve for a longer period than originally planned. Healthy gingival tissue, well-protected tooth structure, and a comfortable patient make the finished restoration easier. Only a well-constructed provisional appliance can assure this result.

REFERENCES

1. Kornfeld M.: *Mouth Rehabilitation,* ed. 2. St. Louis, C.V. Mosby Co., 1974.
2. Amsterdam M., Fox L.: Provisional splinting-principles and techniques. *Dent. Clin. North Am.* 73, March, 1959.
3. Johnston J.F., Mumford G., Dykema R.W.: *Modern Practice in Dental Ceramics,* ed. 1. Philadelphia, W.B. Saunders Co., 1967.
4. Shillingburg H.T., Hobo S., Whitsett C.D.: *Fundamentals of Fixed Prosthodontics,* ed. 1. Chicago, Quintessence, 1978.
5. Donaldson D.: The etiology of gingival recession associated with temporary crowns. *J. Periodontol.* 45:468, 1974.
6. Tylman S.D., Malone W.F.P.: *Tylman's Theory and Practice of Fixed Prosthodontics,* ed. 7. St. Louis, C.V. Mosby Co., 1978.

7. Preston J.D.: A systematic approach to the control of esthetic form. *J. Prosthet. Dent.* 35:393, 1976.
8. Knight R.M.: Temporary restorations in restorative dentistry. *J. Tenn. Dent. Assoc.* 47:346, 1967.
9. Fritts K.W., Thayer K.E.: Fabrication of temporary crowns and fixed partial dentures. *J. Prosthet. Dent.* 30:151, 1973.
10. Braden M., Causton B., Clarke R.L.: An ethylene amine derivative as a temporary crown and bridge material. *J. Dent. Res.* 50:536, 1971.
11. Phillips R.W.: *Skinner's Science of Dental Materials*, ed. 7. Philadelphia: W.B. Saunders Co., 1973.
12. Kramer I.R.H., McLean J.W.: Response of the human pulp to self-polymerizing acrylic restorations. *Br. Dent. J.* 92:255; 92:281; 92:311, 1952.
13. Langeland K., Langeland L.: Pulp reactions to crown preparation, impression, temporary crown fixation and permanent cementation. *J. Prosthet. Dent.* 5:129, 1965.
14. Stanley H.R.: *Human Pulp Response to Operative Dental Procedures.* Gainesville, Florida, Storter Printing Co., 1976.
15. Kazanoglu A., Kim H.W., Sayegh F.: Pulpal response to an epimine plastic. *J. Prosthet. Dent.* 42:183, 1979.
16. Kaiser D.A.: Accurate acrylic resin temporary restorations. *J. Prosthet. Dent.* 39:158, 1978.
17. Federick D.R.: The provisional fixed partial denture. *J. Prosthet. Dent.* 34:520, 1975.
18. Sotera A.: A direct technique for fabricating temporaries using the Omnivac. *J. Prosthet. Dent.* 29:577, 1973.
19. Nayyar A., Edwards W.S.: Fabrication of a single anterior intermediate restoration. *J. Prosthet. Dent.* 39:574, 1978.
20. Silvestri A.R., Gagnon W.N.: Improved temporary restorations of onlay preparations. *J. Prosthet. Dent.* 37:432, 1977.
21. Fiasconaro J.E., Sherman H.: Vacuum-formed prostheses. I. A temporary fixed bridge or splint. *J. Am. Dent. Assoc.* 76:74, 1968.
22. Fisher D.W., Shillingburg H.T., Dewhirst R.B.: Indirect temporary restorations. *J. Am. Dent. Assoc.* 82:160, 1971.
23. Crispin B.J.: The marginal accuracy of treatment restorations: A comparison analysis. *J. Prosthet. Dent.* 44:283, 1980.
24. Krug R.S.: Temporary resin crowns and bridges. *Dent. Clin. North Am.* 19:313, 1975.
25. King C.J., Young F.A., Cleveland J.L.: Polycarbonate resin and its use in the matrix technique for temporary coverage. *J. Prosthet. Dent.* 30:789, 1973.
26. Stein R.S., Glickman I.: Prosthetic consideration essential to gingival health. *Dent. Clin. North Am.* 177, March, 1960.
27. Federick D.R.: The processed provisional splint in periodontal prostheses. *J. Prosthet. Dent.* 33:553, 1975.
28. Barghi N.: The marginal integrity of the temporary acrylic resin crown. *J. Prosthet. Dent.* 36:274, 1976.
29. Jones E.E.: Vacuformed clear resin shells. *J. Prosthet. Dent.* 29:460, 1973.

CHAPTER 11

Interocclusal Records and Cast Articulation

ASTERIOS DOUKOUDAKIS, D.D.S.

THE ORIENTATION OF CASTS on an articulator that will reproduce the mandibular movements of the patient is a fundamental procedure that provides a necessary aid to study the conditions and the problems presented by the patient. Extreme accuracy is required for this procedure or errors can be made that may lead to inappropriate diagnosis and treatment planning or fabrication of faulty restorations. The purpose of cast articulation is to relate the maxillary cast in the articulator to simulate the relation of the maxillary teeth to the temporomandibular joint and then to relate the mandibular cast to the already mounted maxillary cast. Before the articulation, casts should be accurate, without bubbles or voids and with no signs of distortion. They should also have at least three v-shaped orientation grooves in their base.

For the accurate orientation of the maxillary cast a kinematic face-bow, a regular face-bow, or an ear face-bow should be attached to the patient's head. The most reliable and accurate way to locate the centers of rotation and the hinge axis is with the use of the kinematic face-bow. The centers of rotation are located by small opening and closing movements of the mandible and the recording of the styli. With the location of the two centers and the anterior third point of reference, the maxillary arch is oriented to a plane. This relationship is captured by the face-bow and is transferred to the articulator so that the maxillary cast will be mounted at the same position on the articulator. The hinge axis can be located accurately with a kinematic face-bow, although small deviations resulting from operator error can be expected.[1–5]

Although the superiority in accuracy of the kinematic face-bow over the regular face-bow and the ear face-bow is proved,[6, 7] the time required to complete a kinematic face-bow transfer sometimes makes it impractical to use. For this reason a regular face-bow with an arbitrary axis may be the instrument of choice. More recently, ear face-bows[8] have been introduced that are easy to use. Although they do introduce an error with the arbitrary hinge axis, they have proved to be useful.

When the face-bow is removed it is positioned on the articulator and the maxillary cast is mounted in the articulator. This places the cast in the same orientation to the condyles of the articulator as the teeth are to the patient's condyles. The orientation of the mandibular cast to the already mounted maxillary cast should follow. For this an interocclusal registration is needed. There are several methods and techniques for obtaining an interocclusal record using various materials. Unfortunately, there is no technique that does not present problems and there is continuing controversy as to which technique is the most reliable.

According to the materials and the techniques used, interocclusal registrations can be classified into five different catagories: (1) rigid materials; (2) silicone puttys; (3) waxes; (4) registration pastes; and (5) recording devices.

RIGID MATERIALS

Plaster of Paris

This is the oldest material used for the making of interocclusal records. Modifiers have been added to the plaster of paris to control setting time and setting expansion. The modifiers especially help to keep the setting expansion as low as possible and reduce distortions that can otherwise appear in the record. There are several disadvantages associated with the use of plaster as a recording medium. It is brittle and can easily break when retrieved from undercut areas and it is unpleasant to the patient. It can be used when occlusion rims are needed to mount edentulous casts, but normally it is used only to transfer relationships and fabricate matrices for certain laboratory procedures. When used for obtaining an interocclusal record some form of matrix, such as gauze, should be used to direct and maintain the material in the recording area and prevent the flow of plaster to adjacent regions. If breakage occurs during the removal from the mouth, sticky wax should be used to reassemble the pieces.

Impression Compound

Impression compounds are thermoplastic substances that soften under heat and become rigid when cooled. There is no chemical reaction and the material is dimensionally stable after cooling. The material is placed over a flame until it is uniformly heated, softened, and tempered. The use of a water bath is suggested to avoid overheating the material in a flame, which may change its physical properties. After the material has been uniformly softened, it is placed in the mouth and removed when it is completely hardened. If the record is removed before it has hardened, warpage can occur. Impression compound is used for the bite-fork of the face-bow and the fabrication of an anterior deprogrammer. It can also be used as a recording medium for interocclusal records if handled with care.

Autopolymerizing Acrylic Resins

Autopolymerizing acrylic resins have a wide variety of uses in dentistry, including use as a recording medium for interocclusal records. The main advantage of these materials is the rigidity that they demonstrate to eliminate some of the problems dealing with their handling after the recording is made. However, the dimensional accuracy of these materials, because of polymerization shrinkage, is not always acceptable when precise accuracy is required. They also present a serious problem if they engage undercut areas. Autopolymerizing acrylic resins are indicated for use when an interocclusal record is needed for a three or four unit fixed partial denture. In such cases the acrylic resin is applied over the preparation area and is not extended to the remaining teeth in the arch.

Resins are used as the base for an active recording when the functionally generated path technique is used and for the anterior deprogrammer when a centric relation record is required (Fig 11–1). Finally, autopolymerizing acrylic resins are used for the fabrication of clutches that will be used for the recording of mandibular movements with the use of either the pantograph or the minigraph.

WAXES

Waxes are probably the most commonly used material for interocclusal records. They are thermoplastic materials with a low molecular weight. They can be identified as organic polymers that consist of hydrocarbons and complex combinations of organic compounds. Their physical and chemical properties are dependent on their chemical composition and formula. Dental waxes are a mixture of natural and synthetic waxes. This will sometimes cause a variation of properties that result from lack of control in their production. Bite registration waxes are commonly produced from either casting wax or baseplate wax. Waxes are an inexpensive material to use for interocclusal records. Some of their physical characteristics make their use questionable when high accuracy is required. They have a low melting point and the highest coefficient of thermal expansion of all the interocclusal recording materials. As a result of this, they are not dimensionally stable. Their flow, resulting from the application of any static force, is high. This means that they may distort when they are removed from the mouth. Their elastic recovery after deformation is responsible for distortions. This can be reduced by uniform heating before recording and storage of records at low temperatures.

When wax is used for an interocclusal record, it is suggested that type III baseplate wax or types A and B hard inlay waxes be used. The wax should be softened in a water bath for 10 minutes and the record should be chilled after removal from

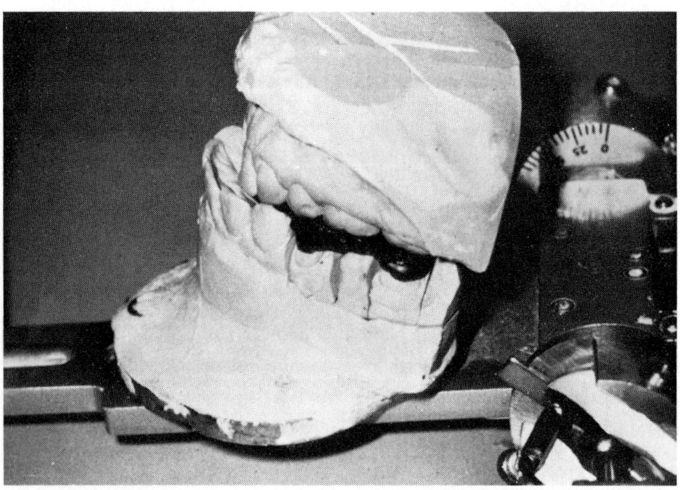

Fig 11–1.—Centric relation record using autopolymerizing acrylic resin and inlay wax. The maxillary cast has been mounted in the articulator with a face-bow and the mandibular cast is positioned in the interocclusal record ready for mounting.

the mouth and stored at low temperatures. The operator should realize that whenever wax is used, inaccurate results may occur from the different parameters that are introduced during the registration and mounting procedures.[9, 10] Some of these parameters are type of wax, thickness of wax, softening technique, pressure, and storage conditions. Careful considerations of these factors are indications of the limitations of wax as an interocclusal recording medium.

SILICONE PUTTY MATERIALS

Silicone putty is a heavy consistency silicone that can be used as a recording medium for interocclusal records. The putty base is mixed with a liquid catalyst that acts as the accelerator for the reaction. The base is a moderately low molecular weight silicone with certain additives that give the proper consistency to the putty. The accelerator reacts with the putty to form the silicone rubber and a byproduct of alcohol. This byproduct is responsible for the dimensional changes of the set material and is the reason silicone putty records are not dimensionally stable. If mounting procedures are not performed immediately, the possibility of error is increased. Addition polymerization putty materials are now available. There is no formation of a byproduct in their chemical reaction and they are dimensionally stable.

There are other problems associated with the silicone putty system. All putty materials are flexible and the record may lack the required rigidity. They also have a tendency to compress and recover when pressure is applied and released. This can invite inaccurate results during the mounting procedures. Trimming of the record with a knife so that only the cusp tips remain is easily and accurately done and may help to reduce the above mentioned problems. It is preferable that a hard putty be used rather than the regular type and the operator should always take into consideration the problems associated with the use of silicones for an interocclusal record (Fig 11–2). These materials have excellent handling characteristics and they do not fracture, tear, or adhere to tooth surfaces.

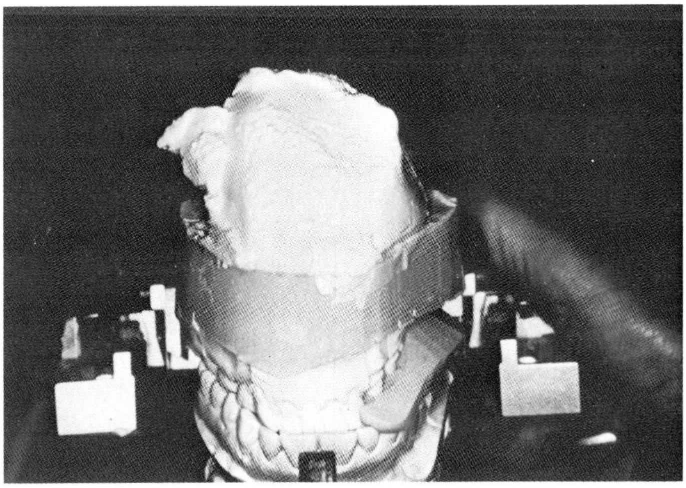

Fig 11–2.—Centric occlusion record using silicone putty. The mandibular cast is being mounted.

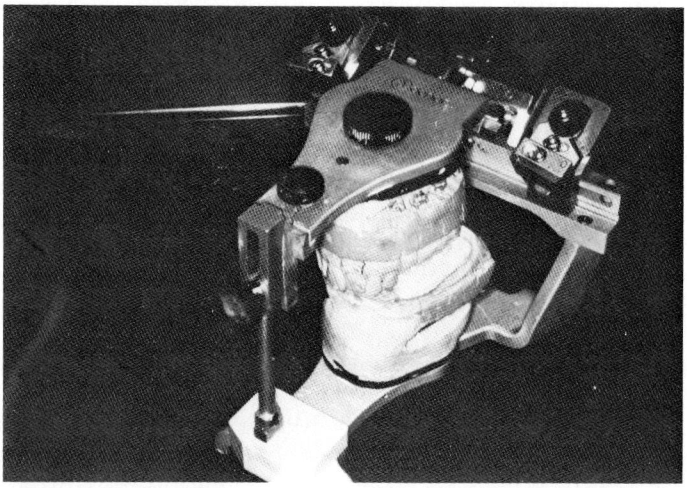

Fig 11–3.—Zinc oxide and eugenol registration paste as a medium for an interocclusal record has been used for the accurate mounting of the mandibular cast.

REGISTRATION PASTES

A commonly used registration material is the zinc oxide and eugenol paste (Fig 11–3). It has the ability to record details well and there is no resistance when the patient closes into the recording material. It is accurate and dimensionally stable. The material is supplied in two tubes that include the base and the accelerator. There are two types of zinc oxide and eugenol pastes: Type I, which is hard, and Type II, which is soft. Equal lengths of base and accelerator are mixed to a homogenous mix. Setting time may vary from 3 to 6 minutes. Altering the base-accelerator

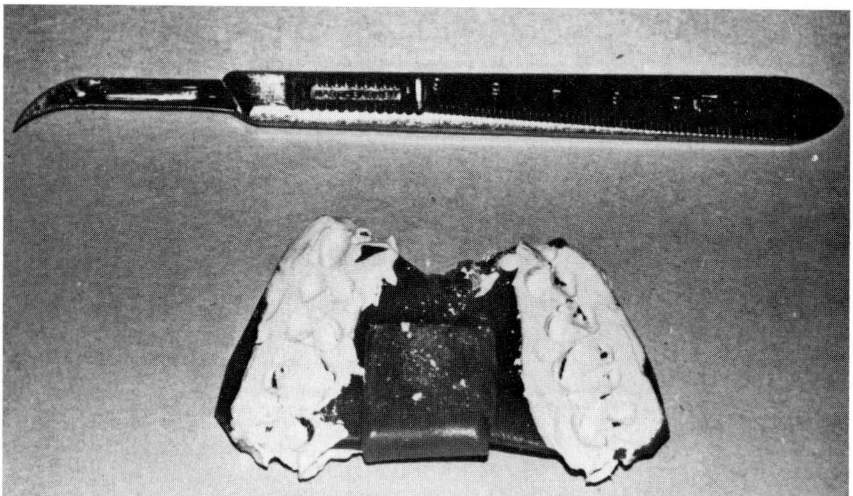

Fig 11–4.—Zinc oxide and eugenol centric relation record with wax as a matrix. The index has been trimmed. Additional registration material may be trimmed away leaving a record of only the cusp tips. This may be necessary to fully seat the working cast in the record.

ratio will alter the setting time but will also alter some of the physical properties of the material. Temperature and moisture can also affect the setting time. The record should be rinsed after removal from the mouth and stored at room temperature. It will be dimensionally unstable in higher or lower temperatures.

Although the material has some excellent clinical characteristics, it also presents some problems when used as a recording medium. The material is not strong by itself and some kind of supporting matrix should be provided. The most commonly used matrix is either a gauze mesh or wax. The hard set material is preferred to the soft set because it sets faster and is more fluid before setting than the soft set material.

The most serious problems with the material are its stickiness and its inability to withdraw readily from undercut areas. Distortion and breakage of the record may occur, especially when excess material is present. Some of the manufacturers have replaced eugenol with substitutes that help to eliminate the problem of stickiness. These registration pastes are superior to the zinc oxide and eugenol pastes in this respect but they still present the problem of removal from undercut areas. A minimum amount of material should be used. Only enough to cover cusp tips of the teeth to be recorded is required (Fig 11–4). Zinc oxide and eugenol paste is a material of choice when a rigid record is required.

RECORDING DEVICES

This category includes any kind of extraoral or intraoral device that can be used to record centric relation or centric occlusion. Among these are graphic tracing devices, electronic devices, the myomonitor, the minigraph, and the pantograph. Some of these devices are discussed in other chapters and each of them has its applications and limitations. Some may be used in place of a face-bow for mounting the maxillary cast and some are used to assist the operator in making interocclusal centric records as well as being the guide for determining articulator settings and adjustments.

RECORDING TECHNIQUES

Several parameters can influence the accuracy of interocclusal records. It is generally accepted that occlusal splints have a beneficial effect when a centric relation record must be obtained. Manipulation of the mandible after the use of an occlusal splint becomes easier because occlusal splints have the ability to relax the muscles.[12, 13] Other authors recommend the use of cotton rolls to separate the two arches before the actual recording.[14] Anterior deprogrammers placed on the two maxillary incisors[15] and made from either impression compound or autopolymerizing acrylic resin, act to guide the mandible to centric relation position. The use of an anterior deprogrammer in the form of a jig, leaf gauge, tongue blade, or cotton roll is highly recommended when centric relation is recoded. However, care should be taken not to exert pressure on the mandible that could possibly displace the head of the condyles posteriorly.

Numerous studies have reported that the most retruded position was recorded when the strongest pressure was applied on the mandible.[16–20] Others have questioned the forced retruded concept of centric recording, and as a result recommend that a light pressure be applied on the mandible in the form of guidance when the record is placed in the mouth. Reproducible and accurate results are attained with the manipulation techniques posed by Dawson[21] who introduced the technique of bilateral manipulation similar to a passive recording technique.[12, 22] The passive recording technique without patient participation and with the help of an anterior deprogrammer is reported as providing the best results when recording centric relation.[5, 22, 23]

The position of the patient during the recording procedure has an effect on mandibular position. In centric relation recording, the most anterior position was recorded when the patient was standing and the most posterior when the patient was prone.[24] Another study reports that condyles may be placed further posteriorly during the night and that centric relation is best recorded during the evening hours.[25]

INTEROCCLUSAL RECORD MATERIAL SELECTION

Errors associated with the use of wax as a recording medium have been reported that indicate that it is the most unpredictable material in use.[10, 11] Several factors such as the softening and cooling of wax, the closing pressure, and the thickness can introduce errors in the recording. In one study, the best results were attained using zinc oxide and eugenol paste or acrylic resin as a recording medium.[26] In the same study, the most unreliable results were obtained with wax registrations. Another study[27] compared the accuracy of two silicone putty and two self-curing resin interocclusal records and indicated that silicone putty records were more reliable although all the materials had some dimensional change over time. Finally, the most accurate results in another study were obtained using the eugenol-free zinc oxide paste or the polyether paste.[28]

It now becomes obvious that there is no single best method or material for obtaining an interocclusal record suitable for all clinical procedures. A clinician should master the use of several techniques and recording mediums to select the appropriate one for a given procedure. A clear distinction should be made as to the

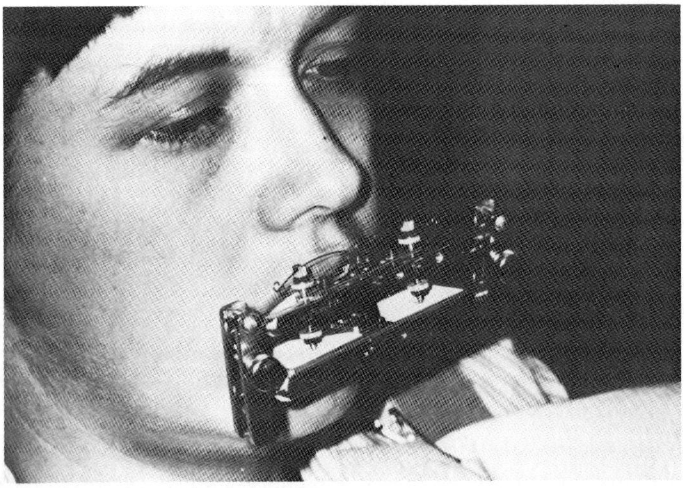

Fig 11–5.—A minigraph extraoral recording device can be used for the accurate determination of centric relation in the double gothic arch tracings and with the help of the transfer vise.

TABLE 11–1.—METHODS FOR CAST ARTICULATION

	CENTRIC OCCLUSION RECORDS		CENTRIC RELATION RECORDS
	Diagnostic Models	Working Models	
Arches with anterior and posterior stops	Hand articulation	Hand articulation	a. Anterior deprogrammer b. Wax or gauze mesh c. Registration paste
Arches with anterior and posterior stops that will receive quadrant preparations unilaterally or bilaterally	Hand articulation	Interocclusal record over the preparation area	
Partially edentulous arches unilaterally or bilaterally			Acrylic trial base with occlusal rims and registration paste

mandibular position we would like to record with our material. The clinician should decide if centric relation or centric occlusion will be recorded and the appropriate record must be obtained for the mounting of the mandibular cast. A pantograph or a minigraph can be used for interocclusal records for either position (Fig 11–5). The following discussion is limited to records obtained without any form of instrumentation. All of the records and materials are summarized in Tables 11–1 and 11–2.

CENTRIC RELATION RECORDS

If centric relation is to be recorded there are two types of records that can be used (Table 11–1). If a full compliment of teeth are present, or at least some opposing posterior teeth bilaterally, an anterior deprogrammer is recommended for use with the recording medium. The anterior deprogrammer can be fabricated from autopolymerizing acrylic resin or impression compound (Fig 11–6). A cotton roll,

TABLE 11–2.—MATERIALS FOR CAST ARTICULATION

PROCEDURE	IMPRESSION COMPOUND	AUTO-POLYMERIZING RESINS	WAXES	SILICONE PUTTY	REGISTRATION PASTES
Face-bow bitefork	X				X (as a reline)
Anterior deprogrammer	X	X			
Functional generated path		X	X		
Centric occlusion over preparations	X	X	X	X	X
Matrix for centric relation record			X		
Recording medium for a centric relation record		X	X	X	X
Record for partially edentulous patient		X	X		X
Clutches for the recording devices		X			
Lateral check bites		X	X	X	X

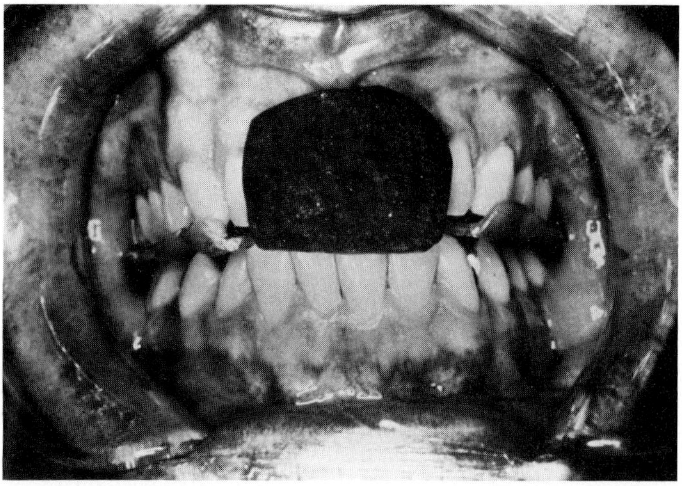

Fig 11–6.—Anterior deprogrammer and wax wafer in place ready for the application of the registration paste.

tongue blade, or leaf gauge can also be used if the clinician is careful not to create a leverage effect that will displace the condyles. The anterior deprogrammer should be adjusted and checked in the mouth. It should provide minimal separation of the posterior teeth while seating the condyles in their fossae. The material of choice for the recording medium is zinc oxide and eugenol, or eugenol-free zinc oxide paste. A matrix must be provided for the recording medium and in most cases wax or gauze mesh is used. Care is taken to use a minimum amount of recording medium, only enough to record the cusp tips (Fig 11–7). Any excess material may flow into undercut areas and fracture or distort when removed from the mouth. The anterior

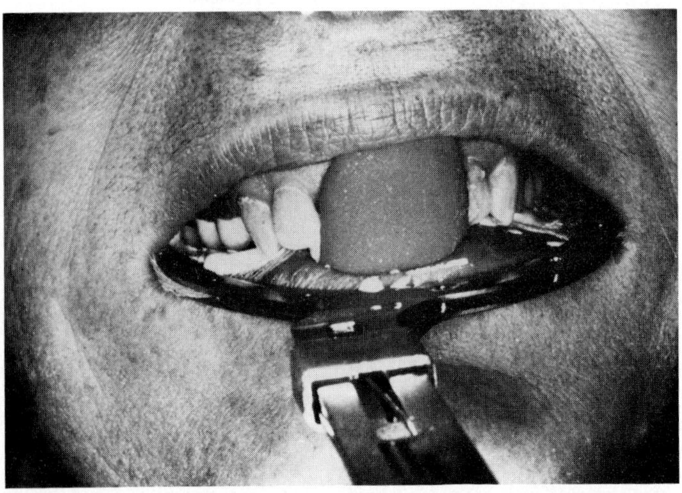

Fig 11–7.—An anterior deprogrammer with zinc oxide and eugenol record in place for the accurate registration of centric relation. Note the minimal amount of registration paste used. A metal frame is used to hold the gauze that supports the zinc oxide.

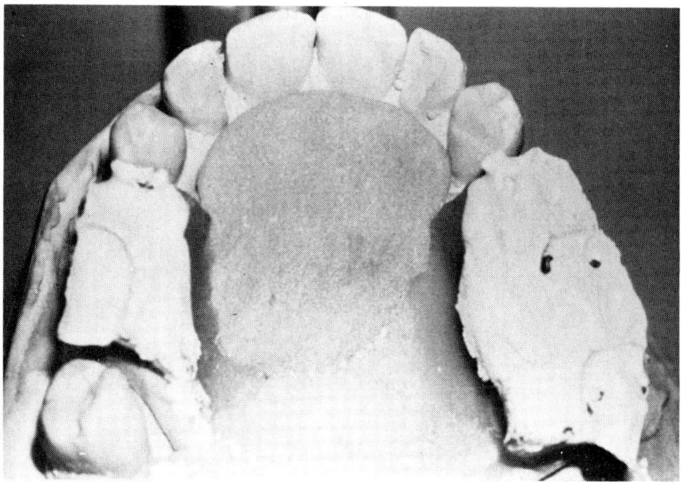

Fig 11–8.—Acrylic trial base with wax rim and zinc oxide and eugenol paste positioned on the maxillary cast for the mounting of the mandibular cast in a partially edentulous patient.

deprogrammer is placed in position in the mouth and the matrix with the recording paste is positioned. With the use of the bilateral manipulation technique the mandible is guided into the proper relation. When the recording material is completely set the deprogrammer and the record are removed from the mouth. The record is trimmed and is ready for the mounting procedures.

If the patient is missing posterior teeth bilaterally or unilaterally, it is suggested that an acrylic trial base be fabricated on the cast over the edentulous areas to be used for the mounting procedure. A wax occlusal rim is placed on the trial base and is carried to the mouth. There should be no contact of the opposing cusp tips on the wax. If contact occurs, the underlying mucosa may be displaced by the pressure. This would result in an open mounting. Zinc oxide and eugenol paste is added on the wax and the record is placed in the mouth. The mandible is manipulated in centric relation and the record is removed when the material has completely set (Fig 11–8).

CENTRIC OCCLUSION RECORDS

Centric occlusion records are usually easier to obtain than centric relation records. If the patient has both anterior and posterior contacting and interdigitating teeth, the best method to obtain centric occlusion is to hand articulate full arch casts with no interocclusal record (Table 11–1). This is probably the most accurate relationship if accurate casts were fabricated. Any recording material could result in an anterior or lateral displacement of the mandible and an incorrect mounting. If the patient has no posterior teeth unilaterally or bilaterally, an acrylic trial base is fabricated and the procedure is the same as described with the centric relation records. The only change is that the patient is instructed to close and there is no manipulation of the mandible by the operator. The operator should be certain that the patient is closing in the maximum intercuspation position. The last category of

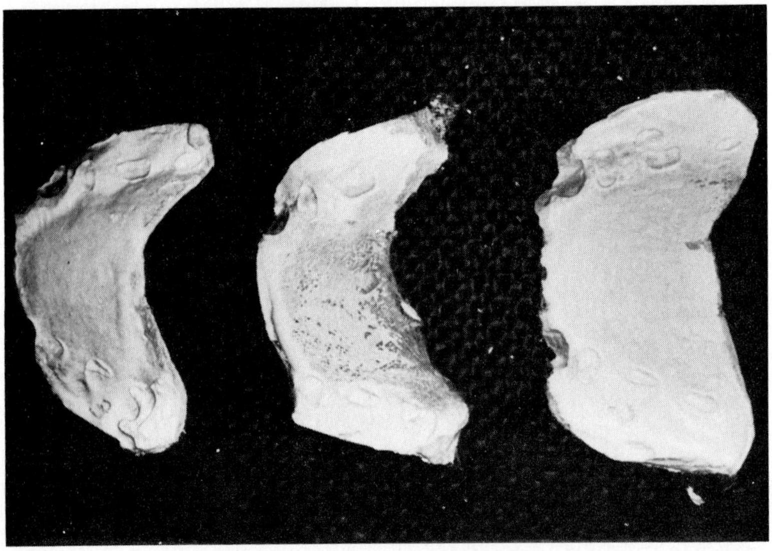

Fig 11–9.—Three centric relation records obtained using zinc oxide and eugenol paste and a gauze mesh as a supporting medium. One record is selected for the articulation of the mandibular cast. If the articulated cast will accept the other two records precisely, centric relation is assured.

centric occlusion record is where quadrant preparations have been completed bilaterally or unilaterally and as a result posterior stops are missing. In such a case, it is imperative that a rigid anterior index is made in centric occlusion before the posterior vertical stops are destroyed in the process of tooth preparation. An interocclusal record is then obtained over the area of the preparation while the anterior index is in place. The record is obtained using a material from the previously described mediums. The operator should have in mind the advantages and disadvantages associated with every material and selection should be based on these facts. The record should only cover the area of the preparation and should not be in contact with the adjacent teeth or tissues.

The discussed methods of obtaining interocclusal registrations have provided good results in the hands of skilled operators. Repetition of the procedure enables most clinicians to achieve consistently accurate results. It is especially important with centric relation records that at least two records be obtained that provide exactly the same relationships. This will assure that centric relation has been captured correctly and accurately and the clinician can proceed with the diagnosis and treatment safely (Fig 11–9). After the fabrication of the interocclusal records the mandibular cast can be mounted on the articulator. Then the articulator can be adjusted to simulate the mandibular movements using the pantograph, the minigraph, or protrusive and lateral check bites.

REFERENCES

1. Lauritzen A.G., Wolford L.W.: Hinge axis location on an experimental basis. *J. Prosthet. Dent.* 11:1059, 1961.
2. Kurth L.E., Feinstein I.K.: The hinge axis of the mandible. *J. Prosthet. Dent.* 1:327, 1951.

3. Knap F.J., Espinoza R.J., Ziebert G.J.: Graphic analysis of hinge motion on the sagittal plane. *J. Prosthet. Dent.* 29:390, 1973.
4. Santos J.L.: *An Electrical Device to Locate the Terminal Hinge Axis* (master's thesis). Ann Arbor, University of Michigan, 1975.
5. Long J.H.: Location of terminal hinge axis by intraoral means. *J. Prosthet. Dent.* 23:11, 1970.
6. Lauritzen A.G., Bodner G.H.: Variations in location of arbitrary and true hinge axis points. *J. Prosthet. Dent.* 11:224, 1961.
7. Aull A.E.: A study of the transverse axis. *J. Prosthet. Dent.* 13:469, 1963.
8. Raxek M.K.A.: Clinical evaluation of methods used in locating the mandibular hinge axis. *J. Prosthet. Dent.* 46:369, 1981.
9. Teteruck W.R., Lundeen H.C.: The accuracy of an ear facebow. *J. Prosthet. Dent.* 16:1039, 1966.
10. Millstein P.L., Clark R.E., Kronman J.H.: Determination of the accuracy of wax interocclusal registrations. *J. Prosthet. Dent.* 25:189, 1971.
11. Millstein P.L., Clark R.E., Kronman J.H.: Accuracy of wax interocclusal registrations. *J. Prosthet. Dent.* 29:40, 1973.
12. Calagna L.J., Silverman S.I., Garfinkel L.: Influence of neuromuscular conditioning on centric relation registrations. *J. Prosthet. Dent.* 30:598, 1973.
13. Celenza F.V.: The centric position: Replacement and character. *J. Prosthet. Dent.* 30:591, 1973.
14. Lammie G.A., Perry H.T., Crumn B.O.: Certain observations on a complete denture patient: Electromyographic observations. *J. Prosthet. Dent.* 8:329, 1958.
15. Lucia V.O.: A technique for recording centric relation. *J. Prosthet. Dent.* 14:47, 1969.
16. Ingervall B., Helkimo M., Carlsson G.E.: Recording of the retruded position of the mandible with application of varying external pressure to the lower jaw in man. *Arch. Oral Biol.* 16:1165, 1971.
17. Helkimo M., Ingervall B., Carlsson G.E.: Comparison of different methods in active and passive recording of the retruded position of the mandible. *Scand. J. Dent. Res.* 81:265, 1973.
18. Federick D.R., Pameijer D.H., Stallard R.E.: A correlation between force and distalization of the mandible in obtaining centric relation. *J. Periodontol.* 45:79, 1974.
19. Kabcenell J.L.: Effect of clinical procedures on mandibular position. *J. Prosthet. Dent.* 14:266, 1964.
20. Ramford S.P., Ash M.M.: *Occlusion*, ed. 2. Philadelphia, W.B. Saunders Co., 1971.
21. Dawson D.E.: *Evaluation, Diagnosis and Treatment of Occlusal Problems.* St. Louis, C.V. Mosby Co., 1974.
22. Kantor M.E., Silverman S.I., Garfinkel L.: Centric relation recording techniques—a comparative investigation. *J. Prosthet. Dent.* 28:379, 1972.
23. Strohaver R.A.: A comparison of articulator mountings made with centric relation and myocentric position records. *J. Prosthet. Dent.* 28:379, 1972.
24. Helkimo M., Ingervall B., Carlsson G.E.: Variation of retruded and muscular position of mandible under different recording conditions. *Acta Odontol. Scand.* 29:423, 1971.
25. Shafagh I., Yoder J.L., Thayer K.E.: Diurnal variance of centric relation position. *J. Prosthet. Dent.* 34:574, 1975.
26. Sindledecker L.: Effect of different centric relation registrations on the pantographic representation of centric relation. *J. Prosthet. Dent.* 46:271, 1981.
27. Millstein P.L., Clark R.E.: Differential accuracy of silicone-body and self-curing resin interocclusal records and associated weight loss. *J. Prosthet. Dent.* 46:380, 1981.
28. Balthazar-Hart Y., et al.: Accuracy and dimensional stability of four interocclusal recording materials. *J. Prosthet. Dent.* 45:586, 1981.

CHAPTER 12

Face-bow Transfer and Hinge Axis Location

ROBERT S. STAFFANOU, D.D.S.

OCCLUSION IS ONE of the most important factors in the practice of dentistry. Indeed, occlusion may be called dentistry's common denominator. No matter what specialty area we are in, the success of our cases depends largely on the management of occlusion. As far back as 1924, Shaw wrote, "The writing cut with precision on the complex pattern of the teeth may indeed be hieroglyphics, but, even so, it was surely no random and meaningless scribbling. More probably it was a real organic language in which the principles of tooth design and mechanism were inscribed, and we might yet succeed in deciphering it if first we took pains to learn its dynamic alphabet and master the elements."[1] For decades we have been trying to learn the dynamic alphabet of mandibular movement and occlusion and to master these elements in the construction of our cases.

We know that all the elements of the gnathostomatic system (muscles, teeth, and condyles), must be in harmony if our cases are going to function successfully. The masticatory mechanism is a sensitive neuromuscular system guided by proprioceptors in the muscles, joint capsule, and the supporting structures surrounding the teeth. All of these structures must work in harmony or the weakest member may become symptomatic. Tooth position always dominates as teeth are the only members of this system that are fixed and will not move or stretch as do the joints or muscles. If there is antagonism within this system, then the teeth, which are the only members that can be readily modified, must be altered to bring them into harmony with the muscles and joint position. If not, as mentioned before, the weakest member will suffer. This may be the teeth through excessive wear, migration, mobility, or loss of supporting structures because of local factors and inflammation. The muscles may be symptomatic and go into spasm as a result of continual occlusal trauma over a long period. Or, frank degenerative joint changes may develop because of occlusal trauma. Occlusion must then be managed properly if we are going to maintain harmony between all the members of this delicate system and keep them working together without antagonism.

In pursuit of this aim, the management and establishment of proper maxillo-mandibular relationships is of vital importance in restorative dentistry. If we can transfer the patient's natural dentition and then simulate its movements on the articulator, we can then construct restorations that will be harmonious to the movements of that patient. The first step in establishing proper maxillo-mandibular relationships is the face-bow transfer.

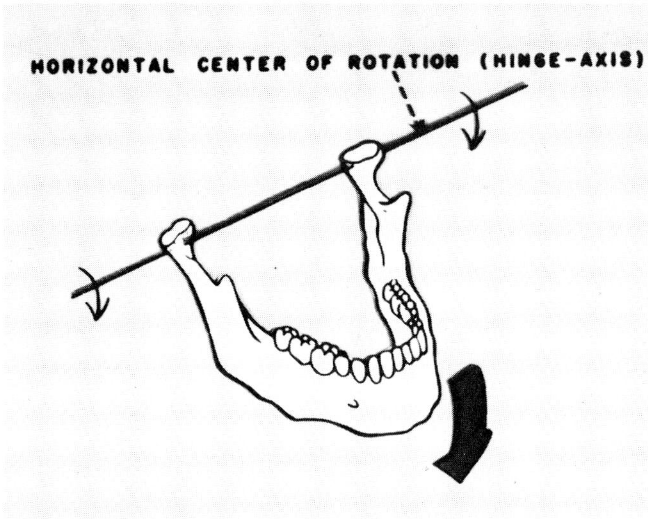

Fig 12–1.—The horizontal (hinge) axis of the mandible is the only axis about which movement takes place in a pure form.

The use of the face-bow is imperative if we are to accurately transfer and subsequently reproduce, or simulate, mandibular movement on an instrument. We know that the mandible rotates about three different rotational axes. These are the horizontal (Fig 12–1), vertical (Fig 12–2), and saggital (Fig 12–3) axes. The only axis about which movement takes place in a pure form is a horizontal or hinge axis of the mandible. This axis, therefore, becomes important and useful to us when trans-

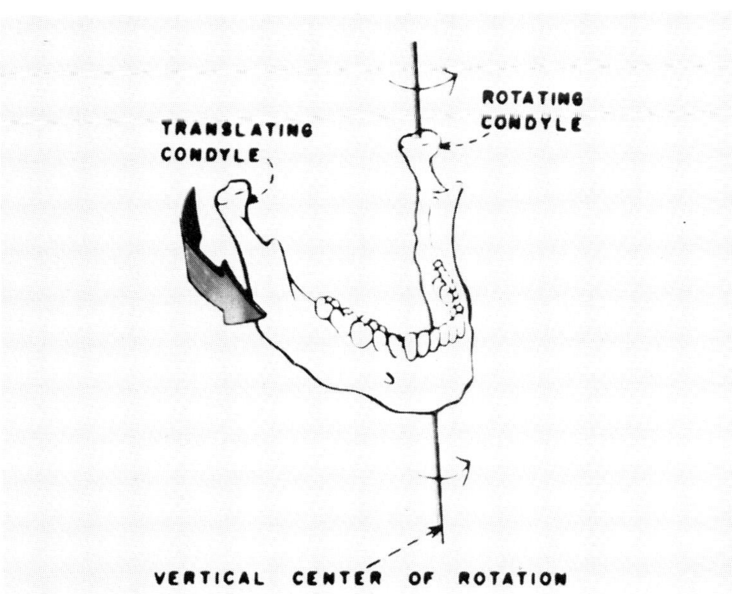

Fig 12–2.—The vertical axis of rotation of the mandible.

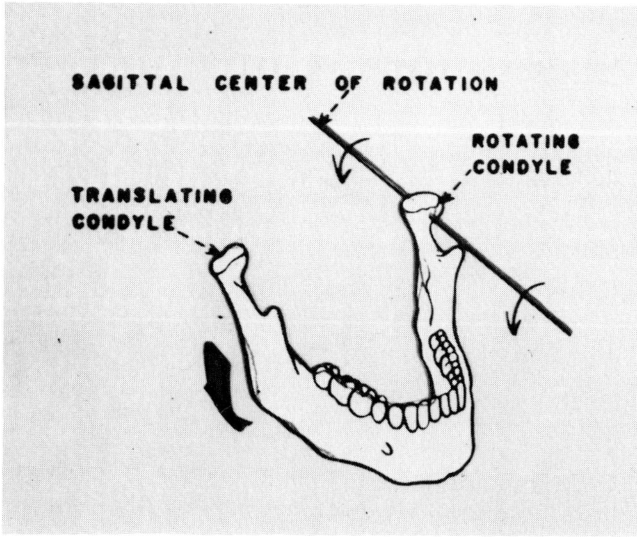

Fig 12–3.—The sagittal axis of rotation of the mandible.

ferring casts of the patient to the instrument in proper relationship. It is this horizontal axis to which we relate the face-bow transfer.

The horizontal hinge axis is an imaginary line connecting the two centers of rotation in each mandibular condyle. To simulate movement and an accurate arc of closure, the maxillary cast must be transferred in the proper relationship from the patient to the instrument with reference to these rotational centers. To transfer a relationship we must first establish a reference plane, or plane of orientation, on which to base the transfer. In other words, we must establish some point, or place, in space to which the maxillary cast can be related. That relationship is then taken from the patient to the instrument. This plane must be permanent and unchanging and it must be consistently relocatable. This is necessary as all subsequent movements of the mandible will be angles related to this plane. If the plane changes, the angles to the plane change, and the articulator settings, as well as the perspective on the case, will also change.

The reference plane that is established is called the axis-orbital plane (Fig 12–4), which corresponds to the Frankfort plane. It is convenient because it is parallel with the floor and gives a consistent perspective of the case from all aspects during construction. To delineate a plane, three points must be located on that plane. The three points chosen are the center of rotation on the right side, the center on the left side, and the infraorbital notch.

By establishing this plane we now have a reference plane against which the maxillary cast and, subsequently, the mandibular cast can be related on an instrument. The face-bow connects these three points to establish the plane. To use these reference points they must in some way be located. The infraorbital notch can be palpated and marked, measured from the medial canthus of the eye, or measured from the incisal edges of the anterior teeth (Fig 12–5,A,B). There are basically three ways in which we can locate and use the centers of rotation, and, therefore,

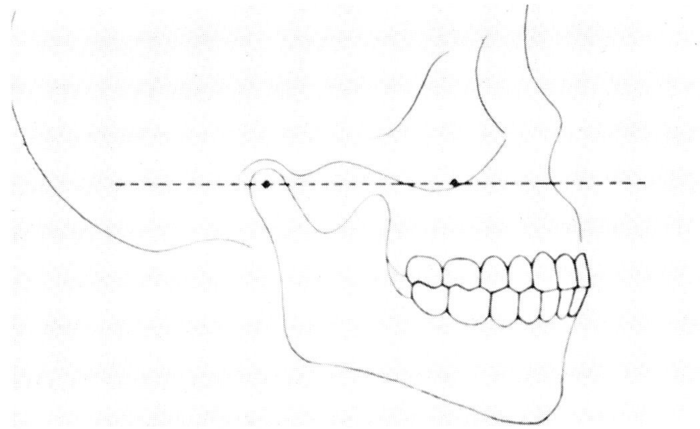

Fig 12–4.—The axis-orbital plane is established by the two centers of rotation, posteriorly, and the inferior border of the orbit anteriorly.

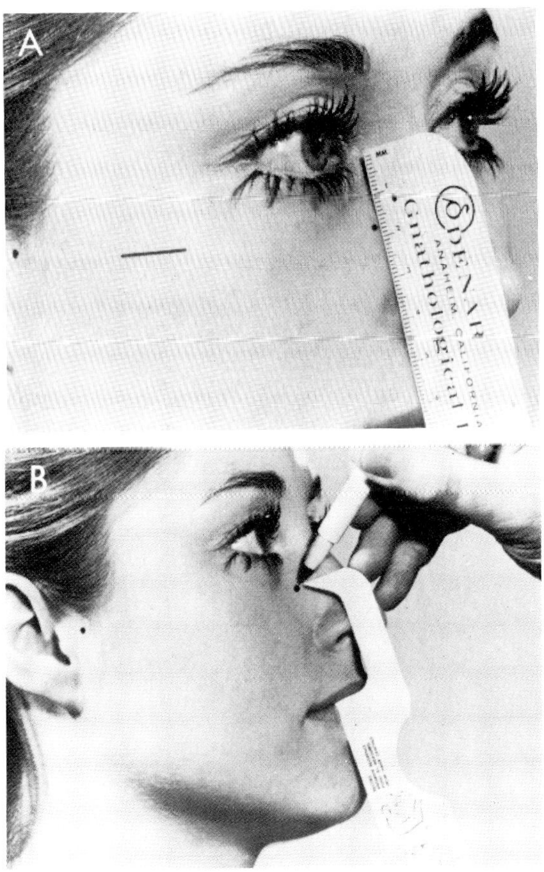

Fig 12–5.—**A,** the anterior reference point can be located by measuring from the medial canthus of the eye. **B,** the point can also be located with reference to the incisal edge of an anterior tooth.

the horizontal hinge axis of the mandible. The first method is by measurement. This is called an arbitrary axis location. In this method, a point is measured 11 to 13 mm anterior from the tragus of the ear toward the outer canthus of the eye. This is the tragus-canthus line (Fig 12–6). The second method, which is also classified as an arbitrary axis location, is the ear face-bow. For this method no measurement is needed. Ear pieces of the face-bow fit into the patient's external auditory canals and automatically determine the axis relationship (Fig 12–7). The third, and probably most technically difficult method of locating the hinge axis, is by actual kinematic location. With this technique a special clutch is rigidly attached to the mandibular teeth. Then, with a special condyle locator arm, the mandible is placed in centric relation and hinged open and closed. The position of the needle is adjusted until it rotates on the hinge axis of the mandible without arcing. The exact technique of this method will be discussed in detail later.

To execute the face-bow transfer, the face-bow is oriented to the patient. Posteriorly, it relates to the center of rotation on each side, either by arbitrary or kinematic means or by ear face-bow. Anteriorly, some type of pointer is oriented to the inferior border of the orbit (Fig 12–8). With these three points establishing the axis-orbital plane, the maxillary cast is transferred onto the articulator. The purpose of any face-bow transfer is to orient the maxillary cast to the instrument. As we mentioned before, to relate a maxillary cast in space it must be oriented to some plane of reference. To establish a plane of reference, three points on the plane must be located or established. The three points that are established or located are: right and left centers of rotation, whether they be arbitrary or exact locations, and the inferior border of the orbit. From these locations the plane derives its name, the axis-orbital plane. This axis-orbital plane is used because it is conveniently parallel to the floor and gives us a good perspective on the case as it is observed and constructed on the instrument. As most articulators are constructed to use the axis-orbital plane as a plane of reference for transferring the maxillary cast, the axis-orbital plane will be parallel with the upper member of the articulator, and the maxillary cast will then be suspended beneath the upper member of the articulator exactly in the manner as the teeth are positioned beneath the axis-orbital plane in

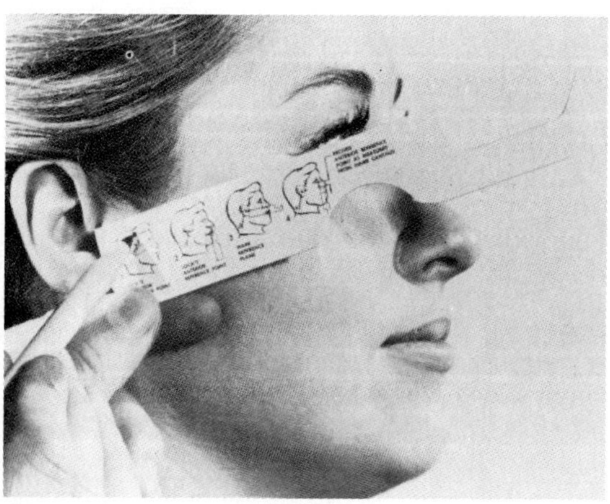

Fig 12–6.—The center of rotation can be arbitrarily located by measurement on the tragus-canthus line.

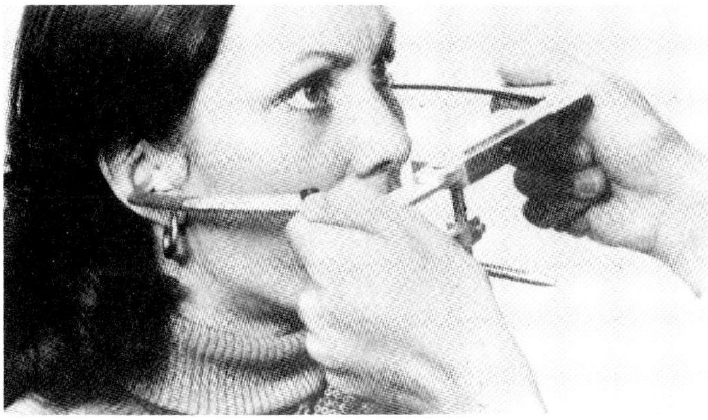

Fig 12–7.—The ear face-bow places the ear locator close to the head of the condyle (the center of rotation) by placement in the auditory canal and pulling gently forward.

the patient (Fig 12–9). By using these consistent points of reference each time, they can be repeated and duplicated. They can be consistently transferred from the patient to the articulator and back to the patient because the same reference points are used each time.

As we mentioned at the outset, the mandible rotates about three axes of rotation. The horizontal or hinge axis is an imaginary line connecting the right and left centers of rotation and is the only one about which we can observe motion in a pure form. The working condyle rotates about a vertical axis rotation during lateral movements. The working condyle also rotates about a saggital axis of rotation during lateral movements. The fact that we can observe motion in a pure form around the hinge axis makes it vital to us when transferring maxillo-mandibular relationships to the articulator.

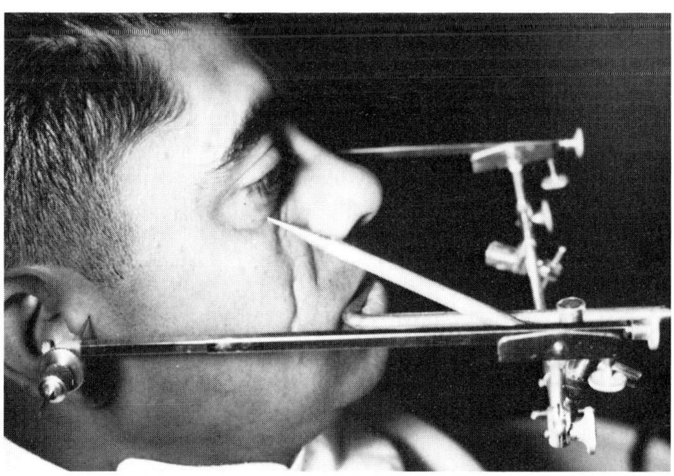

Fig 12–8.—Kinematic location of the hinge axis requires special armamentarium. Regardless of the type of location, three points of reference are needed for the face-bow transfer. Two posterior points (centers of rotation) and one anterior point (infraorbital notch).

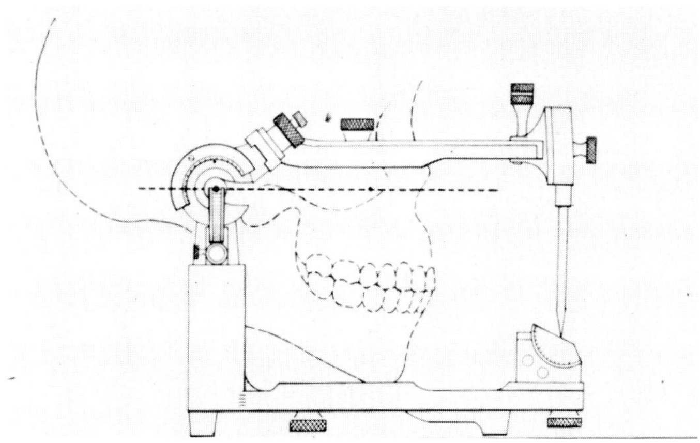

Fig 12–9.—Maxillary cast is suspended under the upper member of the articulator exactly as the teeth are positioned under the axis-orbital plane in the patient.

By placing the condyles in centric relation, the posterior mandibular border position, which is the only duplicatable position of the mandible, we make the hinge axis a constant point to both the maxilla and mandible (Fig 12–10). If the condyle is in a constant position in its relationship to the fossa, then the centers of rotation, the hinge axis, become a constant for transfer of the maxilla as well as the center of the hinge movement arc of the mandible. The maxilla must be placed, spacially, on the articulator the exact distance anteroposteriorly, superioinferiorly, and laterally from the rotational centers as they are in the patient's head. Each tooth is on a different arc of closure, depending on its distance from the rotational center. The rotational center can be thought of as the center of a number of circles. Each tooth, and its corresponding arc, is on a circle with a different radius but with a common center, namely the center of rotation of the mandible. Each circle is larger as its

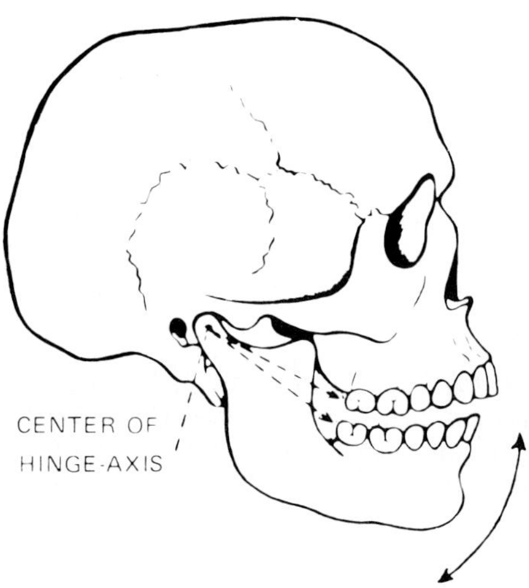

Fig 12–10.—By placing the mandible in centric relation (terminal hinge position) we make the center of rotation (hinge axis) constant to both the maxilla and mandible.

radius from this common center is longer. Each tooth, then, on its arc from the common center will travel a different path to meet its antagonist because of the size of the corresponding segment of the arc of the circle on which it is closing (Fig 12–11). For the teeth to meet properly, each tooth, and its corresponding arc that varies with the size of the circle segment it is on, must be located the exact distance from the center of rotation on the articulator as it is in the mouth. It must also be related laterally and inferiosuperiorly. The face-bow, when used properly, does this for us. By first properly relating the maxilla, the mandible, when properly related, will also be the exact distance from these rotational centers, thus establishing the proper closing arc for any given tooth.

The immovable member of this system, the maxilla, can be referred to as the base of operations. The face-bow transfer suspends this immovable member in space in relation to the axis orbital plane and centers of rotation. By establishing this plane in the patient, using a face-bow to locate three points on this plane, and then transferring this plane to the instrument, we will have the maxillary cast suspended under the upper member of the articulator exactly the same as the maxilla is suspended underneath the axis-orbital plane (Frankfort plane) in the patient's head (Fig 12–9). In essence, we placed the patient's maxilla on the articulator that, when observed in all dimensions, will be in the same relationship as if we removed the tissue from about the patient's face and looked at the patient's maxilla as it is suspended beneath the axis-orbital plane. The axis-orbital plane also becomes the plane of reference for protrusive and lateral movement recordings of the mandible. As the patient makes a protrusive movement, the condyle glides downward and forward over the articular eminence. As the condyles drop to a lower level, with their corresponding centers of rotation within the condyle heads, they form an angle to the axis-orbital plane. The angle that is formed by the downward and forward movement of the condyle and its center of rotation in relation to the axis-orbital plane is referred to as the condylar guidance and this is the angle that will be set on our instrument.

We might next ask what is the significance between locating an arbitrary point and an actual hinge axis location? Unless the actual kinematic hinge axis point is

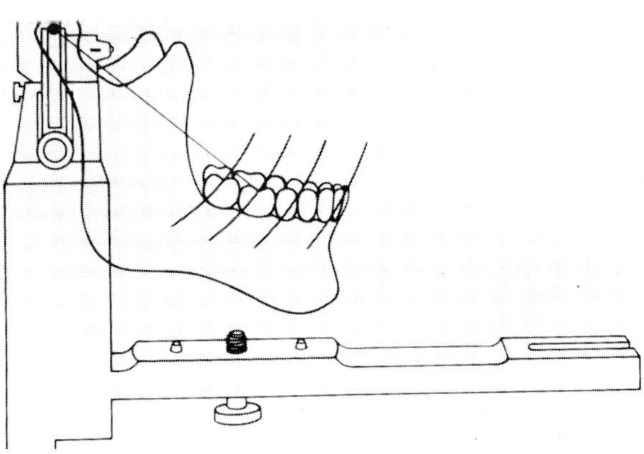

Fig 12–11.—Each tooth is on a circle of a different radius but with a common center (center of rotation). This determines the arc in which teeth close together. Arcs become more vertical toward the anterior of the mouth. Tooth inclines must be compatible with these differing arcs of closure.

transferred to the articulator, there will be some error in the size of the closing circle and we will have different approaching arcs as the teeth meet each other (Fig 12–11). If the teeth do not meet in the same arc on the articulator as in the mouth, we will have incline prematurities or other discrepancies in occlusion when the case is placed in function. Studies by Weinberg[2] have told us that if we can locate an axis point within a 5 mm range of the actual center of rotation of the patient and transfer this to an instrument we will only have .2 mm error in incline contacts in the molar area. This means that when the patient opens and closes we will have minimal error in arc of closure. If we are close to this actual center about which the mandible arcs open and close, we will have minimal discrepancies in inclines as the teeth come together. The further we are from that point the more incline discrepancies we will have and, therefore, the more discrepancy in the occlusion. The closer we can transfer a case and mount a cast in relation to the actual distance from the centers of rotation, the more accurate the closure and theoretically the less refining we will have to do in the mouth. If we are dealing with single restorations, it may not be a problem because there will be other natural teeth to act as guides and the patient can be closed and guided through centric closure and lateral excursions until the new crown or restoration harmonizes with existing teeth. If, however, we are doing multiple restorations and have no natural tooth guides, we must be as accurate as possible in locating this exact center of rotation. This assures that the arc at which the teeth come together on the instrument will be on exactly the same arc as the mandibular teeth are on when they approach in the mouth. Only then can we establish occlusions that are entirely free of deflective contacts.

As we mentioned at the outset, there are three types of face-bow transfers that we can use. The first is a measurement where we measure 11 to 13 mm on the tragus-canthus line. We place a dot and relate the face-bow to that particular point. The second type is the ear face-bow where the ear portions are actually placed in the patient's ears, the patient pulls this as forward as they comfortably can and the transfer is made from this position. The points are automatically located by placing the earpieces in the external auditory meatus. The third method is the actual hinge axis, or kinematic, location.

To do a hinge axis location accurately and exactly, we must have the proper armamentarium. The first step in this procedure is to fasten a clutch securely to the mandibular teeth (Fig 12–12). No flexibility can be tolerated in the system as it must be a rigid extension of the mandible itself. On this clutch a cross-arm and two hinge axis locators are mounted (Fig 12–13). A reference grid, such as graph paper, can be placed on a holder against the patient's skin so there is a background against which to see the movement of the stylus as the patient's mandible is arced open and closed. With this instrument in place, the patient's mandible is placed in terminal hinge position, or centric relation, and then either the patient or the operator guides the mandible slowly through the opening and closing movements (Fig 12–14). While looking at the graph paper in relation to the stylus, the stylus is moved backward or forward and up or down until the stylus rotates about a point without arcing movement as the mandible opens and closes (Fig 12–15). When we can see no extraneous movement in this stylus as the patient opens and closes, we know that we have located the exact hinge axis of the mandible in the centric relation or the terminal hinge position. Terminal hinge position or centric relation is important because this is the only repeatable position of the mandible. It is the

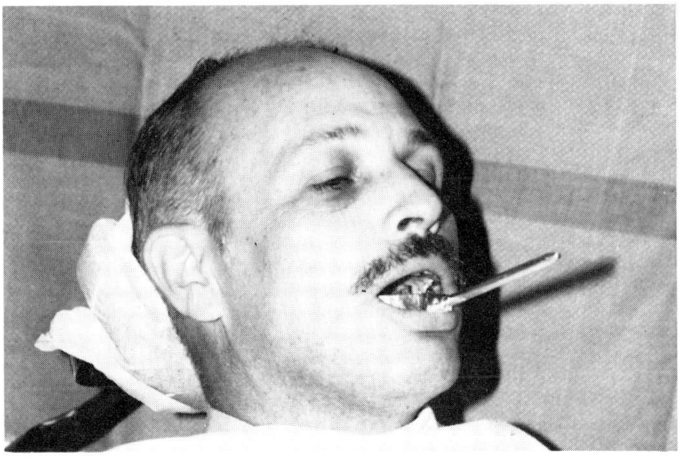

Fig 12–12.—Clutch rigidly attached to mandibular teeth for kinematic hinge axis location.

rear-most, upper-most, mid-most position of the condyle in the glenoid fossa without regard to teeth contact. It is a bone to bone position which gives us consistent relationship between the maxilla and mandible.

Teeth, by the fact that they do not move in their sockets, dictate closure. If the point at which the teeth close is not harmonious with the condyle and muscle position, then we are inviting the problems that were mentioned at the outset. Therefore, the mandible must be placed in the so-called neutral position, starting position, or initiating position of movement. This position is called centric relation. This is the only repeatable position of the mandible and the position from which all movement initiates.

Once the hinge axis has been kinematically located, permanent points may be tattooed in the patient's skin. These will become reference points throughout treatment. Because gravity exerts a pull on the skin, the patient should be placed in a consistent position, an upright postural position with the head away from the head-

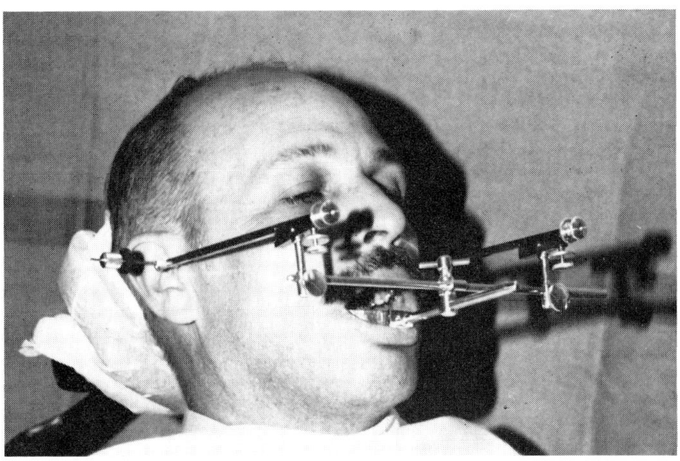

Fig 12–13.—Locator arms with styli attached to clutch.

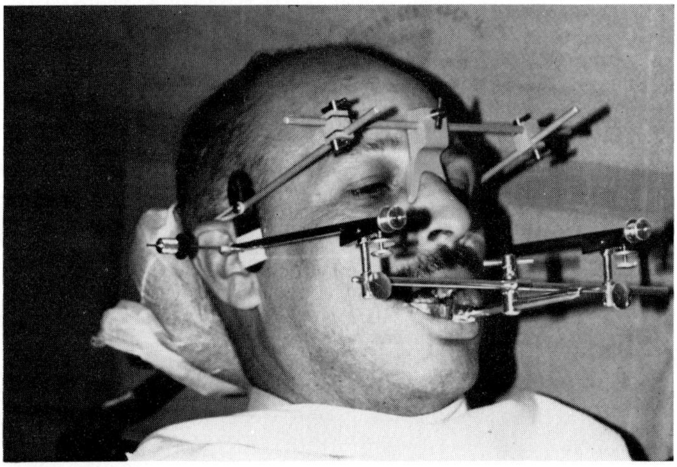

Fig 12–14.—Graph paper is held in place beneath the stylus on a frame supported from the bridge of the nose. The mandible is arced open and closed and the stylus is adjusted up, down, forward, or back until it rotates on a point without extraneous movement.

rest of the chair. If the patient is positioned horizontally, the skin will pull toward the posterior part of the head. If the patient is sitting upright the skin will pull toward the floor. Therefore, we must keep the patient's skin in a consistent position for transfer each time. All of us have a postural position that can be duplicated time and time again, provided there is no damage to the inner ear balance mechanism. This is the position that we should use for consistency. Whether the patient is upright or supine will make a difference on the skin surface of 2 to 3 mm so it should always be marked in the same position (Fig 12–16). The axis itself has not changed but the position of the skin over the axis has changed, so this skin position must be consistent. The most consistent position at which we can place a patient is this upright, postural position with the patient sitting in the chair without head

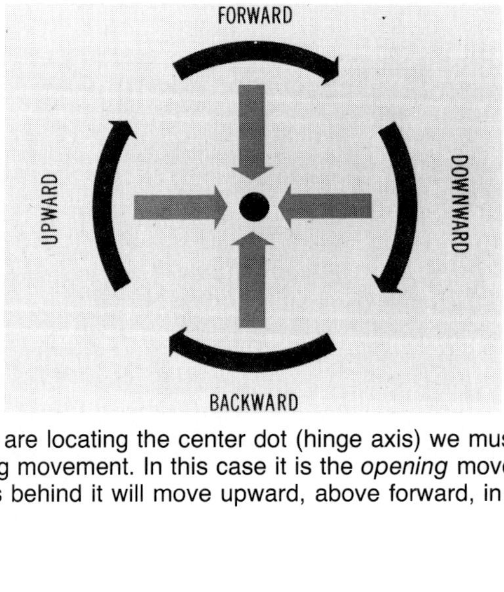

Fig 12–15.—If we are locating the center dot (hinge axis) we must first orient to either the opening or closing movement. In this case it is the *opening* movement. As the patient opens, if the stylus is behind it will move upward, above forward, in front downward, and below backward.

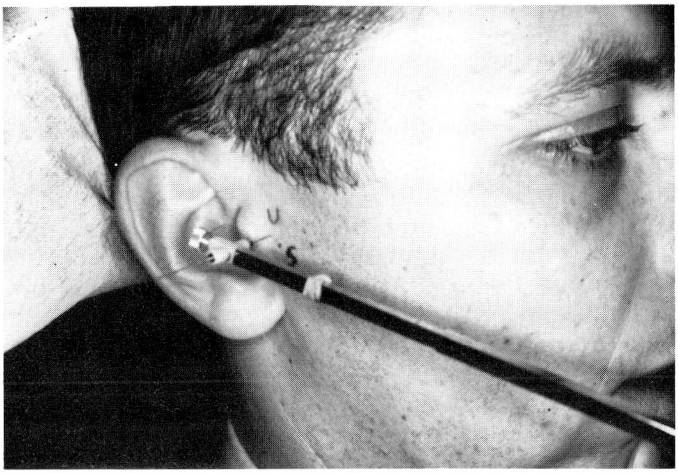

Fig 12–16.—Position is important as the skin will move with gravitational pull. *(U)* indicates the upright position marking and *(S)* indicates the supine position marking. Upright marking is more consistent with regard to skin position.

support. The third point of reference is usually marked at the axis-orbital plane. This can be marked on the skin, a blemish can be used or it can be measured from the corner of the eye or from the incisal edge of the existing teeth. It must, however, be a point that can be exactly relocated for use the next time the case is transferred.

Once these points are marked, we must have a face-bow that will transfer the relationship of these three points to the articulator. A bite fork is placed in the patient's mouth to register the maxillary teeth. This bite fork will suspend the maxillary cast for mounting. The frame is then assembled, the two axis points located right and left posterior, the anterior orbital notch point is located with the orbital pointer of the face-bow, and this relationship is transferred to the articulator. The maxillary cast is placed in the bite fork and with the face-bow oriented the maxillary cast is mounted to the instrument.

When we have mounted the upper cast we must have some means by which to locate the dynamic or mandibular member of the gnathostomatic system. This is usually done with an interocclusal record, which can be of many different materials but wax is used most. With the wax softened the mandible is manipulated forward and back until the patient allows the condyle to drift back into centric relation. The mandible is then closed into the wax with minimal pressure. Generally, the angles of the mandible are supported to prevent any downward displacement of the condyles out of the fossa during the recording procedure. A minimum thickness of wax is used to get the teeth as close together as possible without actually coming in contact. Although we want the minimal amount of material interspersed between the teeth, we do not want the cusps to come in contact, or approach contact. This will initiate proprioceptive guidance and deviate the mandible away from the centric relation position. Because this position is a bone to bone position, it must be taken without letting the teeth come in contact. The wax is interspersed between the contacting surfaces of the teeth so that we can position the condyles in the fossa in the proper position without having guidance from the inclining contacts of the teeth themselves. Generally two or three centric relation records are made.

The first centric relation record is used to mount the lower cast to the face-bow mounted upper cast. Once the lower cast is mounted to the upper cast the second centric relation record is used to compare the position of the first. If both recorded the same position we can assume that the casts are in centric relation because by definition this is the only duplicatable position of the mandible. If we wish to have a further check, we can take the third record and check again. If the third record checks, we can be certain that we have the patient mounted in centric relation. We have duplicated the only repeatable position of the mandible to the maxilla.

A further method of checking centric relation is the split cast technique. With this technique the original study cast is keyed, boxed with masking tape, and a small stone wafer poured against the upper surface of the cast. After the cast is mounted, this is separated (Fig 12–17). The centric relation record is placed over the mandibular teeth, the separated upper cast is placed in the centric relation record (Fig 12–18) and the upper member with its corresponding key (Fig 12–19) is closed into the key on the upper surface of the maxillary diagnostic cast. When these key together they should fit accurately with no space between the base of the cast and the key mounted to the upper member of the articulator (Fig 12–20). Lauritzen[3] has said that we can detect one-five thousandth of an inch of variation with this procedure. This gives us an accurate measure to confirm that we have located and transferred the centric relation position from the patient to the articulator.

Once the upper cast has been transferred to the articulator with the face-bow related to the axis-orbital plane and we have located the mandibular cast to the maxillary with a centric relation record, we have established an arc of centric relation closure on the instrument the same as the centric relation arc of closure on the patient (Fig 12–11). This is important because, if we identify the hinge axis as the center of a circle, each tooth would be on a circle of a different radius as it approaches its antagonist. As you look at these paths of approach, they become more vertical as we go toward the anterior part of the mouth. This is because the anterior

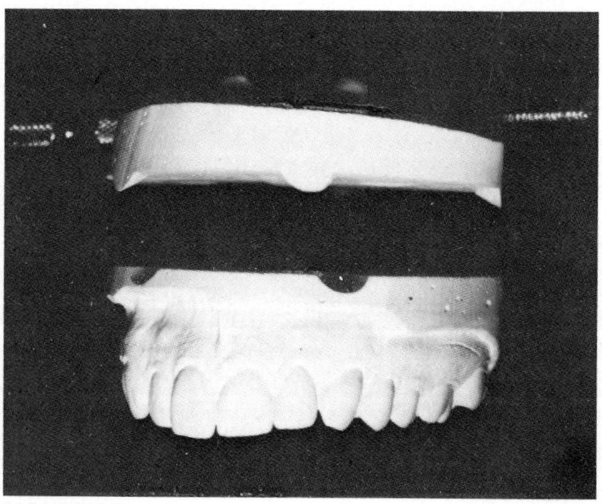

Fig 12–17.—Maxillary cast and wafer with three points of orientation.

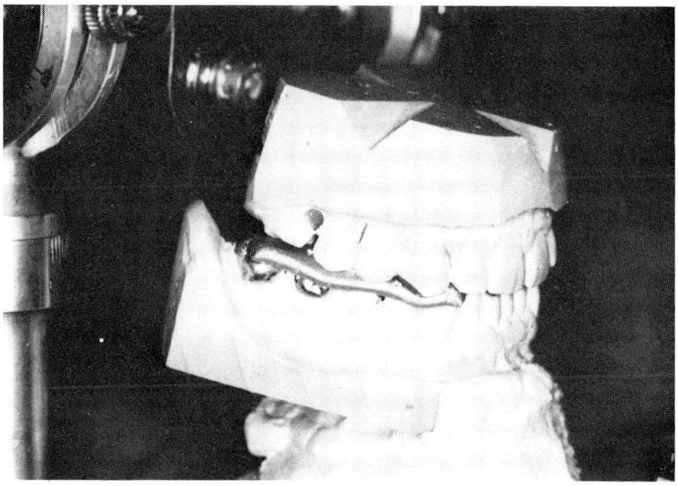

Fig. 12–18.—The upper cast is placed in wax centric relation record. Note V-shaped keying.

of the mouth, being a larger circle with greater radius from the center of rotation, makes any given segment of that circle flatter and creates a more vertical approach. Posteriorly, the circle becomes smaller, and any segment of that circle will have more curvature and be more acute. Therefore, these circles dictate the approach path of the mandibular teeth against the maxillary teeth meaning the incline contacts and cuspal inclines must harmonize to these arcs of closure if there is to be proper occlusion between the maxillary and mandibular teeth.

CONCLUSION

The first step in establishing maxillo-mandibular relationships is the face-bow. The ear face-bow (Fig 12–21,A,B) or the measurement type face bow (Fig 12–22, A–C) may be used. The face-bow is a measuring device used to orient the maxillary

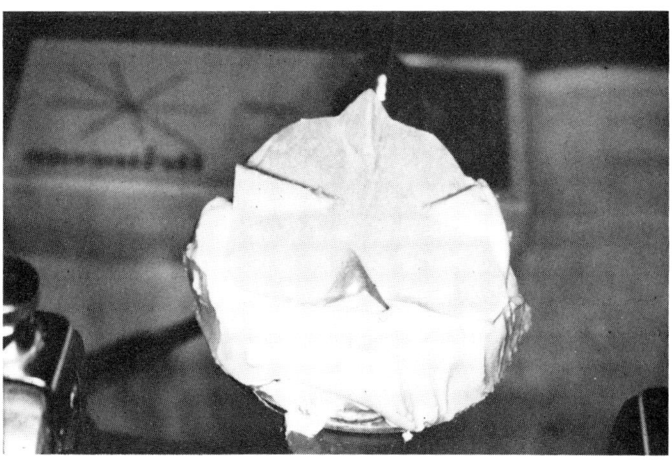

Fig 12–19.—Keyed wafer mounted on upper member of articulator.

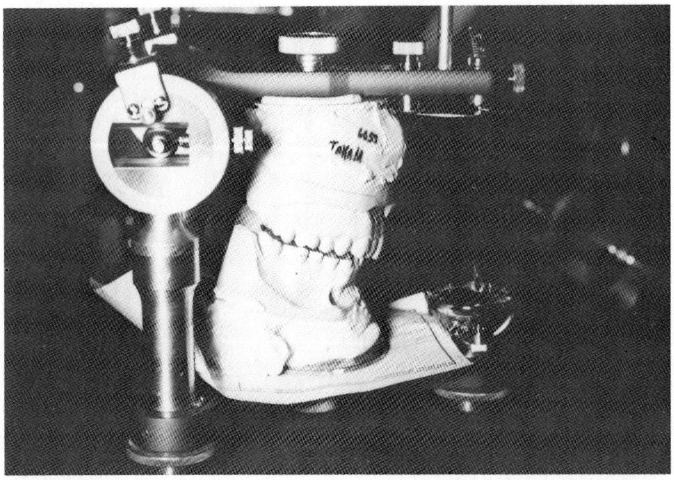

Fig 12–20.—When closed there should be no discernible space between the upper key and the maxillary cast.

cast to the articulator in the same relationship as the maxillary teeth are in the patient's mouth. A plane of reference is established first. It is known as the axis-orbital plane and is formed by the centers of rotation on the right and left, and the infra-orbital notch in the anterior. By locating these three points, we establish a plane that is parallel to the floor (the axis-orbital plane). If this plane is transferred to the articulator, the upper member of the articulator represents this plane. The maxillary cast is suspended beneath the axis-orbital plane of the instrument in exactly the same position that it is suspended on the patient. It will also be related in three dimensions to the centers of rotation. It will be suspended anteroposteriorly a given distance in front of the condyles. The maxillary cast will be suspended laterally in the proper dimension between the condyles of the patient and, correspondingly, of the instrument. It will also be oriented properly inferiosuperiorly in relation to the axis-orbital plane. This orientation is extremely important if the teeth are to close in the correct arcs of closure.

If the teeth are constructed on an articulator that places the teeth farther from the center of rotation and then they are brought back to the mouth, they will be on a smaller arc in the mouth and the teeth will show anterior prematurities, maxillary mesial inclines, and mandibular distal inclines. If the case is constructed on an articulator that has a shorter closing arc than the mouth, when the restorations are placed in the mouth with its longer radius, and therefore longer closing arc, they will have posterior prematurities, maxillary distal inclines, and mandibular mesial inclines. Most arbitrary articulators produce this sort of error. Because the mandible closes on approximately a 3 to 1 arc with 1 mm posterior closure equal to 3 mm anterior closure, it is better to have high spots in the posterior area where there is more tooth structure, or more metal, to adjust in correcting these disharmonies. If the error were in the opposite direction, we would have to remove 3 mm in the anterior of the tooth to close the posterior 1 mm. It is important, then, that this arc of closure be accurate. Studies have shown that if a case is mounted within 5 mm of the actual center of rotation we will only have .2 mm error in the

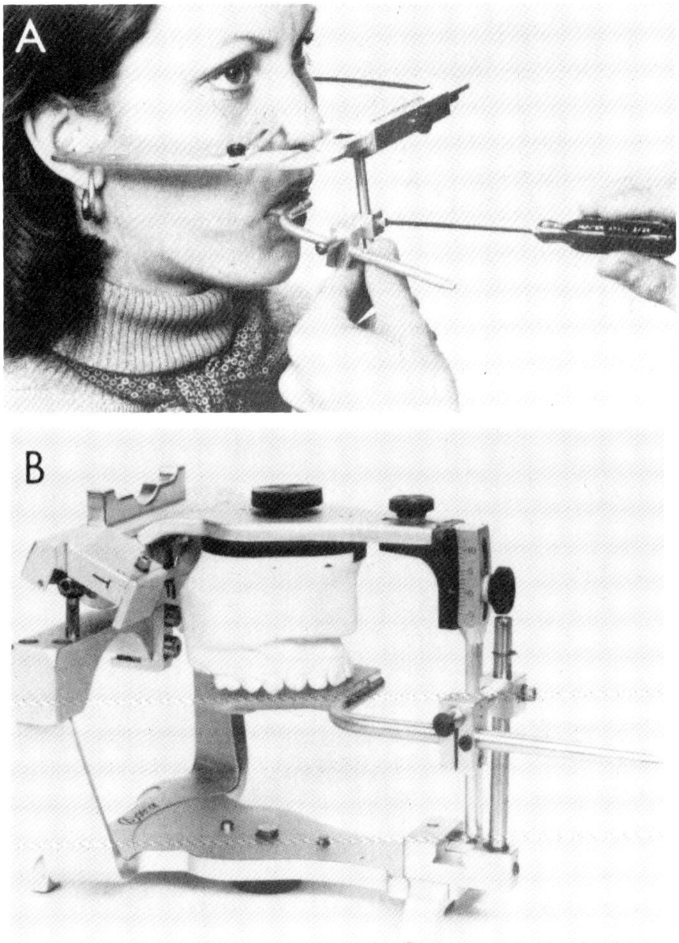

Fig 12–21.—A, the Denar ear face-bow transfer. The bow is attached to the bite fork, the anterior reference point oriented and face-bow locked in position with hex screws and wrench. (Courtesy of Denar Corporation, Anaheim, California.) **B,** the Denar ear face-bow transfer. A special adaptor on the incisal table supports the maxillary cast in the bite fork index for mounting to the upper articulator member.

second molar area.[2] This is the basis of the arbitrary face-bow transfer that does not reproduce the arc of closure exactly, but records what is termed a "segment of the arc of closure." It is usually close to the actual arc of closure. If the arbitrary transfer is within this 5 mm radius limit, on a segment of the arc of closure, and mounted at or close to occluding vertical dimension, we will have little error between the arbitrary and actual closing arcs of the mandible. This is the rationale for the ear face-bow. It will record within 5 mm of the actual center of rotation a high percentage of the time. However, we cannot know if we are within 5 mm of the actual axis unless we kinematically locate it and compare it to the arbitrary location. Regardless of the type of axis location used, the hinge axis, in some form, must be transferred in the terminal hinge position to the instrument. We are accepting

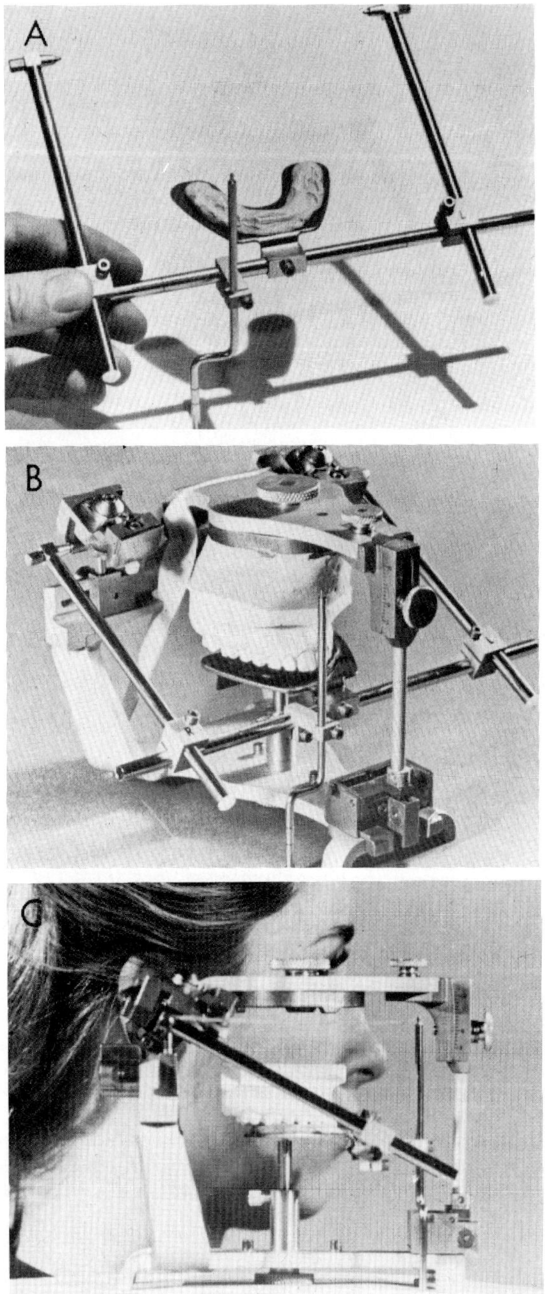

Fig 12–22.—A, the Denar measurement type face-bow. The assembled face-bow removed from patient. (Courtesy of Denar Corporation, Anaheim, California.) **B,** the Denar measurement type face-bow oriented to the articulator. **C,** the maxillary cast is oriented antero-posteriorly, and in all other spacial relationships, to the articulator the same as the teeth are to the patient's head.

centric relation, or the hinge axis, as the starting point of all mandibular movement. If we wish to explore mandibular movement even further we can, after locating this axis, track it through space to trace complete mandibular movement in three dimensions. Any arbitrary transfer to a semi-adjustable instrument will only accurately duplicate hinge movement of the arc of closure. Lateral movements, or translatory movements, are not accurately reproduced. To trace and accurately simulate all translatory movements of the condyle, we must employ a special instrument known as the pantograph. This pantograph is then used to program a special type of articulator that is made to accept three dimensional movement.

REFERENCES

1. Shaw D.M.: Form and function in teeth. *Internat. J. Ortho.* 10:703, 1924.
2. Weinberg H.A.: An evaluation of basic articulators and their concepts. *J. Prosthet. Dent.* 13:622, 1963.
3. Lauritzen A.G., Wolford L.W.: Occlusal relationships: The split-cast method for articulator techniques. *J. Prosthet. Dent.* 14:256, 1964.

CHAPTER 13

Pantography

ROBERT S. STAFFANOU, D.D.S.

USING A FACE-BOW and transferring the maxillary cast to an instrument and then relating the mandibular cast to this maxillary cast with a centric relation record, we can establish an arc of closure on the instrument the same as the arc of closure in the patient's mouth. This is important because each tooth arcs on a circle of a different radius. The hinge axis, or center of rotation, in the head of the condyle is the common center for these circles, or arcs of closure. This means that as the mandible arcs close, each tooth approaches its antagonist in an arc of a different radius. As a result of the differing circle radii, these arcs become more vertical as we approach the anterior and more oblique as we go toward the posterior part of the mouth. This means that as the jaws come together, the inclines have to accommodate for these varying circles or differing arcs of approach. Although we can duplicate these arcs of closure in straight up and down or hinge motion, this has little to do with the lateral movement of the mandible that can be critical in the management and establishment of occlusion in restorations that are to be placed in the patient's mouth.

When we are dealing with simple restorations, such as single tooth restorations or perhaps some three unit fixed partial dentures, and have an intact dentition to work with, we can construct these restorations on a good arc of closure and harmonize lateral excursions in the mouth by using the natural teeth as guides to lateral incline development. In cases where the preparations eliminate all of the occlusion and we have absolutely no natural tooth guides for orientation, new concerns arise. What guidelines do we use in establishing cusp height and ridge and groove direction? When we have no natural teeth, or an unharmonious occlusion, this kind of information can only be obtained by recording the mandibular condyle movement of the patient. The mandible's range of motion has limited border movements. It can only go back as far as centric relation. Centric relation is the posterior border limit of the mandible. The mandible can only go protrusively as far as the protrusive border limit. The mandible can only move to the right or the left as far as the lateral border limits of the mandible.

As the condyles move over their tissue-covered boney controls, certain anatomic designs of posterior occlusal surfaces and anterior lingual surfaces of the teeth are dictated. By understanding these movements and their effects on tooth anatomy and relationships we can more accurately construct occlusally harmonious restorations. We can also analyze articulating instruments more intelligently and be aware of what they will or will not do based on the type of controls they possess.

When we have prepared teeth to eliminate all incline contacts and all occlusal surface contacts, we must establish guides and limits before we can construct a custom-made occlusion. Once the teeth are prepared, the only guides that we have to go by are the condylar determinants of occlusion. These condylar determinants can be recorded on the patient with an instrument called the pantograph. They can then be transferred to a jaw-simulating instrument, an articulator, that can be programmed to reproduce these movements. The pantograph is a three-dimensional mandibular movement recorder. If we accept the pantograph as the instrument that records the most information possible about the patient's mandibular movement, and study and understand the tracings, we can determine these condylar movements and their effect on the tooth morphology. These movements must be visualized in three dimensions to fully understand their effect.

The pantograph must always be related to the hinge axis of the mandible in the terminal hinge or centric relation position. This is the starting point from which all movement takes place. By locating this hinge axis and extending it, via an imaginary line, through the condyles and beyond the patient's skin, we can orient the pantograph to this axis. We can track this hinge axis as it travels through space and as it maintains its constant relationship to the condyles during their corresponding movements (Fig 13–1). We observe this movement oriented to a maxillary lingual cusp that is a stamp cusp and is stationary because it is on the maxillary arch. We imagine this cusp as a fixed stylus (Fig 13–2). We can then move the mandible in relation to this fixed point and see what effects the anatomic controls of the condyles have on the morphology of the tooth surfaces. These condylar movements affect ridge and groove direction, cusp placement, cusp height, mesiodistal spacing of the cusps, and the curvature of the lingual surfaces of the maxillary anterior teeth. Centric relation is the starting point for all movement and is the point at which our pantographic tracing is initiated. When we have no tooth guidance for relationship or when teeth are not harmonious with the condyle paths and must be changed, this is the only indirect method available to determine proper occlusal anatomy for harmonious function between condyles, teeth, and muscles.

The pantograph is assembled and oriented to the patient's hinge axis position

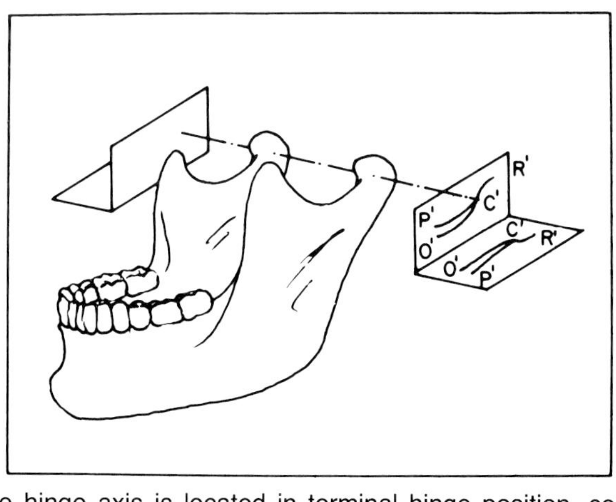

Fig 13–1.—The hinge axis is located in terminal hinge position, centric relation, and then tracked through space as the mandible moves. (Courtesy of Denar Corporation, Anaheim, California.)

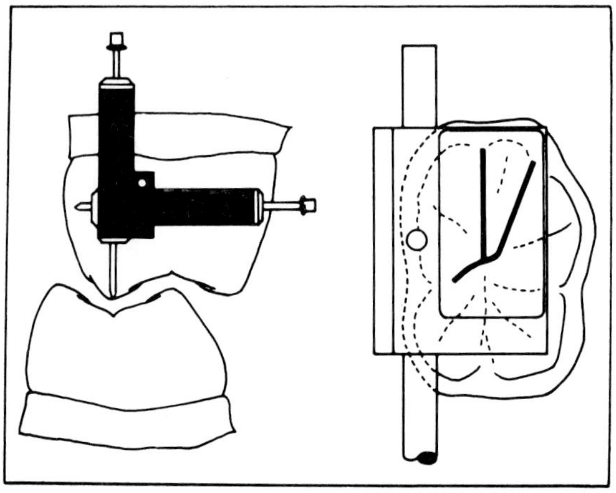

Fig 13–2.—When observing mandibular movement, the upper stamp cusp is a stationary stylus under which the mandible moves and traces the groove pattern on the lower occlusal surfaces. (Courtesy of Denar Corporation, Anaheim, California.)

(Fig 13–3). The teeth are covered with acrylic clutches to negate any tooth guidance in excursive movements. The clutches contact on a central bearing point to allow freedom of movement without tooth guidance (Fig 13–4). The mandible is then placed in centric relation (Fig 13–5). Lines of movement are recorded by styli on pressure-sensitive paper as the mandible moves to the various border positions. Protrusive movement is a straight line that is scribed on the pressure-sensitive paper (Fig 13–6).

The lateral movement of the mandible is referred to as transtrusion. This means movement to the side. Transtrusion has two components: laterotrusion, which is a lateral movement of the working or rotating condyle, and mediotrusion, which is

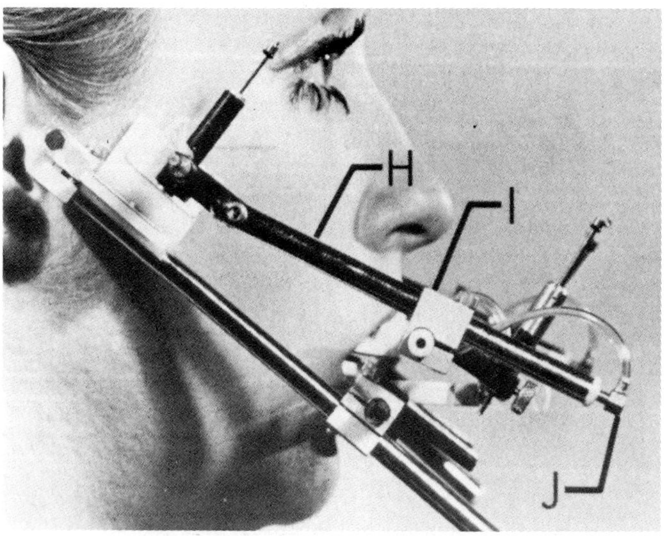

Fig 13–3.—The assembled pantograph is oriented to the hinge axis posteriorly and infra-orbital notch anteriorly. (Courtesy of Denar Corporation, Anaheim, California.)

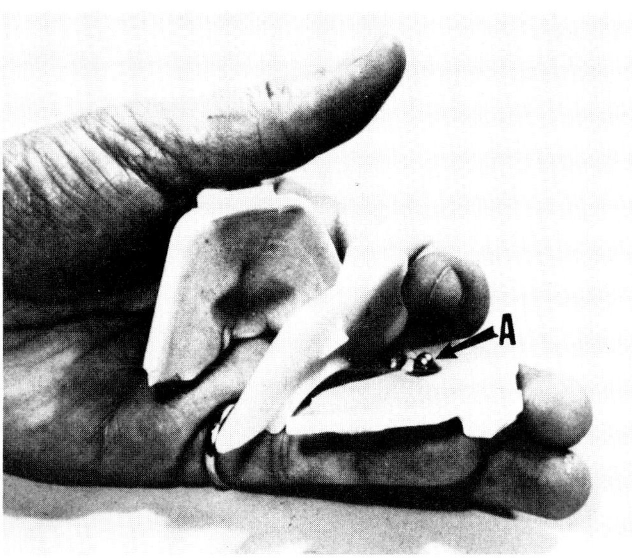

Fig 13–4.—Clutches are constructed to cover the maxillary and mandibular teeth. They contact on a central bearing point ***A*** and support the upper and lower members of the pantograph during recordings. (Courtesy of Denar Corporation, Anaheim, California.)

the medial movement of the balancing, translating, or orbiting condyle (Fig 13–7,A,B). In a lateral movement, the balancing, or orbiting, condyle goes down, forward, and medial. The rotating condyle moves laterally. Because the mandible is a solid bone, the amount that the balancing condyle moves medially determines how far the rotating condyle will move laterally. This lateral movement of both the rotating and the balancing condyles is known as Bennett movement or side shift of the mandible.

If we examine this side shift of the mandible more closely, we will find that there are actually three controls that govern Bennett movement or mandibular side shift

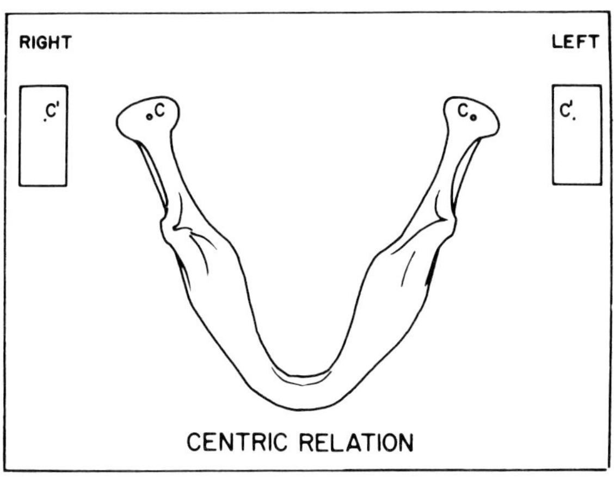

Fig 13–5.—Centric relation is the rearmost, uppermost, and mid-most unstrained position of the condyle in the glenoid fossa. It is the starting place for all movement. (Courtesy of Denar Corporation, Anaheim, California.)

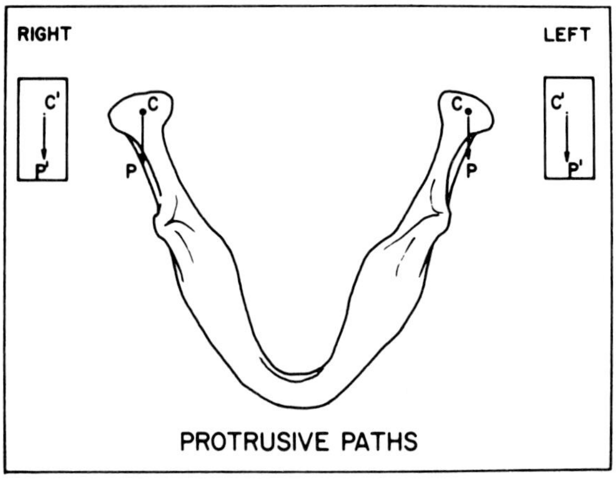

Fig 13–6.—The protrusive tracing will be a straight line on the horizontal table. (Courtesy of Denar Corporation, Anaheim, California.)

(Fig 13–8). The first control is on the balancing side. This is the medial wall, or so-called inner curbing, of the glenoid fossa on the balancing side. This is the side that shows mediotrusion. The amount of medial movement of this balancing condyle will dictate the amount of lateral movement of the rotating condyle on the opposite side. This medial wall configuration also determines one other phenomenon known as immediate side shift. Certain individuals will have an immediate shift to the working or rotating side before the orbiting condyle begins to translate down, forward, and medial. This is thought to be a result of a bracing action whereby the muscles contract to splint the working condyle in the fossa and stabilize it while the orbiting condyle translates. If this inner curbing or medial wall allows, the mandible may shift slightly to the rotating side preparatory to the translating movement.

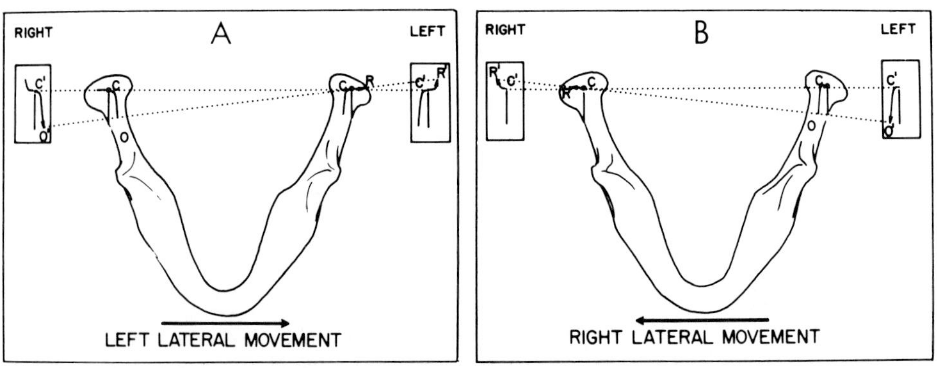

Fig 13–7.—A, lateral movement is called transtrusion and has two components: The working condyle travels outward, or laterally (laterotrusion), and the balancing condyle travels downward, forward, and medially (mediotrusion). (Courtesy of Denar Corporation, Anaheim, California.) **B,** during a right lateral movement the left (balancing) condyle travels downward, forward, and medially along the medial wall of the glenoid fossa. The angle it forms with the protrusive path is called the Bennett angle. The right condyle travels laterally (C′-R′). (Courtesy of Denar Corporation, Anaheim, California.)

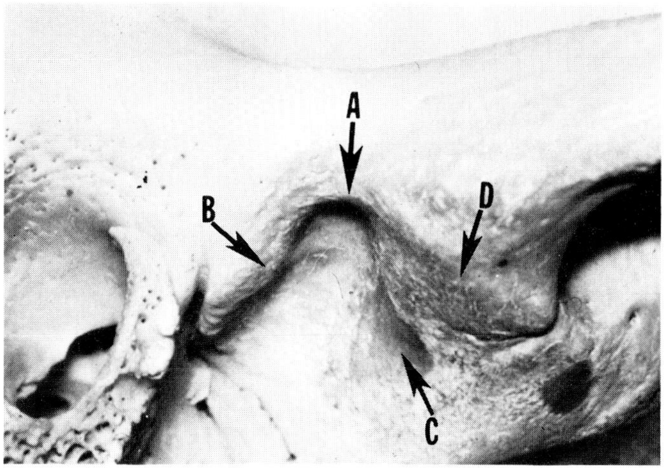

Fig 13–8.—Side shift is influenced by three controls: the superior wall *(A)* and the posterior wall *(B)* on the working (rotating side) and by the medial wall of the glenoid fossa *(C)* on the balancing side. *(D)* denotes the articular eminence involved in the protrusive path.

Based on these facts, we can classify lateral movement and lateral side shift in five basic patterns: progressive side shift, immediate side shift, early side shift, distributed side shift, or a combination of progressive, distributed, and early side shift (Fig 13–9). The immediate side shift movement must be accommodated in our restorations to avoid damaging lateral forces that are delivered to the tooth (Fig 13–10). Movement of the mandible is usually most critical during the first 4 mm of movement, as beyond this point the patient is usually beyond functional range.

The foregoing factors are dependent on the medial wall configuration of the glenoid fossa on the balancing side. This movement affects the buccolingual sulcus width, cusp height, and groove placement. As previously mentioned, there are

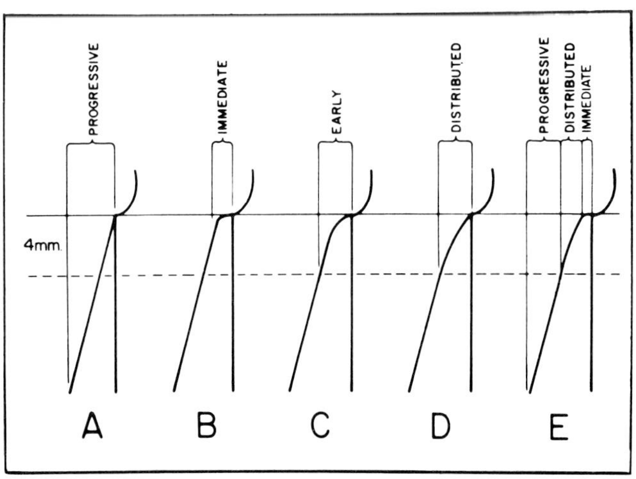

Fig 13–9.—Side shift of the mandible can follow several different paths during lateral movement. (Courtesy of Denar Corporation, Anaheim, California.)

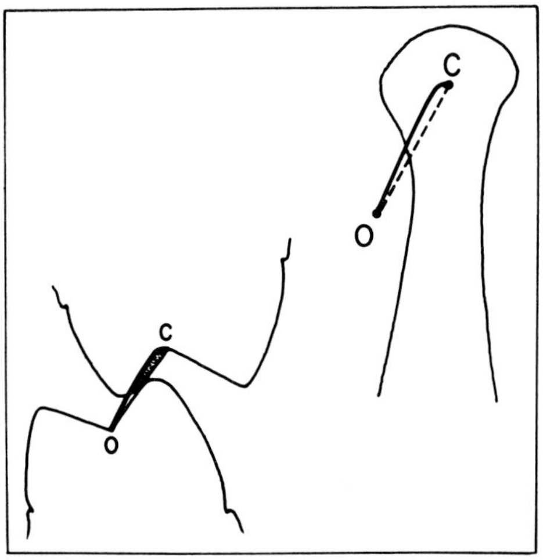

Fig 13–10.—Immediate side shift must be accommodated in the shape of the tooth inclines to prevent damaging lateral stresses. (Courtesy of Denar Corporation, Anaheim, California.)

three controls governing Bennett or side shift of the mandible. We have discussed the first, which is the medial wall of the glenoid fossa on the balancing side. The other two controls are the rotating, or working, side controls. These are the superior wall of the glenoid fossa and the posterior wall of the glenoid fossa on the rotating side (Fig 13–8). These controls govern the rotating condyle direction in conjunction with the amount of lateral movement and are governed by the medial wall on the balancing side. The superior wall effect is seen in the frontal plane. As the rotating condyle moves laterally, the superior wall of the glenoid fossa on the rotating side may deflect the condyle either up, which is called laterosurtrusion, straight laterally, which is laterotrusion, or downward, which is called laterodetrusion (Fig 13–11). This movement will, of course, affect cusp height. The greatest effect from this control is when surtrusion is present, since the influence of surtrusion is to bring the opposing arches closer together as the mandible travels further laterally in the working relationship. This means that if the patient has surtrusion in their movement pattern it must be incorporated into the restorations in the mouth in the form of shorter cusps. If it is not accommodated, destructive tooth contact will occur.

Semi-adjustable instruments will only allow straight laterotrusion and therefore will not be accurate for a patient with surtrusion. Laterosurtrusion dictates shorter cusps, particularly on the working side. This is because the effect is always greatest on the teeth that are closer to the control. As the control is the superior wall on the rotating sides, the teeth are affected the most on the rotating condyle side. Laterosurtrusion also requires greater lingual concavity of the lingual surfaces of the maxillary anterior teeth. As the rotating condyle shifts laterally, it may not go up or down, but rather in straight laterotrusion. This means that the condyle moves straight laterally with no upward or downward deflection. This means the cusps can be longer than if laterosurtrusion was present. Laterodetrusion indicates that as the working condyle travels laterally its corresponding superior fossa wall deflects it

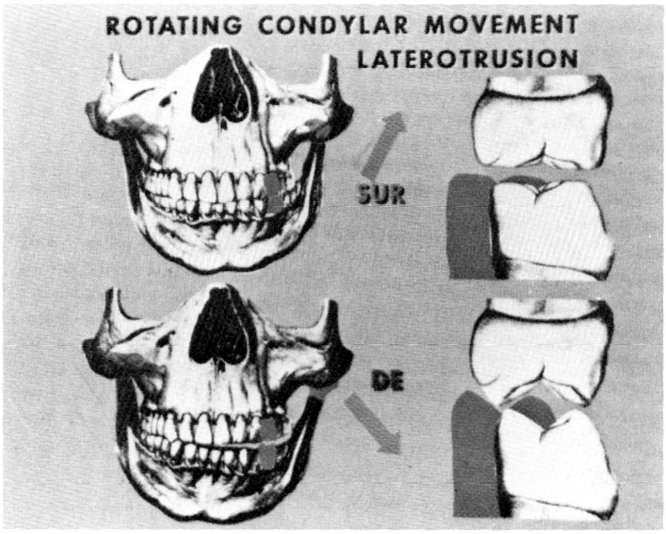

Fig 13–11.—Surtrusion and detrusion are controlled by the superior wall on the working or rotating side. Surtrusion requires shorter cusps than detrusion. (Courtesy of Denar Corporation, Anaheim, California.)

downward, causing the opposing arches to become further apart as they move laterally. This will allow longer cusps on the teeth than either laterosurtrusion or laterotrusion. If the patient has a laterodetrusion in lateral movement pattern and we construct restorations on an instrument that does not reproduce this particular movement, no problems are generally created. Semi-adjustable instruments only simulate a laterotrusive pattern that develops cusps that are lower than those that could be accommodated by the laterodetrusive movement. This means that when restorations are placed in the mouth they will clear in lateral excursion by an amount greater than they did on the articulator and provide a little extra amount of disclusion in a properly controlled case. Laterodetrusion requires less lingual concavity of the lingual surfaces of the maxillary anterior teeth.

The posterior wall effect is on the rotating side and is seen in the horizontal plane. As the condyle moves laterally, the posterior wall of the glenoid fossa on the rotating side may deflect the condyle anteriorly. This is called lateroprotrusion. If it deflects backward it is called lateroretrusion (Fig 13–12). This movement affects ridge and groove direction on the occlusal surfaces of the posterior teeth. Its main effect is on the balancing and working escape grooves of the teeth. Lateroretrusion causes the working and balancing grooves to be more mesial on the lower arch, lateroprotrusion causes the working and balancing grooves to be more distal on the lower arch, and laterotrusion will place them somewhere between these two (Fig 13–13). Lateroretrusion and lateroprotrusion affect the mesial and distal spacing of the cusps on the posterior teeth by virtue of their effect on ridge and groove direction. Lateroprotrusion requires more lingual concavity of the maxillary anterior teeth, lateroretrusion less.

By dissecting side shift of the mandible a little more thoroughly, we can restate that there are three controls over the side shift of the mandible. The first is on the balancing side, the medial wall or inner curbing of the glenoid fossa. This controls

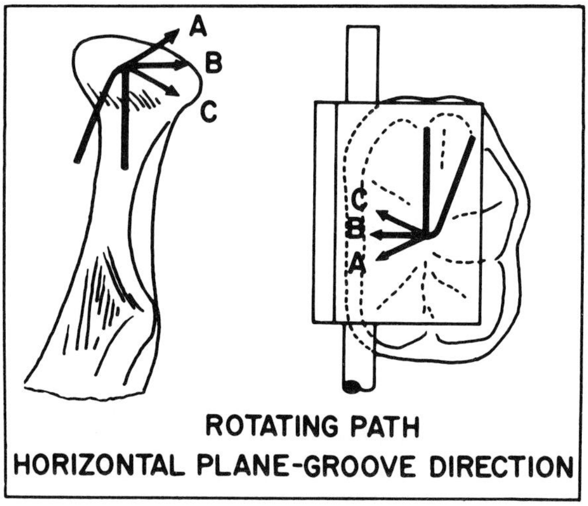

Fig 13–12.—Retrusion and protrusion are controlled by the posterior wall on the working or rotating side. In relation to our fixed upper point, grooves are more mesial on the lower with retrusion *(A)* and grooves are more distal on the lower with protrusion *(C)*. *(B)* denotes straight laterotrusion. (Courtesy of Denar Corporation, Anaheim, California.)

how much the entire mandible will move laterally. How much this balancing condyle moves medially on the balancing side will dictate the amount that the rotating condyle moves laterally on the rotating side.

On the rotating side we have two controls on the condyle movement. The first control is from the superior wall, which can deflect the condyle upward, straight laterally, or down. We also have an effect from the posterior wall of the fossa, which can deflect the condyle backward, straight laterally or forward. We can now put all of these movements together in combination to develop an even more complex pattern of movement. As the rotating condyle moves laterally it may shift laterally,

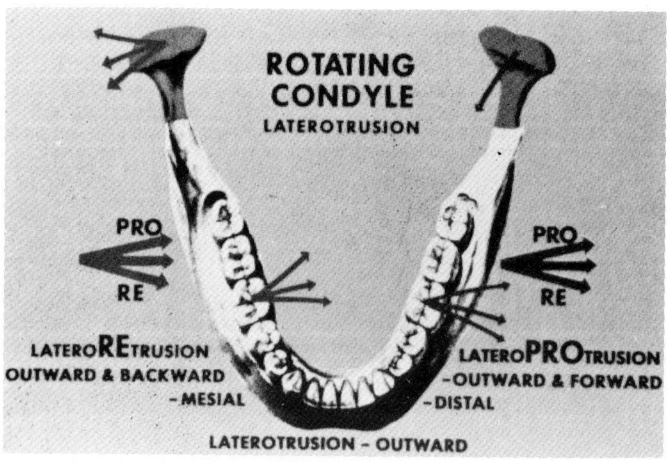

Fig 13–13.—Retrusion and protrusion affect the working escape groove (lingual groove) of the mandibular teeth. Their corresponding effect is also seen on the balancing (buccal) escape grooves. (Courtesy of Denar Corporation, Anaheim, California.)

backward (lateroretrusion), or up (laterosurtrusion). By the same token, as it shifts laterally, it may go laterally, forward, and up. Or, it may go laterally, forward, and down. This becomes a complicated movement that has pronounced effects on the ridge and groove direction, upon cusp height and cusp placement. The only way to gather this information is to record it with a pantographic tracing and subsequently use this pantographic tracing information to program a fully adjustable instrument.

At this point we can make some definite statements about side shift of the mandible.

1. The more side shift, the more mesial are the working and balancing grooves on the mandibular teeth;
2. The less side shift, the more distal are the working and balancing grooves on the mandibular teeth;
3. The greater the side shift, the shorter the cusps *must* be and the more lingual concavity needed on the maxillary anterior teeth;
4. The less the side shift, the longer the cusps *may* be and the less lingual concavity needed on the maxillary anterior teeth;
5. The more lateroprotrusion, the more distal the working and balancing grooves on the lower teeth;
6. The more lateroretrusion the more mesial are the working and balancing grooves on the mandibular teeth;
7. With a laterosurtrusion, the shorter the cusps *must* be on the working side and more lingual concavity is necessary on the maxillary anterior teeth; and
8. With laterodetrusion, the longer the cusps *may* be on the working side and less lingual concavity is necessary on the maxillary anterior teeth.

This is all information that significantly affects the occlusion of restorations and about which we would know nothing unless we actually trace and analyze these jaw movements. As mentioned previously, perhaps with single or simple quadrant restorations, we can gain enough guidance from existing natural tooth inclines to occlusally harmonize these restorations. We must assume that the existing natural tooth inclines are harmonious and acceptable for our restorative purposes. When we undertake cases in which we are restoring all, or nearly all, of the patient's occlusion, we cannot afford to be "just close." We must be as accurate as possible so that there is minimal discrepancy when the restorations are placed in the mouth. If the relationships are grossly inaccurate we have no orientation or guides to follow and we will be merely guessing to correct them. When we have no natural tooth guidance, or tooth guidance that is incompatible with muscle and joint function, we must rely on the information from condylar movement to tell us what our ridge and groove direction, cusp height, fossa width, side shift effect, lingual concavity of the maxillary teeth and arc of closure must be for the given case. The only way to obtain this information is with the pantographic tracing. It is a necessary tool for occlusal reconstruction, diagnosis of mandibular movement criteria, or a learning device for understanding mandibular movement.

TECHNIQUE

Pantographic recording and articulator programming is done before active preparation of the teeth for restoration is begun. Patient comfort, stability of the recording apparatus on the teeth, and observation of diagnostic information on the subsequently mounted diagnostic casts make this approach necessary. To obtain the tracing, clutches must first be constructed to cover the existing natural teeth. These clutches can be constructed from preformed or universal metal clutches, cast metal, or acrylic. The acrylic is usually the most expeditious means. These clutches are constructed so that they contact only a central bearing point during centric closure and eccentric movement. They are constructed with minimum thickness so that vertical dimension is increased as little as possible. It is essential that the two clutches do not contact, other than on the central bearing point, during closure and excursive movement. The clutches are retained by frictional fit or cementation to the teeth with a zinc oxide and eugenol impression material. No movement of the clutches whatsoever can be tolerated.

Once the clutches are stable, the pantograph is assembled and supported on the clutches. The first step is to locate, kinematically, the hinge axis of the mouth. Once this hinge axis has been located in the terminal hinge position it is usually permanently marked or tattooed on the patient's skin. This then becomes a permanent reference for future transfers of the case during construction. The pantograph will be oriented to these marks just as the face-bow is for recording and transfers (Fig 13–14). These landmarks orient the pantograph to the axis-orbital plane. The pantograph is then assembled on the clutches in preparation for recording (Fig 13–3). Pressure-sensitive paper is then placed under the six movable recording styli. There are two horizontal recording plates anteriorly and one vertical plate and one horizontal plate on each side posteriorly. The patient is placed in the terminal hinge position, the styli activated to mark the position on the pressure-sensitive paper (Fig 13–15). The styli are raised, the patient allowed to protrude, and then placed in centric relation again to recheck the position. If the position is the same as the previous mark, we assume that it is accurate.

Starting at centric relation the patient is instructed to protrude the mandible, keeping the central bearing point in contact throughout the movement. At the end of the movement, the styli are raised and the patient returns to centric relation. The styli are air activated with a button control that raises and lowers them simul-

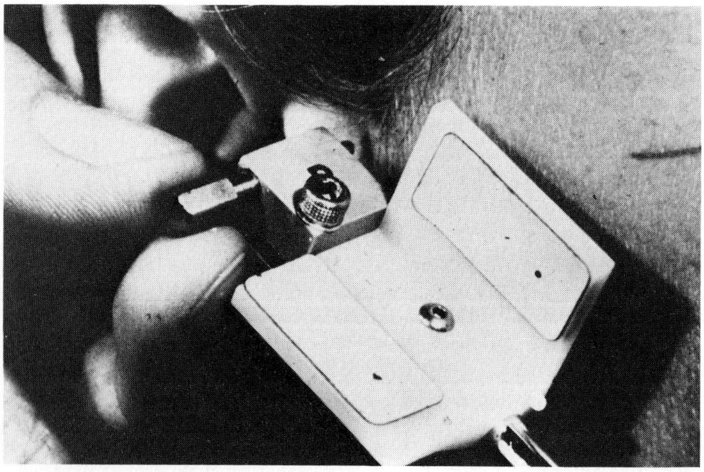

Fig 13–14.—Pantograph styli are oriented to the hinge axis mark for recording and transfer. (Courtesy of Denar Corporation, Anaheim, California.)

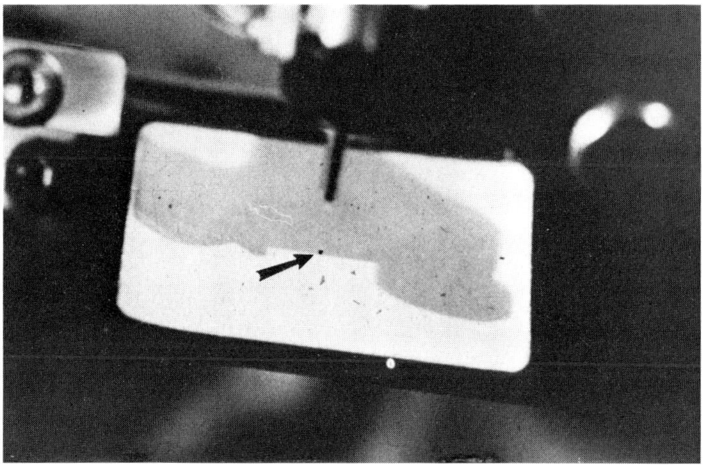

Fig 13–15.—The centric relation mark must be repeated exactly to verify this position. (Courtesy of Denar Corporation, Anaheim, California.)

taneously. Starting at centric relation the patient is instructed to make a lateral movement (Fig 13–16). As the patient makes this lateral movement, gentle pressure is applied on the angle of the mandible to make certain that the full range of side shift is recorded. At the end of this lateral movement the styli are raised and the patient returned to centric relation. The same procedure is repeated for the opposite side. At this point the tracing is complete (Fig 13–17). With the styli raised, the tracings are covered with celluloid overlays to preserve the tracing. Once again the patient is guided to centric relation the all styli are checked to make sure they are on the appropriate centric relation mark. Maintained in this position, the upper and lower members of the pantograph are joined together. Again, make

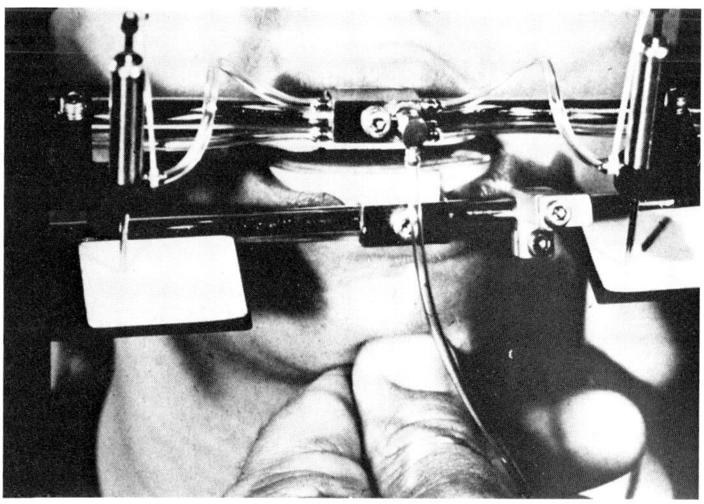

Fig 13–16.—The tracing is made as the patient is guided toward the border of the movement being recorded. The styli are raised before the patient returns to centric relation. (Courtesy of Denar Corporation, Anaheim, California.)

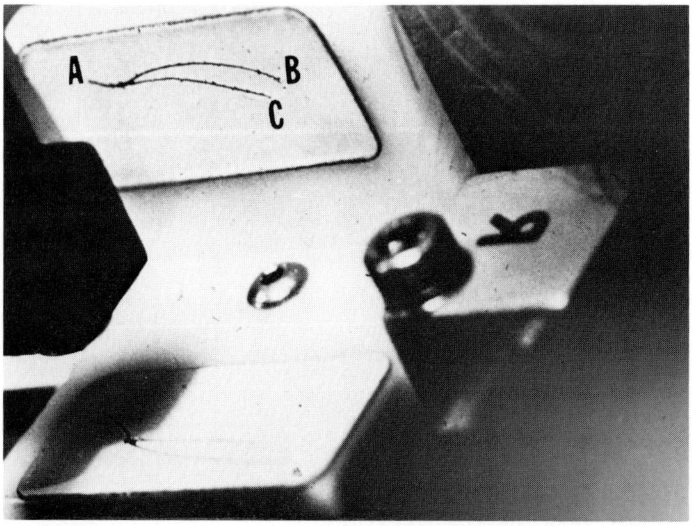

Fig 13–17.—Completed vertical plate tracing: *(A)* working (rotating) condyle movement; *(B)* balancing condyle movement; *(C)* protrusive condyle movement. The angle formed between lines *(B)* and *(C)* is called Fisher's angle. (Courtesy of Denar Corporation, Anaheim, California.)

sure the styli are correctly positioned and the orbital indicator is properly adjusted (Fig 13–3). The pantograph is carefully removed from the mouth and oriented to the articulator. The orientation is the same as that of the face-bow, the axis-orbital plane. With the pantograph properly oriented the maxillary and mandibular clutch are rigidly attached to their respective articulator members. After they are attached, the upper and lower pantograph members are released. With the panto-

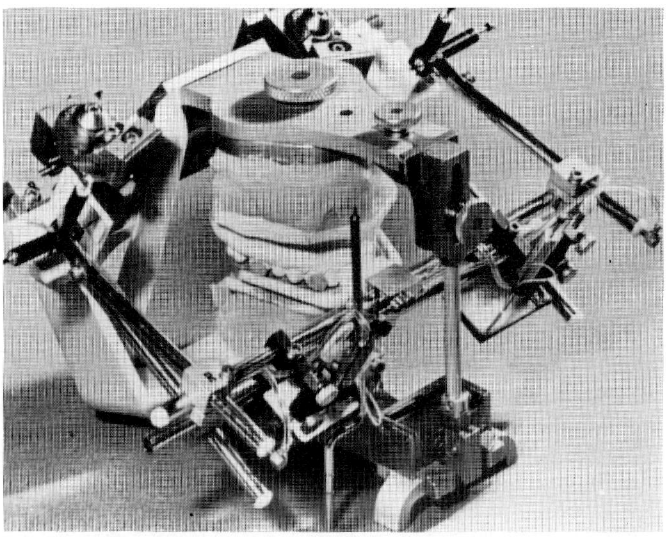

Fig 13–18.—Once the upper and lower clutches are rigidly attached to their respective articulators' members, the instrument is programmed with the information recorded on the pantographic tracing. (Courtesy of Denar Corporation, Anaheim, California.)

graph supported by the attachment of the maxillary and mandibular clutches, the articulator is set so that during its eccentric movements the pantograph styli follow the recorded lines (Figs 13–17 and 13–18). When the instrument is set, we can say that it will simulate the movements actually recorded and transferred from the patient. All condylar movement recorded from the patient will be programmed into the articulator for use during construction of the planned restoration.

CHAPTER 14

Articulators

ROBERT S. STAFFANOU, D.D.S.

ARTICULATORS ARE devices that represent substitutes for the maxillary and mandibular jaws of the patient and, with varying degrees of accuracy, simulate mandibular movement. With the proper technique we can, in essence, place the patient's mouth on the laboratory bench for construction of dental restorations. The accuracy of the articulator is reflected in the occlusal contact of the opposing teeth. The articulator provides a means to develop an adequate occlusion of the teeth that will harmonize with the patient's jaw movements. No restoration can function satisfactorily unless the occlusion is properly organized and developed. The mouth presents difficult access to fabricate restorations. We are always competing with muscles, cheeks, tongue, saliva, and reflexes for access, visability, and manipulation. As it is impossible to carry out certain intraoral procedures because of these imposed restrictions, it is necessary to transfer the mouth to the laboratory bench for ease and convenience of construction.

The device with which this is done is the articulator. For the articulator to accurately simulate jaw movement, the casts must be properly transferred to the instrument with the aid of a face-bow. The articulator must be capable of being programmed to the patient's jaw movements. Articulators that will accurately simulate all jaw movements are known as fully adjustable articulators. Since fully adjustable instruments are time-consuming to program, compromises are often accepted and articulators that simulate some, but not all, movements are used. To evaluate what any given instrument will or will not do, we must have some criteria with which to compare them. For an articulator to be fully adjustable the following criteria must be met.

1. It must open and close on a horizontal (hinge) axis in the sagittal plane;
2. It must move and adjust laterally in a horizontal plane about a vertical axis;
3. It must move and adjust in the frontal plane about a sagittal axis;
4. It must adjust to simulate the patient's articular eminence curvature;
5. It must adjust to the patient's facial width or intercondylar distance; and
6. It must adjust for amount, direction, and timing of lateral condylar movements on both the working and balancing sides. Timing refers to the exact path the condyle takes from centric relation to a given border position.

If we accept the above as the maximum amount of information that can be programmed into an instrument, we then have appropriate criteria with which to judge the adjustability of any instrument. An articulator that accepts anything less than the above stated criteria will not reproduce all jaw movements. Based on these criteria we can measure the ability of any instrument to simulate some, all, or none of the patient's jaw movements. Articulators, then, can be classified and catagorized according to their ability to reproduce varying degrees of jaw movement. There are four basic catagories.

1. Arbitrary;
2. Positional;
3. Semi-adjustable: (a) condylar shaft, (b) arcon; and
4. Fully adjustable: (a) checkbite, (b) sophisticated checkbite, (c) gnathological, (d) functionally generated path.

Arbitrary Articulators

Arbitrary instruments, as the name implies, are constructed to accept two casts arbitrarily mounted without any type of transfer orientation (Fig 14–1). They are small and much narrower than the intercondylar width of most patients. The casts cannot be oriented anteroposteriorly, laterally, or inferiosuperiorly in relation to the articulator condyles with the face-bow transfer. The best they can do is accept a static centric occlusion position. Any movement away from this static position will be inaccurate.

Recently, an arbitrary articulator has been developed that will accept a face-bow transfer (Fig 14–2). This improves the condylar orientation and places the casts close to the mandibular arc of closure. Preset, nonadjustable lateral, and protrusive guidances make eccentric movements that are less than exact. Arbitrary articulators do not simulate any type of eccentric jaw movement. Only one arbitrary instrument places the casts in a face-bow orientation to simulate the mandibular arc of closure. Eccentric movements are inaccurate and based on anatomic averages.

Positional Articulators

The only positional articulator in use today is the Verticulator* (Fig 14–3). This instrument is made to be used with the functionally generated path technique. This

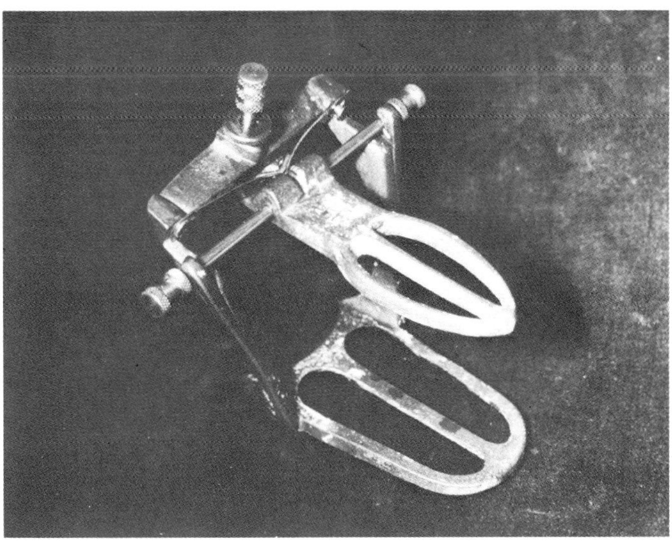

Fig 14–1.—An arbitrary crown and bridge articulator (Stephens). Intercondylar distance is too narrow and the casts are too close to opening and closing axis.

*J.F. Jelenko Co., New Rochelle, NY 10802.

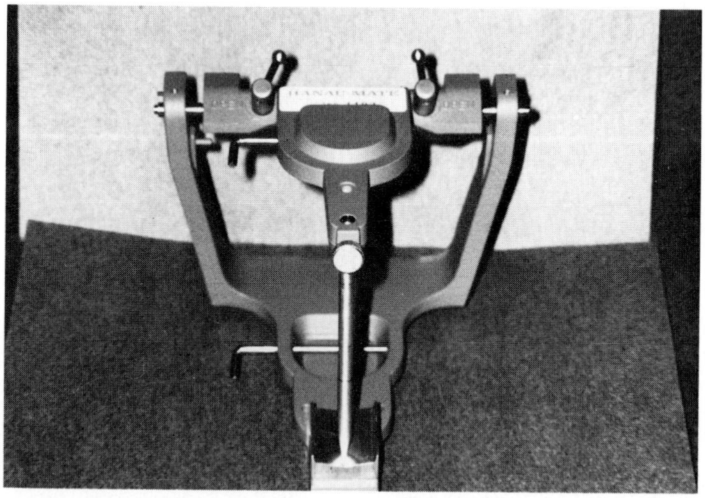

Fig 14–2.—Frontal view of Hanau-Mate, an arbitrary articulator that will accept a face-bow transfer. (Courtesy of Teledyne-Hanau, Buffalo, New York.)

instrument does not have an opening and closing axis nor is it capable of lateral movements. The functionally generated path chew-in record is a static representation of dynamic movement and, therefore, only the static instrument is needed. The lateral and protrusive movements are incorporated in the chew-in record that provides the basis for occlusal anatomy and makes this procedure workable.

Semi-Adjustable Articulators

Moving to the next level in articulator sophistication, the semi-adjustable instruments are the first that begin to meet some of the criteria previously set forth as

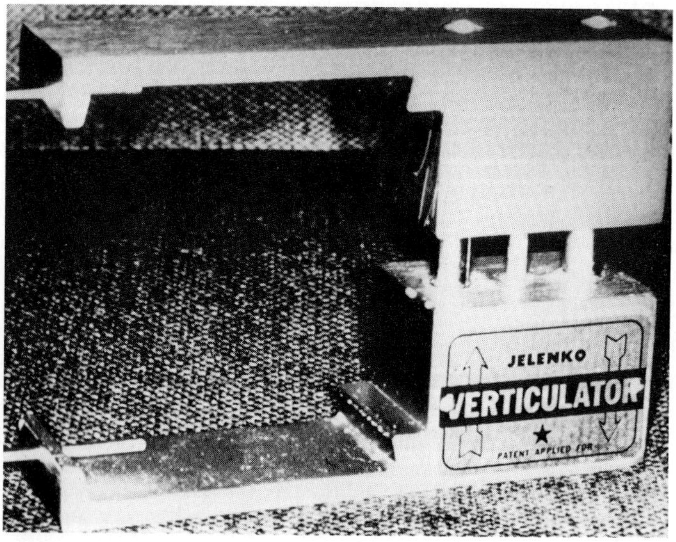

Fig 14–3.—The Jelenko Verticulator is used with the functionally generated path technique. There is no axis closure (Courtesy of J. F. Jelenko, New Rochelle, New York.)

requirements of a fully adjustable articulator. They will all accept either an arbitrary or a kinematic face-bow. This relates the maxillary cast with reference to the axis-orbital plane and at the correct distance anteroposteriorly, laterally, and inferosuperiorly to establish a correct arc of closure (Fig 14–4). All semi-adjustable instruments will establish an accurate opening and closing arc. This will satisfy the first requirement to rotate about a horizontal axis. All semi-adjustable instruments have some type of adjustment for Bennett angle. All eccentric movements on semi-adjustable articulators remain on a straight line. We know from pantographic tracings that most patient's jaw movements are not straight line. Many patient's lateral movements are curvilinear. The straight line movement is a shortcoming of the semi-adjustable instrument.

The protrusive pathway on these articulators is also a straight line, but the patient's articular eminence is curved. This is not always a problem because the straight line path of the articulator allows the teeth to pass closer on the instrument than they will when the patient moves over the curved pathway. Although the distance between the teeth will then be greater in the patient, a degree of tolerance has been established and cuspal collision will be avoided. If the teeth would pass closer together during the patient's movement than they did on the articulator, problems of cuspal interference could develop. As long as the error is in the other direction no problem will exist.

Semi-adjustable instruments have varying ranges of adjustment for intercondylar distance. Some have none, whereas others have preset ranges (small, medium, large) (Fig 14–5). This moves the center of rotation closer to the same width as in the patient to make lateral movements in the vertical axis rotation more accurate. Semi-adjustable instruments allow only a progressive laterotrusion in relation to mandibular side shift. They will adjust for Bennett angle on the balancing side, which corresponds to the medial wall of the glenoid fossa (Fig 14–5). As the balancing condyle travels downward, forward, and medially along this path it allows the working condyle to drift straight laterally. We know from pantography that

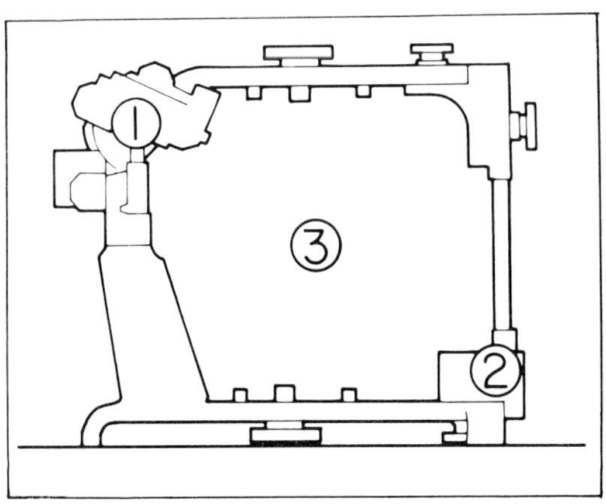

Fig 14–4.—Semi-adjustable articulator must provide for *(1)* an adjustable condylar guidance and Bennett angle, *(2)* an adjustable incisal guidance, and *(3)* for the mounting of casts that are oriented with a face-bow to position them laterally, anteroposteriorly, and superoinferiorly to the axis-orbital plane. (Courtesy of Denar Corporation, Anaheim, California.)

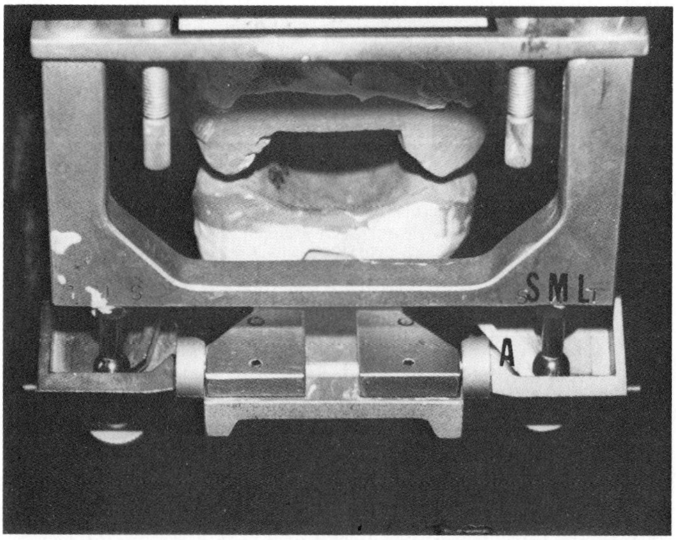

Fig 14–5.—This inverted Whip-Mix articulator is an example of a preset small, medium, and large intercondylar distance adjustment instrument. Adjustment is done by removing the condylar posts and replacing them in the threaded holes designated *S* or *L*. *(A)* is the Bennett angle adjustment.

some patients have surtrusion-detrusion or retrusion-protrusion or a combination thereof during lateral movement of the rotating condyle. Because these instruments will not adjust for these types of movements, they are not always accurate in their reproduction of lateral pathways. This is a shortcoming and can result in inaccuracies for certain patients.

Semi-adjustable articulators are of two basic designs. These are called the arcon type (Fig 14–6) and the condylar shaft or slot type (Fig 14–7,A,B). The arcon principle refers to the "articulated condyle" concept and thus the name arcon. This means that the condyle is on the mandibular member of the instrument and the glenoid fossa is on the maxillary member, just as in the human skull. With this construction the fossa and its articular eminence will remain in a constant relationship to the upper member of the articulator and therefore to the axis-orbital reference plane throughout all degrees of opening. The condyle movements will also coincide with the patient's movements when observed on the articulator. Additionally, there is more latitude in setting the articulator when the condyle balls are not confined to an enclosed track as with the condylar shaft or slot instrument.

On shaft or slot type articulators the controls are reversed (Fig 14–7,B). The condylar guidance, which represents the articular eminence of the fossa, is on the lower member and the condyle balls are on the upper member. With this design, whenever the upper member, which coincides with the axis-orbital plane, is opened or closed the condylar guidance angle will be increased or decreased. Because the fossa is on the lower member it is immovable in relation to the upper member of the articulator. This means that the case must be mounted and maintained at the same vertical dimension if the condyle guidance is to remain constant. Although this can be done with complete denture bite rims, it is difficult to do with

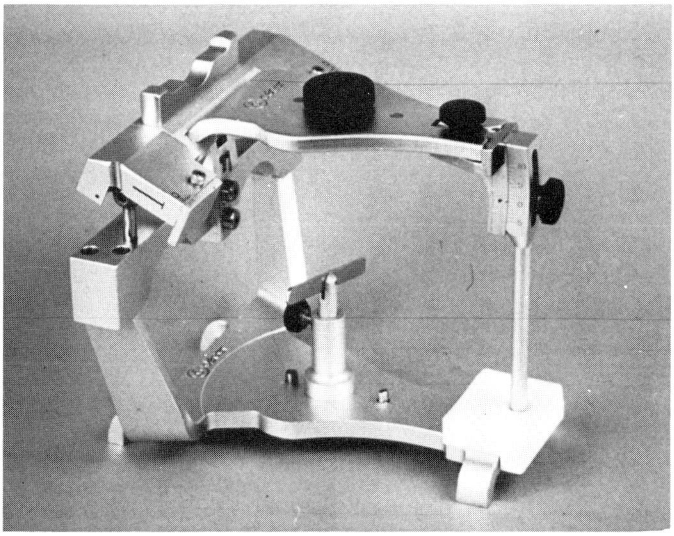

Fig 14–6.—The Denar Mark II is an arcon type semi-adjustable articulator. This instrument will accept a face-bow transfer and an arbitrary or kinematic hinge axis transfer. It has adjustable condylar guidances and Bennett angle guidance, and an immediate side shift adjustment. It does not adjust for intercondylar distance. (Courtesy of Denar Corporation, Anaheim, California.)

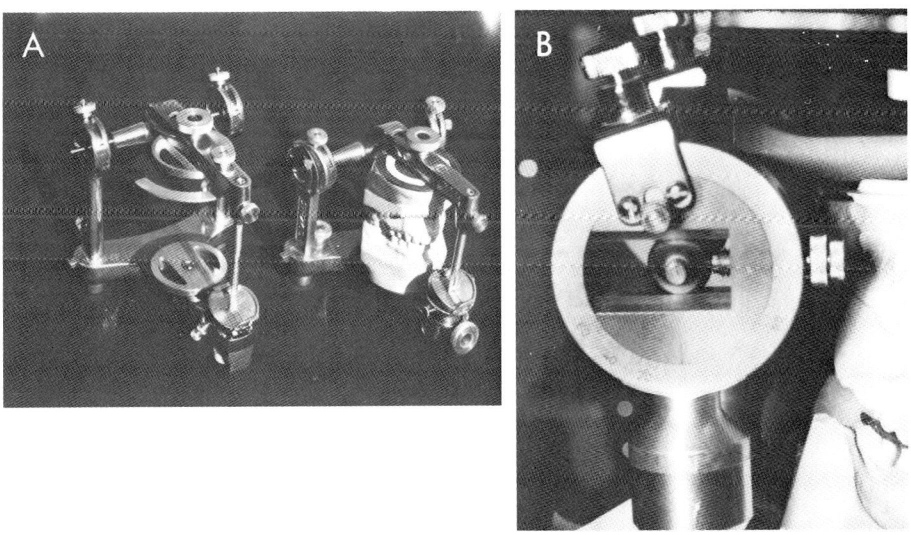

Fig 14–7.—**A,** Hanau semi-adjustable articulators are an example of the slot type instruments and will adjust for Bennett angle and condylar guidance. They will accept a face-bow transfer mounting, but will not adjust for intercondylar distance. **B,** in the slot instrument, the condyle ball is on an anterior stop instead of a posterior stop like the arcon instrument. This reverses the movement from the direction in which it takes place in the patient. Whereas the occlusal effect of the two instruments is not greatly different, it is confusing to study mandibular movement on the slot type instrument. The slot also limits the articulator acceptance of lateral checkbites.

an interocclusal record over natural teeth. This means that every time the case is re-mounted, a new condylar guidance record must be made to achieve maximum accuracy.

Because the condyle ball is locked within a track or slot, it will not accept lateral checkbites as freely as will the arcon instrument. Within its range of adjustment, the overall anterior movement simulated by the condylar shaft instruments is probably not greatly different from that of the arcon instrument. It is, however, a confusing instrument to the novice. This is because the movements on the instrument are the reverse of what is happening in the patient. For example, instead of the balancing condyle moving downward, forward, and medially as in the mouth, it moves backward, upward, and laterally on the condylar shaft instrument. Arcon instruments more closely simulate the actual mandibular movement patterns of the patient and have a higher acceptance of lateral checkbites because the condyle ball is not restricted in a slot. Both instruments will reproduce an accurate arc of closure, adjust for Bennett angle on the balancing side, and allow straight laterotrusion for the working condyle movement but neither adjust for movement timing. Some semi-adjustable instruments adjust for intercondylar distance, but others have no allowance or depend on preset ranges of adjustment. Intercondylar distance probably has less effect on occlusion than the other factors as long as it is close to the facial width of the patient.

All semi-adjustable instruments have some type of adjustment for lateral and protrusive incisal guidances. To set the protrusive incisal guidance, the anterior teeth are placed in an end to end position and the guidance raised horizontally until it touches the incisal pin. To set the lateral incisal guidance, the casts are moved laterally to the end-to-end position of the canines and the lateral wings are raised until they touch the incisal pin (Fig 14–8). With the guidances thus set, the casts can be moved across each other without cast wear taking place. If the casts

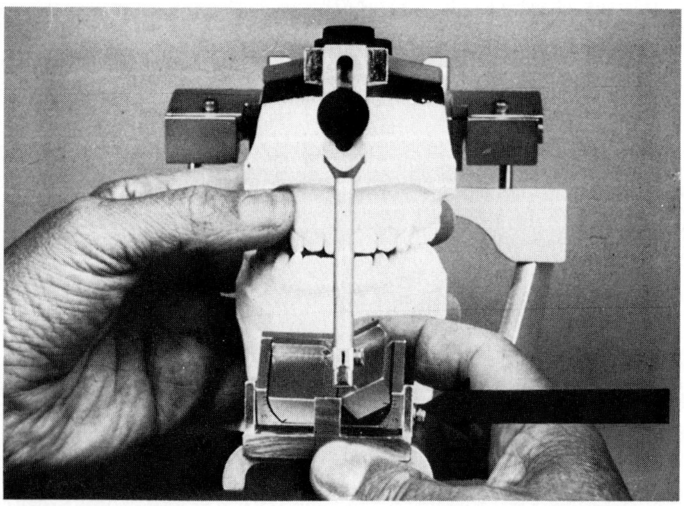

Fig 14–8.—The right lateral incisal guidance is set by placing the right canines in an end-to-end position and raising the lateral wing until it touches the incisal pin. The left wing is set in the same manner. The protrusive guidance table is set with the casts protruded to an end-to-end central relationship.

wear and abrade, the vertical dimension of the case is reduced. Incisal guidance prevents this from happening. We should remember that incisal guidance is a variable factor and should be determined before restoration is begun. Once incisal length is established and the articulator incisal guidance set, it becomes a guide constant for construction of the case along with the condylar guidance. The incisal guidance adjustment holds this incisal dimension for us regardless of whether we are constructing crowns, fixed partial dentures, or removable prosthetic restorations.

Semi-adjustable instruments are set with static centric and eccentric checkbites. The lower cast is related to the face-bow mounted upper cast with a centric relation record and the lower cast is mounted. Additional checkbite records made at or near the lateral border position are used to set the condylar element inclinations. The position at which the checkbite is made will be related in the articulator as a straight line guidance from the centric relation. The instrument guidance, which is straight, adjusts from centric relation to the point of the checkbite. The path, which connects these two points in the articulator, is a straight line (Fig 14–9). We know, from pantography, that the patient's condyle usually follows a curvilinear path from centric relation to a border position (Fig 14–10). The exact path that the mandible traces from centric relation to the given border position is called "timing" of the movement. Semi-adjustable instruments, because they are relating only two points in space, will not simulate "timing" of mandibular movements. They may adjust for amount and direction of the movement but have no information about the character of the path between centric relation and the border position of the mandible. This missing information could be important in establishing an atraumatic occlusion. Therefore, if the articulator is to simulate all movement as to amount, direction, and timing, we must accurately trace the movement and transfer it to an instrument that will accept it. This can only be accomplished with a fully adjustable articulator.

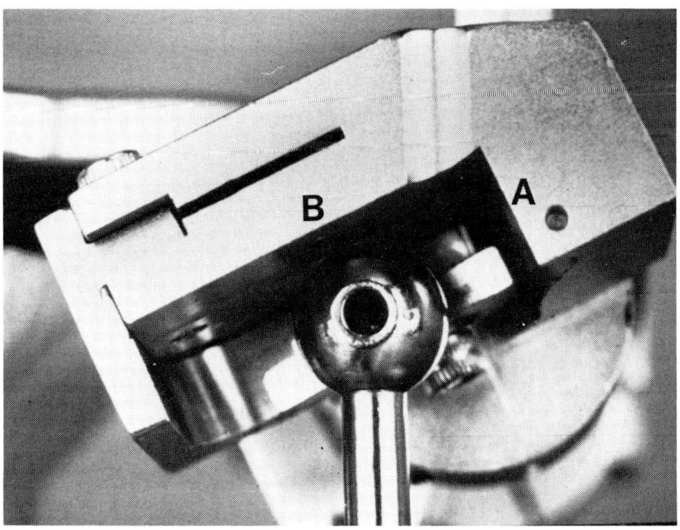

Fig 14–9.—With the lateral checkbite record between the mounted casts the fossa housing is rotated until it touches the condyle ball of the articulator at point *B*. As it connects only 2 points, centric relation at point *A* and right lateral at point *B*, it is a straight line guidance.

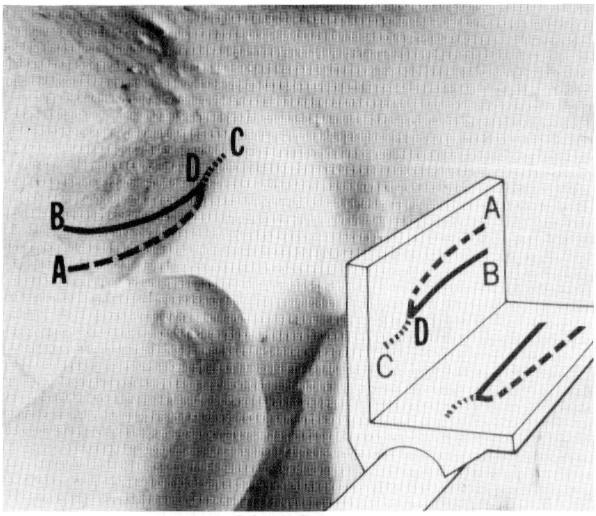

Fig 14–10.—The actual millimeter by millimeter path taken by the condyle from centric relation to a given border position is known as the "timing" of the movement. *D,* centric relation. *A,* the balancing movement over the medial fossa wall guidance. *B,* protrusive movement over articular eminence. *C,* the lateral working condyle movement over the posterior and superior fossa wall guidances. Semi-adjustable instruments only connect two points, centric relation and eccentric positions, with a straight line guidance, and are not capable of reproducing the timing of the movement. A pantographic tracing represents an infinite number of lateral and protrusive checkbites.

Fully Adjustable Articulators

Fully adjustable instruments will meet all of the six previously listed criteria. To do this they must adjust independently in three planes of movement. Some do this by mechanical means and others by guidance pathways that are custom ground.

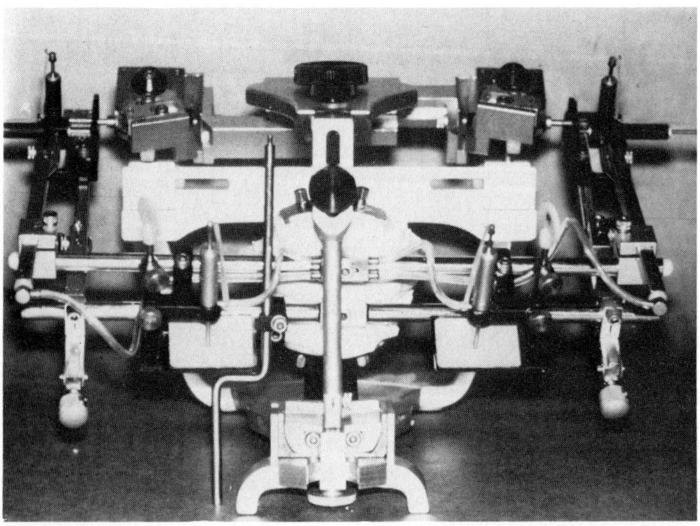

Fig 14–11.—Denar D5A fully adjustable instrument with pantograph attached. The fully adjustable instrument, programmed with a pantographic tracing, will reproduce "timing" of mandibular movement in addition to amount and direction of a given movement.

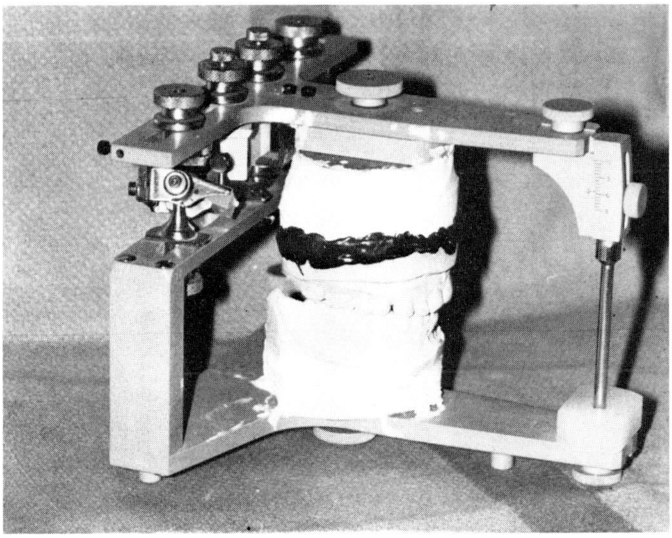

Fig 14–12.—The Stuart fully adjustable articulator can also be programmed to reproduce all facets of mandibular movement.

Regardless, they will adjust infinitesimally to the pantographic tracing. We can truly simulate all facets of mandibular movement with these instruments (Figs 14–11 and 14–12).

Another type of fully adjustable instrument, not programmed with the pantograph, is the functionally generated path instrument. It records via a maxillary and mandibular clutch supported by a central bearing point. There are four cutting blades embedded in the maxillary clutch that are close to, but not contacting, the mandibular clutch. A special autopolymerizing acrylic resin is placed under each of the four styli and a path is generated to include all border movements of the man-

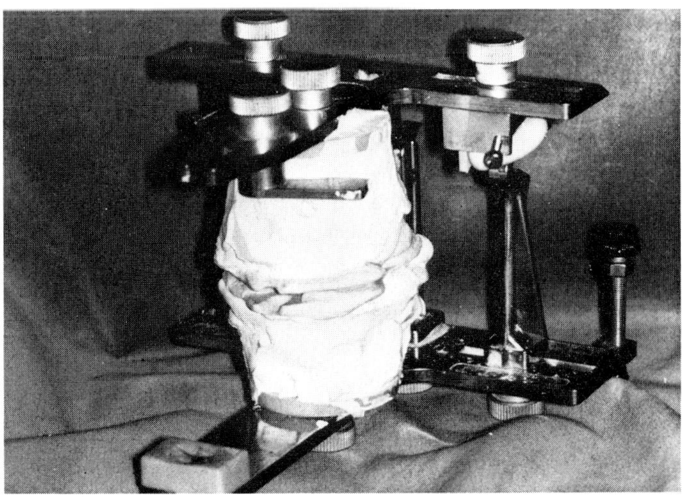

Fig 14–13.—The TMJ instrument is a fully adjustable instrument because it enables custom condylar elements and a custom incisal guide table to be fabricated for each patient. A special patient clutch with multiple styli develops the controls to make this fabrication possible.

dible. The result is four separate arrow point tracings into which is incorporated mandibular movement. The maxillary clutch is transferred to the instrument by the face-bow. The mandibular clutch is oriented with the cutting blades in the apices of the four tracings that correspond to centric relation. Both clutches are rigidly attached to the upper and lower members of the articulator, respectively (Fig 14–13).

This instrument has no preformed or mechanical fossae. Instead, it has a three-walled "mud cup" into which the condyle elements of the lower member extend. A special autopolymerizing acrylic resin is placed into this three-walled box or "mud cup." By keeping the styli of the upper clutch rigidly seated into the tracings of the lower clutch the members are moved over each other so that the styli retrace the entire arrow-point tracing generated by the patient. As this is happening, the condyle elements of the lower member are forming a fossa and articular eminence

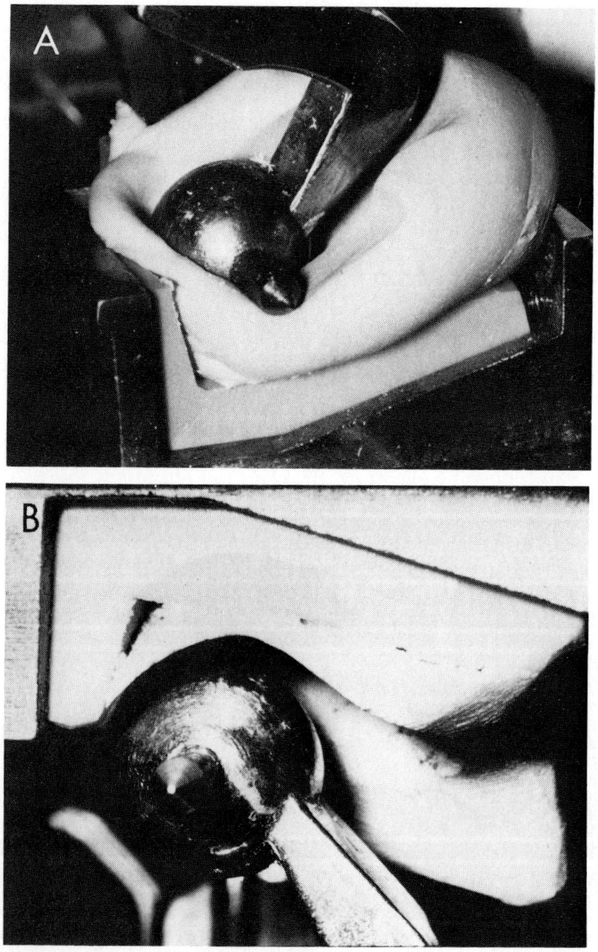

Fig 14–14.—A, autopolymerizing resin is placed in the "mud cups" of the fossae. With the cutting blades firmly within the lower clutch tracings, the articulator is moved through the border movements of the tracing while the condyle balls custom form the fossae. **B,** excess material is trimmed, leaving a fossa with all guidance walls and paths.

out of the soft plastic in the "mud cup" (Fig 14–14,A). This is continued until the resin cures. The excess is trimmed off and the fossae that are formed contain the movement criteria generated in the intraoral tracing (Fig 14–14,B). These articulators are accurate when properly used and programmed. They do not have the double check capacity that is provided with the pantographic tracing. When the articulator is set with the tracing, the settings can be rechecked by retracing the pathway. We can also observe the character of the movements that may be of diagnostic value. With these instruments, however, once the resin in the fossae has polymerized, no further accurate refinement is possible.

SUMMARY

Articulators have varying degrees of accuracy and movement reproduction. All articulators, other than the fully adjustable, have shortcomings in their ability to simulate all jaw movement. Articulator selection must therefore be based upon the degree of accuracy needed for a given restorative situation. In a mouth that has an intact dentition with an abundance of tooth guidance, a fully adjustable instrument is not needed if we are constructing simple restorations. We could use an instrument for fabrication that would be close, but not entirely accurate, in simulating movement. The restoration could then be taken to the mouth and harmonized meticulously in all excursions using the natural teeth for guidance. If we are restoring all or nearly all of the patient's occlusion and have no remaining accurate natural inclines for reference, we must capture as much information from the patient as possible and transfer it to a fully adjustable instrument. Only then can we accurately reconstruct and rehabilitate a complete dentition. We must gain all the information possible to place restorations that will function atraumatically and in harmony with the patient's jaw movements.

CHAPTER 15

The Working Cast and Removable Dies

ARUN NAYYAR, D.M.D.

A GYPSUM CAST with removable dies is usually used to fabricate a cast prosthesis by the indirect technique. Meticulous tooth preparation, tissue management, and an accurate impression are prerequisites for the development of a cast that is the replica of the patient's teeth. The transformation from an impression to a final working cast requires modification of the replica cast together with interpretation of supportive information provided by the dentist. All this has an impact on the success or failure of the final prosthesis and every improvement of the working cast enhances the capability of a technician to provide a superior prosthesis with fewer chairside adjustments.

Before techniques for the fabrication of working casts with removable dies are discussed, it is important to understand the criteria for a removable die, the type of impression material used, and its compatibility with the die material. The procedures described are suitable for casts for the fabrication of metal, metal-ceramic, or all ceramic restorations.

CRITERIA FOR A WORKING CAST WITH REMOVABLE DIES

A dentist's or technician's preference often dictates the technique used for the development of a working cast with removable dies. The removable die is an accurate reproduction of the prepared tooth and can be repeatedly returned to its original relationship in the working cast. It is used to fabricate the wax pattern and finish the margins. When the removable die is seated in a cast that has been accurately mounted on an articulator, a restoration with correct form, contacts, and occlusion can be made. The cast is then known as the working cast. The criteria for an acceptable working cast with removable dies include:

Working die surface and preparation margins

1. The working die should be an accurate reproduction of the prepared tooth.
2. Prepared surface and margins are bubble-free.
3. Gingival margins are clearly visible for wax-up.
4. Trimmed die representing tooth structure at least 0.5 mm apical to the prepared margins is mandatory.

Working die stability

1. The die(s) are removable and return precisely to their original position.
2. Seated die(s) cannot be moved mesiodistally or faciolingually.

3. Working cast may be inverted with no movement of the die(s).

Dowel pin and saw cuts

1. Dowel pin(s) are located in the center of the die.
2. The dowel pin is firmly luted to the gypsum base.
3. Saw cuts are parallel or have maximum convergence of 6 to 8 degrees toward the base.
4. Saw cuts do not cut into dowel pins.
5. Saw cuts do not destroy
   (a). the pontic area.
   (b). teeth in the contralateral segment.

Interface between first and second pour

1. The area of the second pour, where the die seats, is an exact replica of the die base and dowel pin.
2. The interface between the two pours is closed and is debris- and bubble-free.

Second pour for model base

1. The second pour adapts around the dowel pin.
2. The dowel pin channel is free of debris and bubbles.
3. The tip of the dowel pin is exposed a maximum of 2 to 3 mm at the base of the second pour and is easily accessible.

SELECTION OF DIE MATERIAL

The choice of die material is made before the impression procedure. The die material can be gypsum, epoxy resin, or copper or silver plate.[1] The preferred die material is type IV gypsum. Some dentists prefer silver[2, 3] while others prefer epoxy dies.[4] Measurement of the scraping resistance of die materials shows that silver dies are the most resistant, followed by epoxy and type IV gypsum.[5]

The Electroformed Silver Die

The use of electroformed silver dies is limited to the nonaqueous elastomeric impression materials. Other impression materials are incompatible for plating.[6, 7] Electroformed silver dies are known to give excellent clinical results[3] and their accuracy compares favorably with gypsum and epoxy dies.[5, 8–10] Silver dies are reported to be 0.07% to 0.23% smaller than the master die from which the impression was made.[6] The casting technique must be suitably corrected to compensate for the dimensional change with these dies. The hard silver dies are preferred for fabrication of porcelain jacket crowns. The polysulfide,[8] silicone,[10] and vinyl polysiloxane[7] materials are suitable for silver electrodeposits but polyethers are not.[7] The impression material and the electrodeposit can contribute to die inaccuracy.[7, 11] The silver plating technique is expensive, time consuming, and not popular for routine die fabrication.

The Epoxy Resin Die

Epoxy resin material is being successfully used by some commercial labs and dentists.[4] The dies have a higher scrape resistance than type IV gypsum dies.[5] Epoxy dies are reported to be undersized[12] and their compressive strength is less than that of gypsum dies. The material has a long setting time, continuous polymerization shrinkage, and is incompatible with some impression materials.[12, 13] Two studies found an epoxy die material to give consistently good results[4, 14] whereas another found it unsuitable for precision fixed prosthodontic procedures.[13]

The Type IV Gypsum Die

The most popular die material is type IV gypsum. It is accurate, inexpensive, requires minimal equipment, easy to manipulate, and compatible with all impression materials.[1] Gypsum is susceptible to surface abrasion during carving but its abrasion resistance can be improved by 100% by adding a gypsum hardener to the mix.[15, 16] Further improvement is possible by treating the die and margins with a fine film of cyanoacrylate.[1, 5, 16]

Type IV gypsum die material has a setting expansion of 0.1% or less,[1] which is somewhat negated by containment in the impression.[17] The material is suitable for routine fixed prosthodontics. Gypsum die material is available in several colors. Contrasting colors of die material and wax are an aid during the trimming and waxing of margins.

The following techniques utilize type IV gypsum as the die material.

Preparing the Impression

Saliva or blood residue on any elastomeric impression is rinsed off with cool water. Failure to do this results in a cast with poor surface details (Figs 15–1 and 15–2). Hydrocolloid impressions must be rinsed with cold water. Avoid using the air-water syringe, because some are equipped with a water heater, and warm water will distort the hydrocolloid impression. The excess water is shaken from the hydrocolloid impression and it is soaked in 3% potassium sulfate solution for 15 minutes.[16, 18, 19] This improves surface details,[17] accelerates setting, hardens the stone surface,[18] reduces formation of the hemihydrate on the surface of the stone,[19] and produces a superior die.

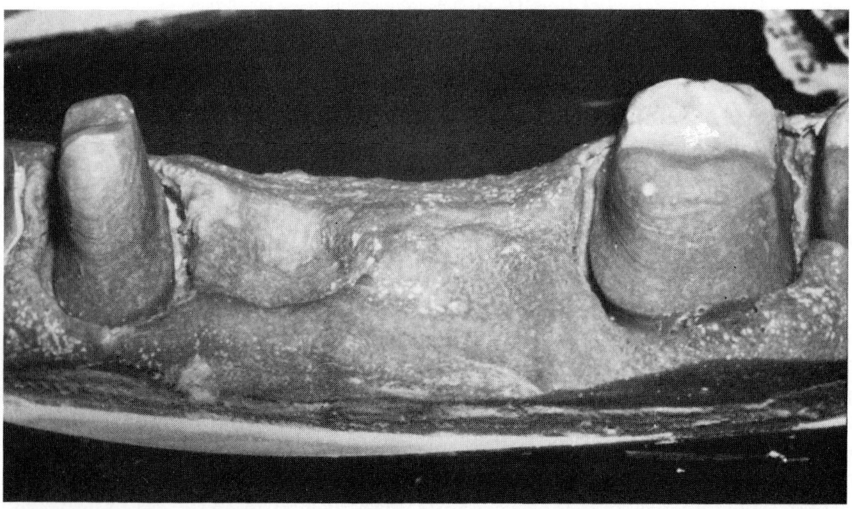

Fig 15–1.—When saliva or blood residue is not washed off, the resulting cast has poor surface detail. This cast was made without rinsing the impression.

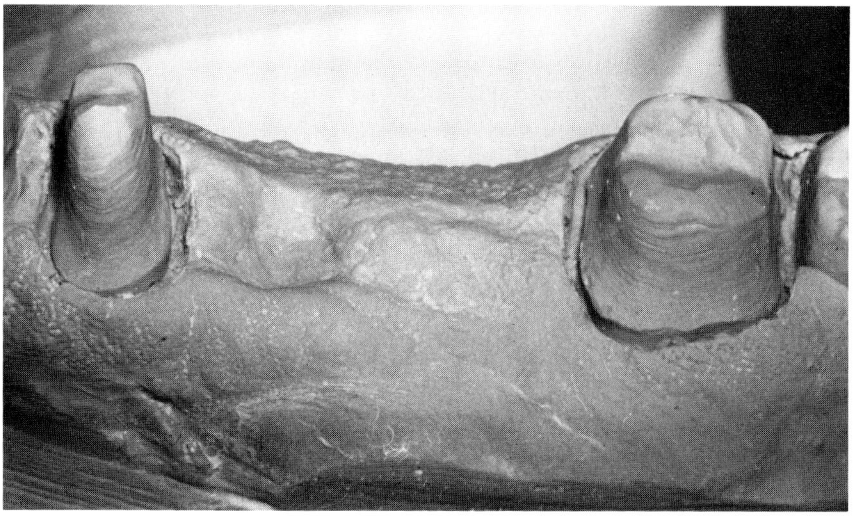

Fig 15–2.—This cast of the same prepared teeth was made from an impression that was carefully rinsed and cleaned.

Casting the Impression

The polysulfide or silicone impressions should be poured immediately after removal from the mouth. Polyether impressions have good shelf life but are known to absorb water if allowed to remain on the impression surface. The vinyl polysiloxane has no dimensional change after setting. The material is known to give off hydrogen and if poured immediately after removal will cause pitting on the surface of the stone cast. Consequently, it is best to wait a minimum of 30 minutes before making the pour. Some manufacturers recommend a longer wait. The correct water-powder ratio of the gypsum die material is important for pouring all impressions.

Impression materials with a high contact angle have a greater tendency toward entrapping air bubbles in the stone cast. The contact angle of impression materials was measured[20] to be approximately 92° to 98° for silicone, 67° to 77° for polysulfides, 50° for polyether, and 40° for hydrocolloid. Another study showed that incorporating nonionic surfactants in the silicone and polysulfide mix increases its wettability.[21] However these additions should best be left to the manufacturers and are not suitable for routine clinical use.

Before making the final impression, the dentist must know the technique by which the working cast and removable dies will be made. The die technique has a direct impact on how the impression is managed (this is discussed later). Only the technique of pouring a mix of type IV gypsum die material into the impression is presented here. The armamentarium for casting the impression is:

1. preweighed type IV gypsum die material;
2. vacuum mixing unit and accessories;
3. vibrator;
4. mixing spatula;
5. premeasured gypsum hardener liquid or room temperature water;

6. no. 4 paint brush; and
7. humidor.

For a full arch impression, 100 gm of type IV gypsum die stone is mixed with 18 cc of Stalite* gypsum hardener liquid.[15, 16] Some materials have a gypsum hardener incorporated in the powder and are mixed with measured water instead of hardener liquid. The liquid is poured in the plastic mixing bowl and the gypsum material sprinkled over it. The mix is hand spatulated until all the powder is wet. Then the material is mechanically spatulated at 30 pounds per square inch (psi) vacuum for 30 seconds. This should result in a homogenous, creamy, bubble-free mix.

The no. 4 paint brush is used to pick up the gypsum mix and gently vibrate it into the distal end of the impression (Fig 15–3). The impression tray is vibrated and the mix creeps forward as the tray is gently tipped mesially. The mix is allowed to slowly laminate the impression, tooth by tooth. If the impression is filling too fast, the tray is tipped distally to hold back the material. As the teeth begin to fill, additional gypsum mix is added at the original starting point. If there is any concern of a possible air bubble, the impression is inverted and the mix vibrated out. This leaves a thin film of gypsum over the impression material, the bubble is eliminated, and the casting procedure can be continued. The option of rinsing out the entire mix with water and starting over is at the discretion of the operator.

After the impression of the teeth is covered, a spatula is used to carry material to fill the rest of the impression. The remaining mix is used to build up the base of the cast. The minimum height of the cast should be 10 to 15 mm from the border of the tray (Fig 15–4). This buildup prevents fracture of the cast during removal

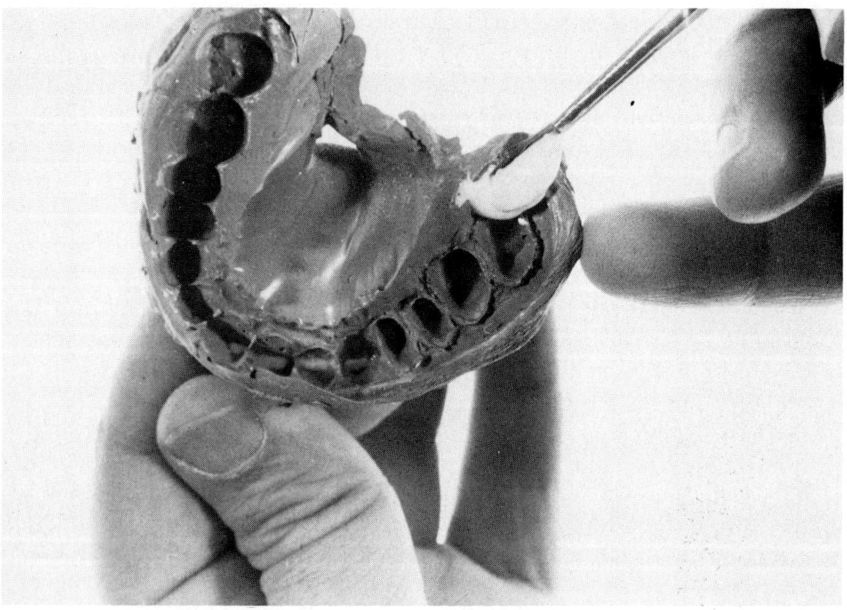

Fig 15–3.—The impression tray rests on the vibrator and the no. 4 paint brush is used to apply the die material. Note the finger rest of the hand holding the paint brush that helps to control the flow of the die stone.

*Buffalo Dental Manufacturing Col., Inc., Brooklyn, NY 11201.

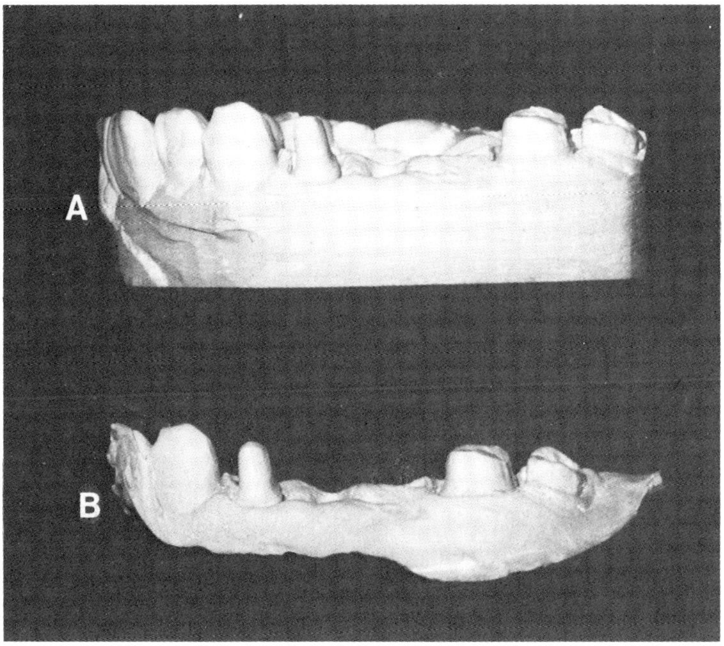

Fig 15–4.—The base of the first pour should be at least 10 to 15 mm thick as illustrated by cast A. This prevents accidental fracture of the cast during removal from the impression and subsequent procedures. It would be quite difficult to remove cast B from the impression as well as use it to fabricate individual dies.

from the impression. After the gypsum mix has its initial set, excess stone is trimmed away and the cast is allowed to set in a humidor. The impression should not be inverted as this is known to cause slumping and distortion of the cast.[22] The impression should be supported by the impression tray and not by any excess impression material extending from the heels. This prevents compression and distortion of the elastic impression material from the weight of the tray and stone. The cast is separated from the impression after one to two hours. The longer the delay, the stronger the cast. It is important for hydrocolloid impressions to be separated at one hour. Rubber base impressions can be left overnight. After 24 hours, the cast is completely dry and has reached its final strength.[1] It is now ready for fabricating removable dies.

REMOVABLE DIE SYSTEMS

The removable die is a replica of the prepared tooth and is used for the fabrication of a cast restoration by the indirect technique. Working casts with removable dies are a standard laboratory procedure, and operator preference influences the technique used in developing the removable die. The removable die techniques that will be discussed are: the dowel pin technique, the Typadon* tray technique, and the Di-Lok** tray technique.

---

*Typadon Co., 1937 34th W., Seattle, WA 98101.
**Lactona Corp., 1330 Industry Rd., Hatfield, PA 19440.

The dowel pin system (Fig 15–5) is the most popular and widely used technique. Other systems use manufactured plastic trays in which the dies are positioned (Fig 15–6). Any of the three techniques is suitable for making removable dies. The accuracy of various die systems has been measured,[24–27] but none were found to be superior. All removable dies show a vertical and horizontal distortion within a range that is acceptable for laboratory and clinical use.[27]

The Dowel Pin Technique

There are two ways that dowel pins can be positioned in the working cast. One is to position the dowel pin in the impression before the gypsum material is poured and sets[28–36] and the other is to cement the dowel pin in the gypsum cast after it is separated from the impression.[37] The second technique is gaining popularity and is routinely used in commercial laboratories. An advantage of this technique is that it encourages the dentist to pour the impressions immediately after removal from the mouth thereby ensuring accurate working dies and makes it possible for the technician to fabricate the removable dies at any later convenient time.

Removable Dies with Dowel Pins Imbedded in Unset Gypsum

Traditionally, dowel pins have been positioned in the impression, the cast poured, and the gypsum allowed to set around the dowel pins. This technique has several modifications, some of which are:

1. The impression is marked, poured, and the dowel pin positioned freehand in the setting gypsum;
2. The dowel pins are positioned over the impression with matches, clips, needles, or bobby pins[22, 28–35] and then the impression is poured; and
3. Using a commercial device such as the Oxydental* pin setter, positioned over

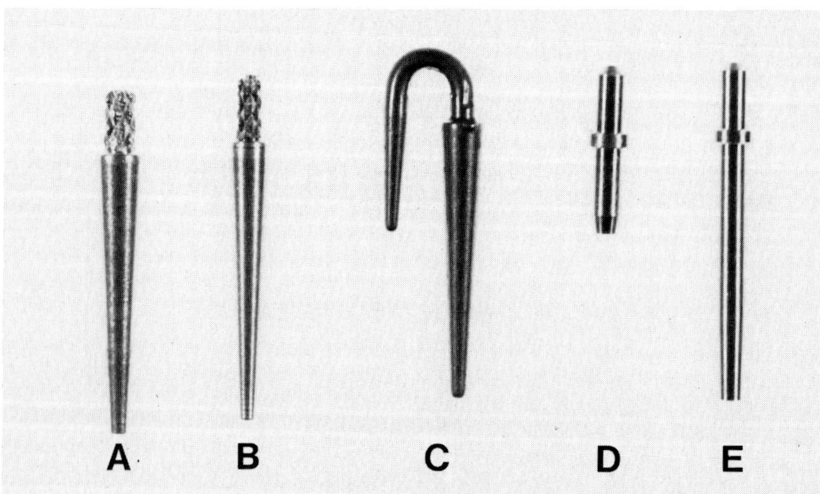

Fig 15–5.—Dowel pins are available in several shapes and sizes. Conventional dowel pins, large and small **(A)** and **(B),** J-pin **(C),** short index pin **(D),** and long pin **(E).** Pins **(D)** and **(E)** are used with the Pindex system.

*Oxy Dental Products, Inc., 6 Hoffman Pl., Hillside, NJ 07205.

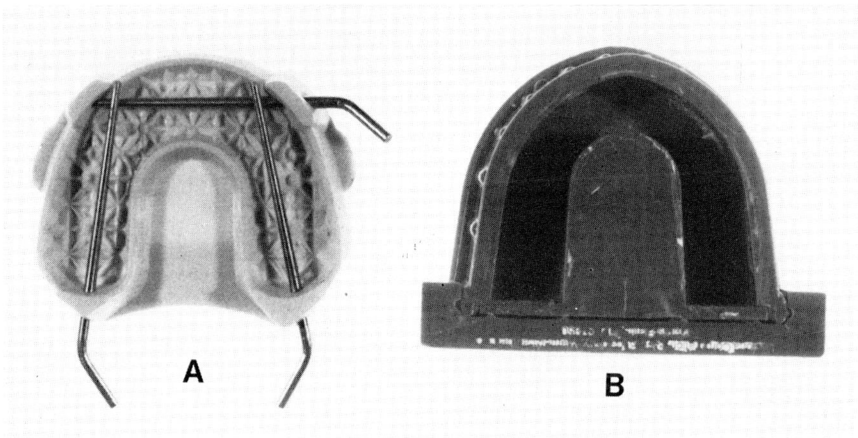

Fig 15–6.—The Typadon **(A)** and Di-Lok tray **(B)** are manufactured plastic trays designed for fabrication of removable dies.

the impression, the impression is poured with gypsum and the dowel pins are lowered into the unset material.[36]

Although the results achieved by any one of the above mentioned techniques is acceptable, the procedures discourage immediate pouring of the impression. In addition, proper dowel pin alignment and depth are sometimes difficult to attain.

Removable Dies Using Cemented Dowel Pins

When using the cemented dowel pin technique the impression is cast and the gypsum is allowed to harden. The cast is separated, holes are drilled in its base, and dowel pins are cemented using cyanoacrylate resin. This technique ensures the proper alignment of each dowel pin and die. There is no urgency to place the pins before the die stone sets, so the technician can make the removable dies at a convenient time.[37] The armamentarium for cemented dowel pins and working cast base is:

1. red and blue (nongraphite) pencils;
2. arbor band and chuck;
3. red handle Bard Parker knife with no. 25 blade;
4. boley gauge;
5. no. 6 or no. 8 round bur (HP);
6. dowel pins;
7. cyanoacrylate resin;
8. kerr boxing wax strips and sticks;
9. paint brush no. 4;
10. acrylic floor wax, gypsum separating medium, or 50% green soap;
11. type IV gypsum in a different color from the die, gypsum hardener liquid, and plaster mixing accessories; and
12. die saw.

Die and Working Cast Base Technique

1. Final impressions are rinsed, dried, and cast in type IV gypsum die material using the casting technique discussed earlier, and placed in a humidor,

2. The gypsum is allowed to set for more than one hour and then the cast is separated from the impression;

3. The cast is allowed to dry and reach its final strength by leaving it in a humidor overnight;

4. The facial and lingual borders of the dry cast are trimmed with an arbor band. A U-shaped trimmed cast is made (Fig 15–7) with a slight occlusogingival taper on the lingual wall and the facial wall vertical to the base. The faciolingual width of the trimmed cast should be about 15 mm;

5. A line is marked 10 mm apical to the gingival margins of the preparations and the entire base of the cast is trimmed to this line. The entire base should be flat and the segment below the proposed removable segment smoothed with a knife. The working cast is trimmed with arbor bands rather than a model trimmer because slurry water on the dies could alter the margins;

6. The removable segments of the cast are identified by drawing parallel lines on the facial and lingual surfaces of the cast (Fig 15–8). These lines serve as a guide for making the saw cuts;

7. The facial line is joined with its corresponding lingual line across the base of the cast. Now each removable segment has been identified and pin placement becomes an easy task;

8. A boley gauge is used to locate the center of each removable die segment and marked on the base (Fig 15–9). This identifies the placement of the dowel pins. Dowel pins are located below the occlusal center of each prepared tooth. The number of removable segments is dependent on operator preference. Besides removable working dies, the pontic area and one tooth on either side of the preparation should be removable. This helps in wax-up and finishing;

9. Depending on the diameter of the head of the dowel pin, a no. 6 or no. 8 round bur is used to drill a hole in the base of the cast. The hole should be slightly deeper than the length of the knurled portion of the dowel pin. The holes are drilled in the center of each die segment and made parallel to the vertical lines drawn on the facial aspect of the cast. Consequently the holes are parallel to the path of removal of the future removable dies (Fig 15–10);

10. An orientation groove is made facial and lingual to the pin holes with the

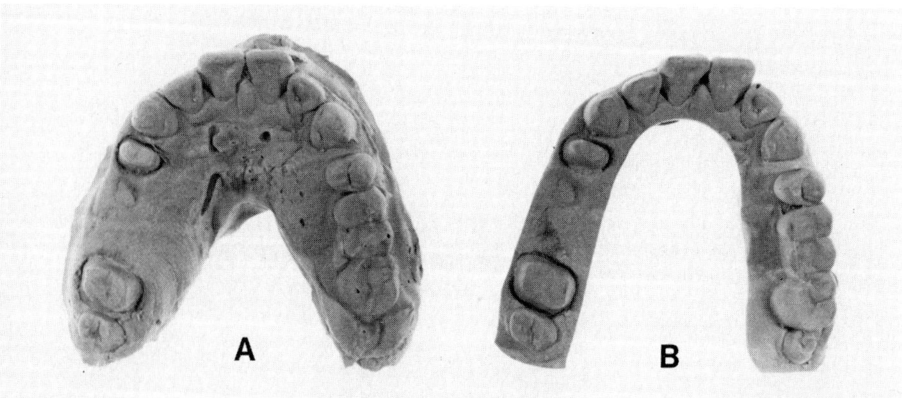

Fig 15–7.—The facial and lingual borders of the first pour **(A)** are trimmed to make it U-shaped **(B).** Width of the trimmed cast is approximately 15 mm.

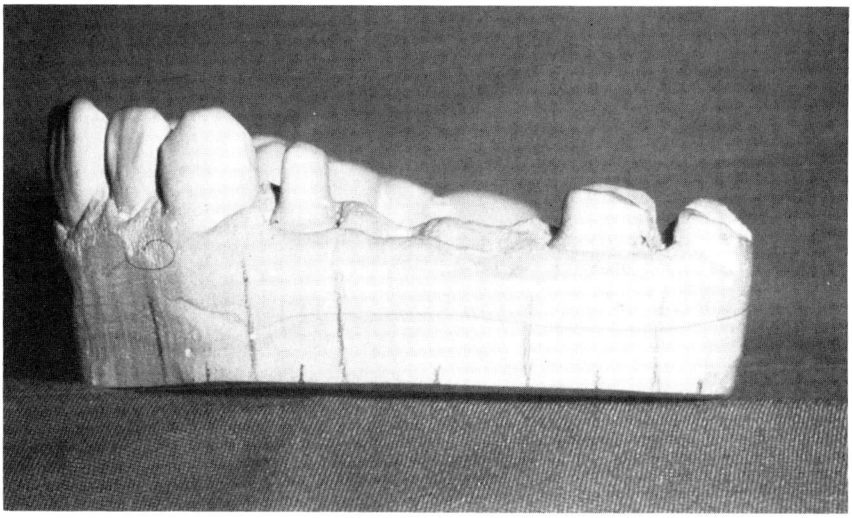

Fig 15–8.—The entire base of the working cast is reduced to 10 mm from the gingival margins. The base should be flat and smooth. Removable segments are individually identified. The parallel lines serve as a guide for making the saw cuts.

round bur (Fig 15–11). The grooves extend the length of the removable segment and have no undercuts. Two to three large, nonparallel, retentive undercuts are made in the remaining portion of the base (Fig 15–12);

11. Each channel is custom machined with a separate dowel pin. The knurled head of the dowel pin acts as a reamer and creates a snug fit. The skirt at the base

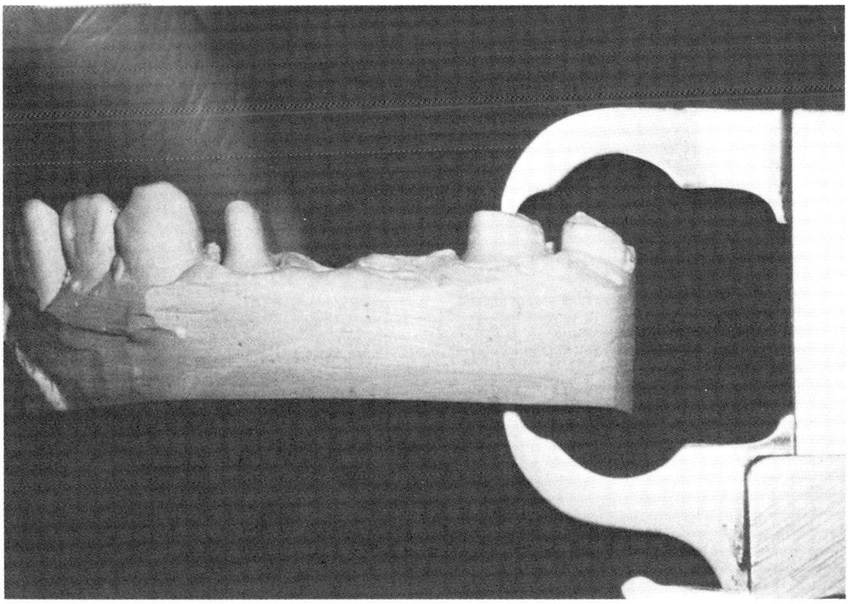

Fig 15–9.—A Boley gauge helps locate the center of each abutment or other removable segment.

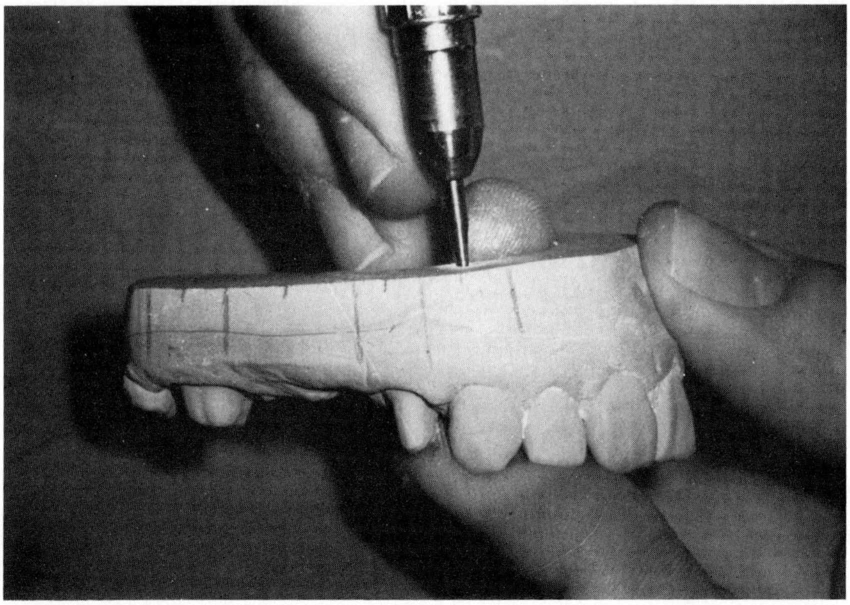

Fig 15–10.—Holes for dowel pins are drilled in the base of the cast. Each hole is parallel to the line of draw and has a diameter and depth slightly greater than that of the knurled segment of a dowel pin.

of the knurled portion of the dowel pin must touch the stone base (Fig 15–12). The dowel pins and holes are cleaned with compressed air;

12. The dowel pins are arranged according to the proposed insertion sequence. With the cast absolutely dry, cyanoacrylate is applied to the knurled portion of the dowel pin, which is then seated in its corresponding hole. To facilitate die orien-

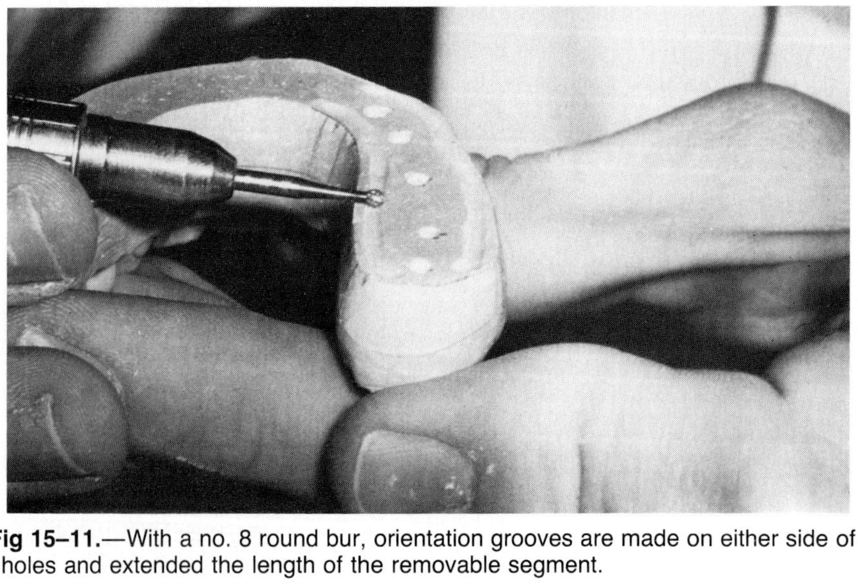

Fig 15–11.—With a no. 8 round bur, orientation grooves are made on either side of the pin holes and extended the length of the removable segment.

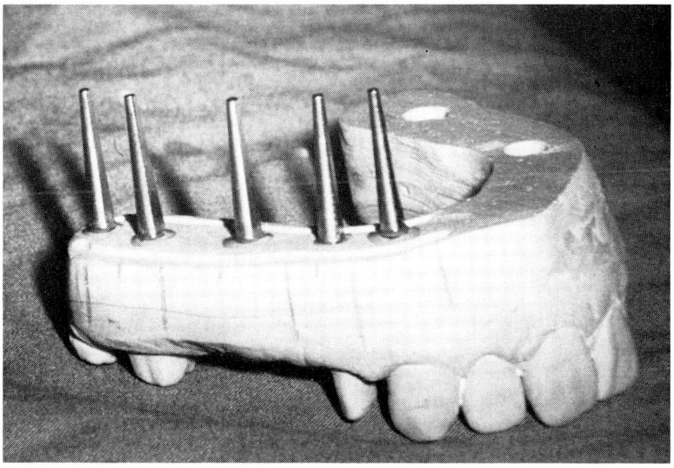

Fig 15–12.—Nonparallel retentive holes are cut on the opposite side of the arch. The dowel pins are cemented with cyanoacrylate resin. They are aligned with each other and are parallel to the path of removal of the working die. The flat portion of the dowel pin faces mesially for easy die orientation. The knurled segment of the dowel pin is completely imbedded in the base.

tation, the flat portion of the dowel pin should face mesially (Fig 15–12). The pin should be held parallel to the faciolingual and mesiodistal axes of the die segment for approximately 15 seconds, until the cement sets;

13. Rope boxing wax is flamed to make it sticky and is then wrapped around the facial and lingual walls of the removable die segment of the cast. The wax is placed 3 mm from the lingual border of the base and flush with the facial border (Fig 15–13). Sheet boxing wax strips are used to box the entire working cast (Fig 15–14). The top edge of the boxing wax strip should be 2 mm lower than the ends of the dowel pins. To prevent accidental leakage of plaster from the second pour onto the stone dies, the wax should be in intimate contact and sealed to the cast;

14. The removable segment of the base is painted with a separating medium. Commercially available gypsum separator, acrylic floor wax, or green soap half diluted with water works equally well. Vaseline should not be used because of its film thickness. Traditionally, the second pour is made in type II gypsum model plaster. This creates a weak base, and the dowel pin channels are susceptible to easy abrasion and subsequently unstable and inaccurate dies are made; and

15. This problem can be avoided if type IV gypsum die material of a contrasting color to the first pour (Fig 15–15) is used for the base. This is far superior to plaster or cast stone because it provides a more accurate and stable base for the dowel pins and removable dies. When the second pour is made care is taken to avoid resting the working dies on the vibrator.

Sectioning the Working Cast

After the second pour has set, the working cast is ready for sectioning into removable die segments. The parallel lines, originally drawn on the facial and lingual walls of the cast, help to guide the saw cuts (Figs 15–8 and 15–16).

The working cast can be sectioned with a hand or motorized saw. The motorized

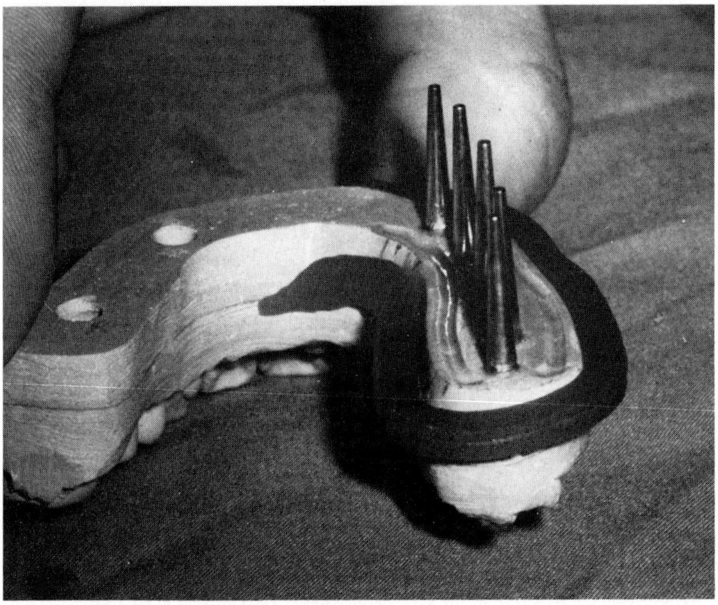

Fig 15–13.—The facial and lingual walls of the removable segment of the working cast are lined with rope wax. The wax is placed 3 mm from the lingual border of the base and flush with the facial border.

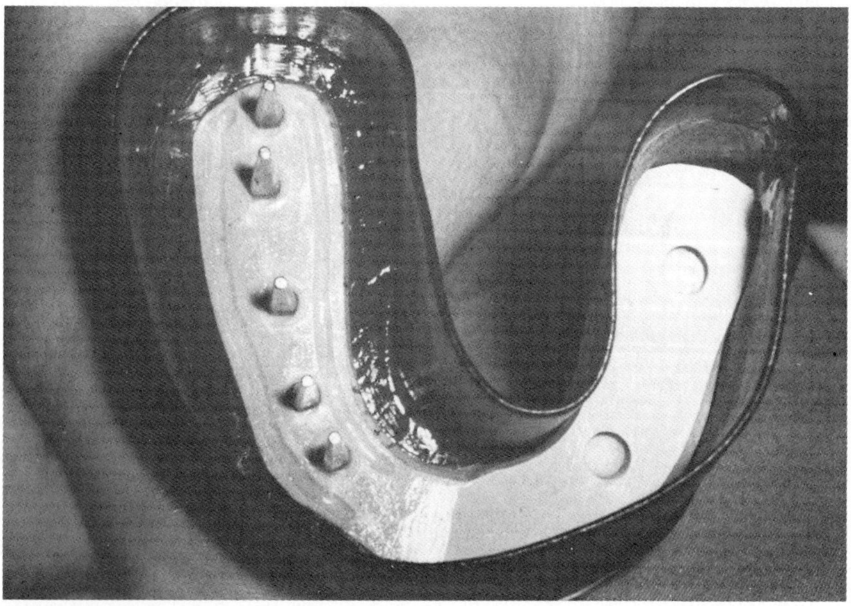

Fig 15–14.—Separating medium is painted over the removable segment of the working cast and it is boxed, leaving the dowel pins extending 2 mm above the top edge of the boxing wax.

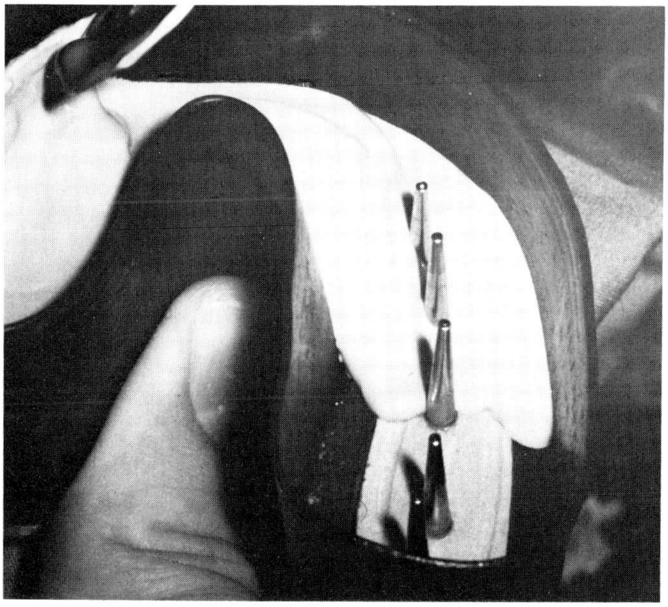

Fig 15–15.—The second pour is made with a different colored type IV gypsum die material. The boxed cast is filled from the nonremovable end and the gypsum is allowed to slowly flow into the grooves and around the dowel pins.

saw is expensive and suitable for commercial laboratories. Its ultra-thin blade sections the gypsum precisely and accurately. The usual method of sectioning dies is with a hand saw. A thin, wide blade is preferred because it reduces flexure and twisting while cutting. The saw blade is attached so it will cut in a pulling stroke. The saw cuts are extended 0.5 mm into the second pour. After all the segments have been sectioned, the dowel pins are tapped on the end and each section is separated from the second pour (Fig 15–17). Any residue is blown from the channels and the sectioned units with air. The unit is reassembled and each segment is checked for precise seating with no gap between the first and second pours of gypsum (Fig 15–18).

Trimming the Working Dies

A critical phase in developing a good cast restoration with proper physiologic contours is when the working die is trimmed.[38–40] This should be the dentist's responsibility but it is often relegated to the technician. Whenever possible, the preparation margin and 1 to 2 mm of tooth surface apical to it should be recorded in the final impression. This is generally possible with proper tissue retraction (Fig 15–19,A,B). The armamentarium for trimming and preparing the die is:

1. round or inverted cone acrylic trimming bur (HP);
2. no. eight round bur (HP);
3. red handle Bard Parker knife with no. 25 blade;
4. red pencil with a sharp point;
5. paint brush;
6. gypsum slurry water;

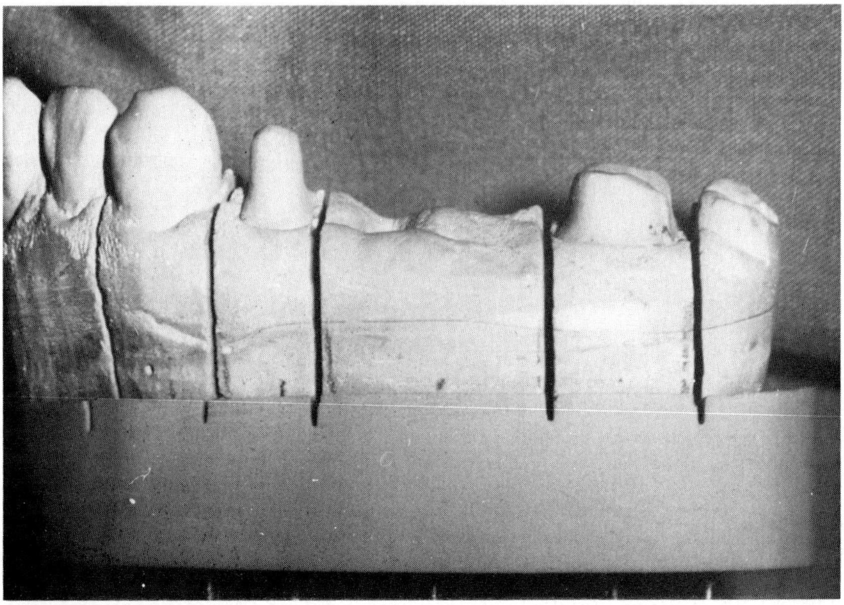

Fig 15–16.—Parallel lines on the facial and lingual aspects of the cast help to align the saw blade for sectioning the dies.

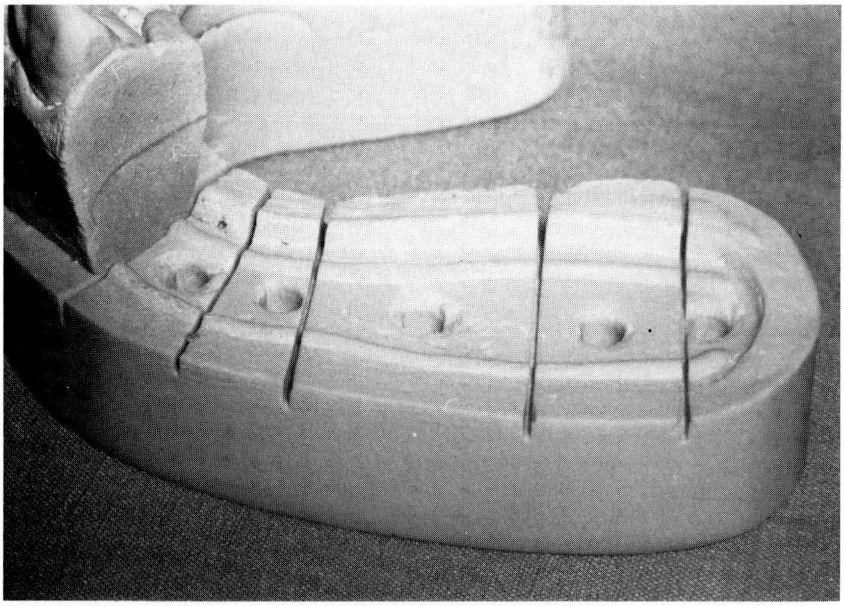

Fig 15–17.—With the dies removed, note that the flat portion of dowel pins face mesially and the orientation grooves are clean and definite where the two pours separated.

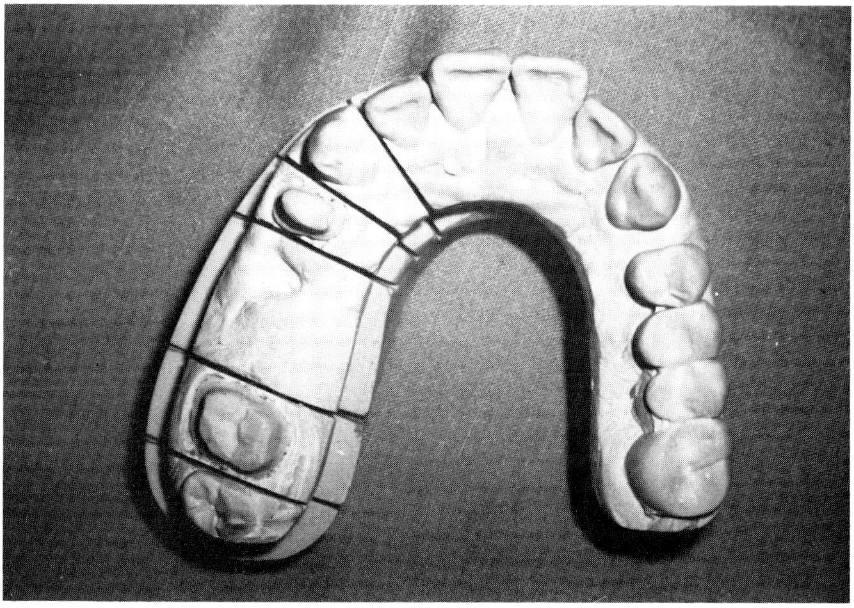

Fig 15–18.—The working cast with removable dies. Each segment can be easily removed and completely reseated.

7. stereo zoom microscope (10X) or magnifying loops; and
8. air syringe.

The following steps constitute proper die trimming technique.

1. The gypsum die is ditched with a round or inverted cone acrylic trimming bur. The reduction is made 3 mm apical to the preparation margin (Fig 15–20) and should be of a conservative depth;
2. A no. 8 round bur is used to undermine the replica of the gingival tissue;
3. The cervical margins of the gypsum die are lightly moistened with a supersaturated gypsum slurry water using a paint brush. This procedure softens the gypsum without dissolving the critical margins and reduces the possibility of chipping the die margins;
4. The Bard Parker knife blade is used to carefully cut away the gingival tissue stone and expose the cervical margins (Fig 15–21). The undermined stone should break clearly, exposing excellent topography of the natural tooth structure apical to the margins;
5. A stereo zoom microscope or high magnification loops should be used to read the prepared margins. The area cervical to the margins is trimmed to an emergence angle comparable with the root of the tooth; and
6. A sharp, nongraphite pencil is used to identify the preparation margins. A color that has an extreme contrast with the die stone and that is easily discernible is used. The pencil tip is held over the margin and brought in contact at a 5-degree angle (Fig 15–22). The pencil tip is rotated around the preparation much like a surveying rod. High magnification makes correct identification and marking of the prepared margins easier.

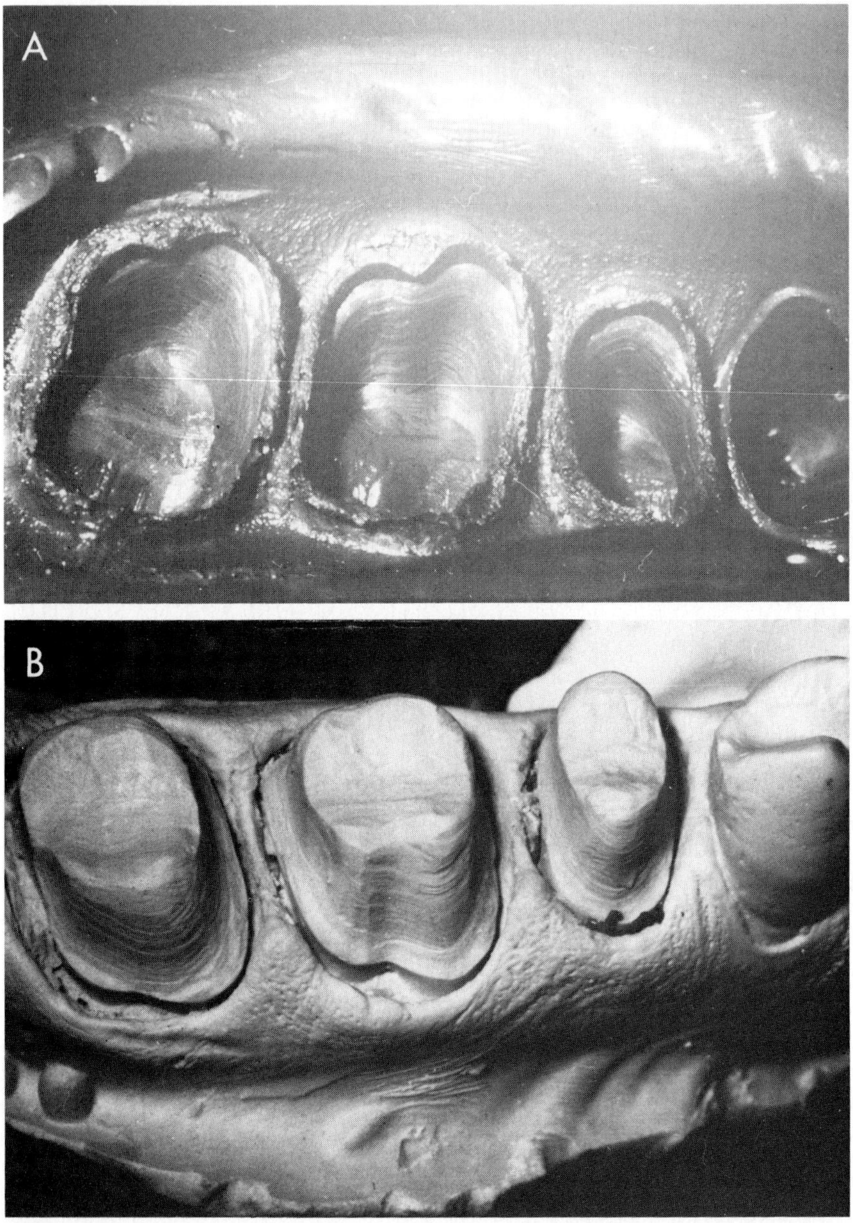

Fig 15–19.—**A,** a final impression of teeth with proper gingival retraction yields good working dies. **B,** replication of the preparation margin and tooth structure apical to it aids in die trimming which helps develop proper emergence angles on the restorations.

USE OF DIE-SPACERS AND HARDENING FILMS

The film thickness of zinc phosphate cement under cemented crowns has been reported to be 90[41] to 143 μ.[42] By applying a paint-on die spacer to the surface of the stone die, internal relief of the casting is possible and the film thickness of a cemented crown can be reduced to near 40 μ. The use of die spacers is becoming

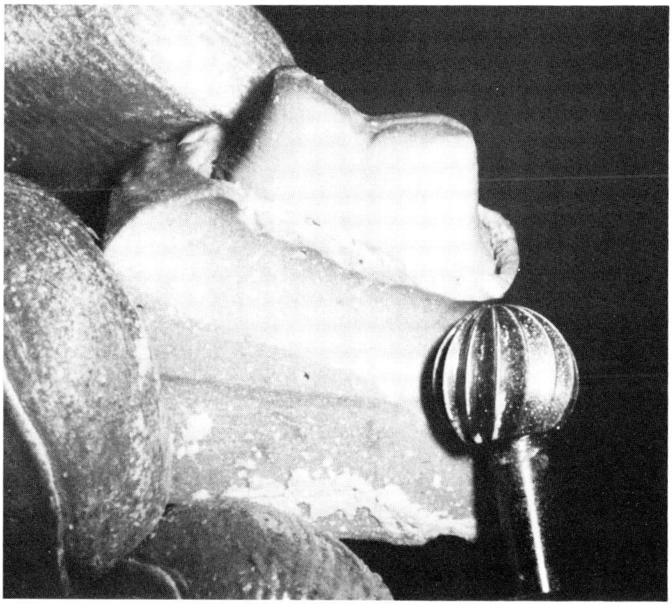

Fig 15–20.—A round acrylic trimming bur is used to ditch the die 3 mm apically to the gingival margin of the preparation to a conservative depth.

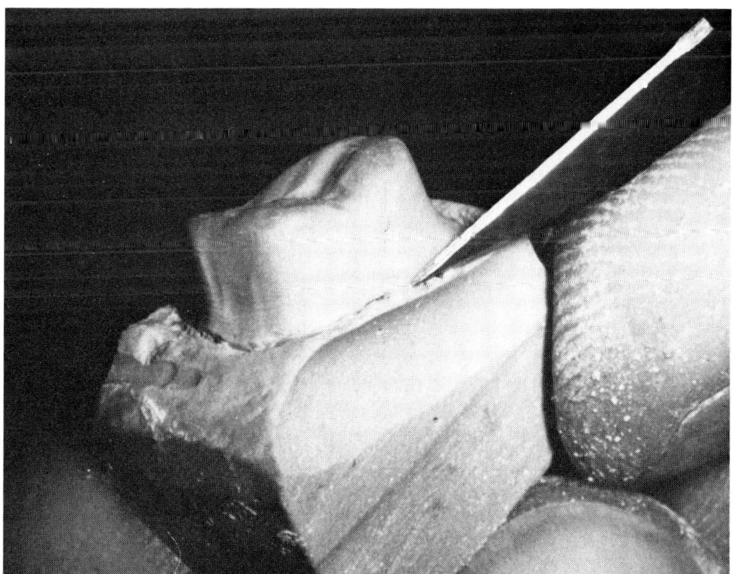

Fig 15–21.—A sharp blade is used to cut away the stone replica of the gingival tissue after using the round bur.

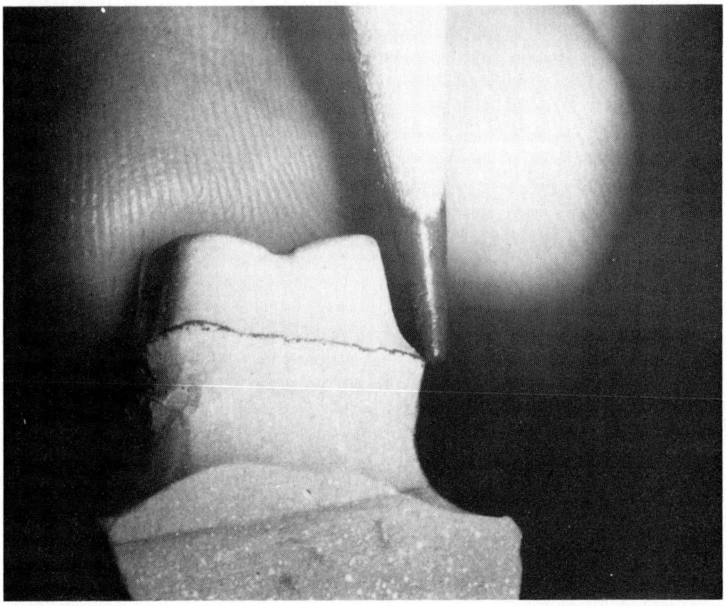

Fig 15–22.—The largest diameter of the trimmed die is at its gingival margin. This area is identified by marking it with a nongraphite pencil of a contrasting color.

a standard laboratory procedure and the film thickness of different paint-on die spacers has been reported (Fig 15–23). Successful relief of 20 to 40 μ is possible by varying the number of coats applied to the die.[43]

Die Spacer Technique

1. The Blue Cement Spacer* requires two coats for approximately 20 μ of relief and four coats for 40 μ of relief;
2. The die spacer should be kept at the correct dilution. It has a tendency to evaporate and thicken rapidly. The manufacturer supplies a thinner;
3. The occlusal and axial surfaces of the die are painted stopping 0.5 mm short of the preparation margins. A no. 0 sable hair brush is suitable for applying the die spacer;
4. Each coat of die spacer is allowed to dry completely before applying a subsequent layer; and
5. After the fourth coat has dried, the bur marks and topography of the die should still be clearly visible through the paint. If they have been obliterated, the paint was applied too thick and should be removed with the thinner and the procedure repeated.

Hardening Films

Margin abrasion of gypsum dies during wax carving is possible. A protective coating of cyanoacrylate resin has been found to be effective in improving the surface hardness and abrasion resistance of the gypsum die margins. The film thickness

*Belle de St. Claire, Van Nyes, CA 91408.

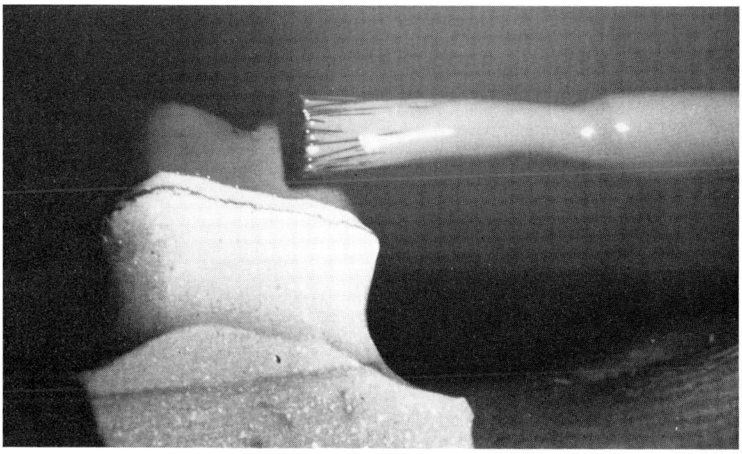

Fig 15–23.—Blue Cement Spacer yields approximately 10 microns of relief for each coat up to six coats. The die spacer is applied with a fine sable hair brush. Care should be taken to avoid pooling the liquid on any surface of the die. Spacer should be kept at least a half mm away from the margin of the preparation.

of Eastman 910** cyanoacrylate resin has been measured to be one micron, provided the material is air-blown immediately after application.[44]

A cotton tipped applicator is used to lightly paint cyanoacrylate cement on the margins of the preparation (Fig 15–24). Excess cement is immediately air-blown dry.

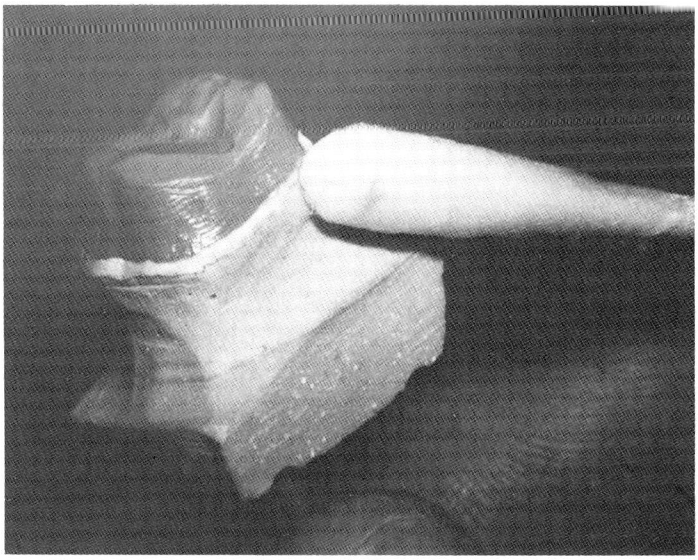

Fig 15–24.—The cyanoacrylate resin is applied with a cotton tip applicator. Any excess resin is blown away with air immediately after application.

**Eastman Kodak Co., Rochester, NY 14603.

ARTICULATION OF THE WORKING CAST

Diagnostic casts are mounted on an articulator in the retruded contact or centric relation position. A face-bow transfer orients the maxillary cast in its correct relationship. The working casts are mounted in the intercuspal or centric occlusion position. The rationale for selecting the above position is discussed elsewhere.

The Opposing Cast

There are numerous techniques that describe the accuracy of working casts made with elastomeric impression materials, but little mention is made of the accuracy of the opposing cast. Conventionally, the opposing cast is made from an alginate impression. Alginate impressions are known to distort more than elastomeric impression materials. Consequently, when two casts of different dimensional accuracy are articulated with an accurate interocclusal record, some degree of inaccuracy in the mounting will be evident. It is preferable to make both casts from a similar impression material. This procedure deserves serious consideration when multiple castings are planned.

Mounting the Working Cast

The occluding surfaces of both casts are examined carefully and any occlusal artifacts that may prevent correct and complete articulation are removed. The distal extension of both casts are checked to make sure there are no interferences. The palatal area of the working cast is blocked with a sheet of wax that is sealed to the lingual aspect (Fig 15–25). The working cast is articulated with the previously mounted opposing diagnostic cast and stabilized with wood applicator sticks (Fig 15–26). The articulator is closed to make sure that the working cast is not interfering. The exposed tips of the dowel pins are covered with wax sticks and the rest of

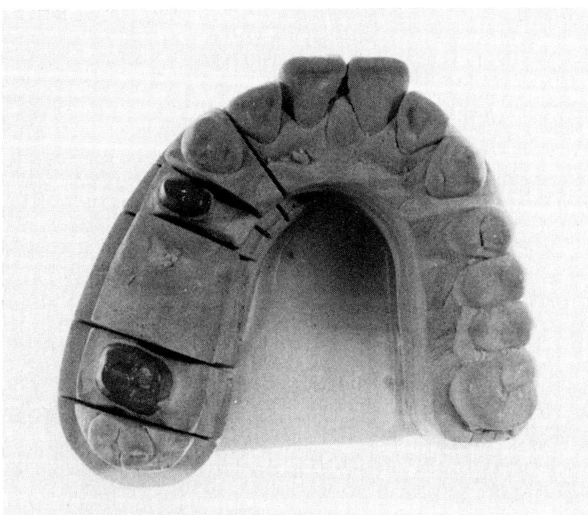

Fig 15–25.—The working cast with removable dies properly trimmed, painted with die spacer, margins marked, and coated with cyanoacrylate resin is ready for mounting and fabrication of the prosthesis. Note the wax sheet in the palatal area that prevents the mounting plaster from contacting the dies.

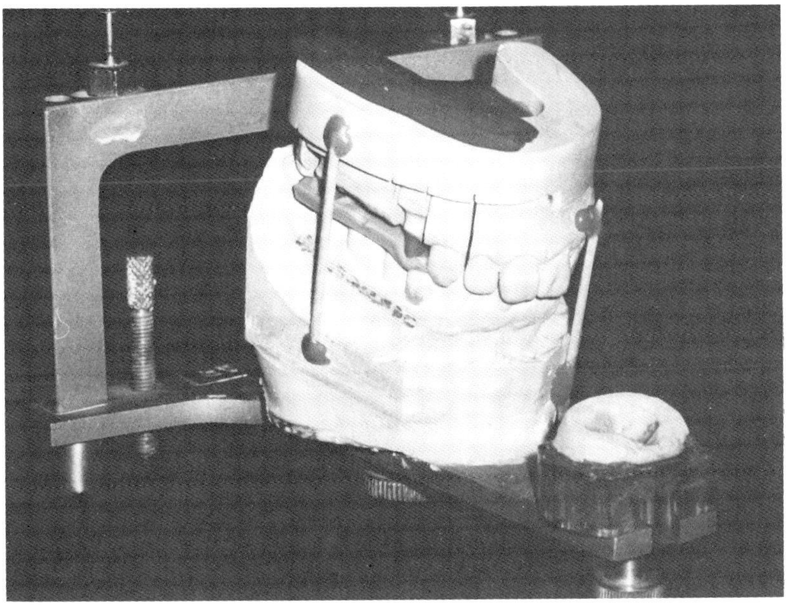

Fig 15–26.—Wooden applicator sticks attached with sticky wax ensure stable articulation during the mounting procedure. Note the wax covering the ends of the dowel pins to provide access after mounting with plaster.

the gypsum base is moistened with water for better adhesion with the mounting plaster.

If remount procedures are anticipated, the base of the cast is notched at this time and separating medium is applied. If remounting is not planned, it is especially important to ensure that once the cast is mounted it will not separate from the mounting plaster. When mounting the working cast with an interocclusal record made in the intercuspal relation, the guide pin is set at zero. Mounting plates are tightened and a mix of mounting plaster is made with correct water-powder ratio. The mix is applied over the moist surface of the working cast. Plaster is also applied to the mounting ring and the articulator is closed. The upper member of the articulator is gently tapped until the incisal pin touches the guide table. Any excess material from near the dowel pins is removed. If the mounting procedure is managed correctly, there is little possibility of the plaster accidentally flowing into the dowel pin canals or over the prepared teeth.

COMMERCIAL DOWEL PIN PLACEMENT SYSTEMS

Two commercial dowel pin systems, where the dowel pins are cemented after the cast has been recovered from the impression, are available. They are the Pindex* and the TDI** systems. The dowel pin technique described earlier in this chapter is suitable for all clinical situations and is appropriate for use in a small laboratory. For high production work the use of a commercial dowel pin placement

*Whaledent Int., New York, NY 10001.
**Apm-Sterngold, Stamford, CT 06904.

system is most appropriate. The concept of using cemented dowel pins is the core of both techniques, but neither is superior to the other. The Pindex system uses a short and a long dowel pin (Fig 15–5), each with its own plastic sleeve.

The working cast is trimmed and the base flattened similar to the technique described earlier. The dowel pin holes are then located and drilled in the base with the aid of a centering device and a motorized drill. Two holes are drilled for each removable segment, one lingual and one facial. Cyanoacrylate cement is used to cement a short pin in the lingual hole. A long pin is cemented in the facial hole.

Plastic base-formers are available that may be filled with a gypsum mix and then the working cast seated into them. The entire technique is well described in the literature provided by the manufacturers. These systems merit serious consideration for high volume use. They are efficient, cost effective, and produce consistent results.

REMOVABLE DIES FROM PREFORMED TRAY SYSTEMS

Although the dowel pin system is considered the most popular technique, alternative die systems are available. The Typadon tray or the Di-Lok tray (Fig 15–6) can be successfully used to make removable dies of an equivalent quality to the dowel pin dies. Both of these trays are referred to as keyed matrix systems. Operator preference dictates the choice of the die system used in the laboratory.[20, 45, 56]

Keyed Matrix Die Technique

1. For both preformed tray systems, the gypsum cast is poured as before, removed from the impression and trimmed to conform to the shape of the tray;
2. Both systems permit a single pour for the impression and the base at the same time if care is taken. This encourages the dentist to pour both the impression and the base;
3. When the die stone is set, all excess is trimmed away so that the base contacts only the keyed portion of the tray (Fig 15–27); and

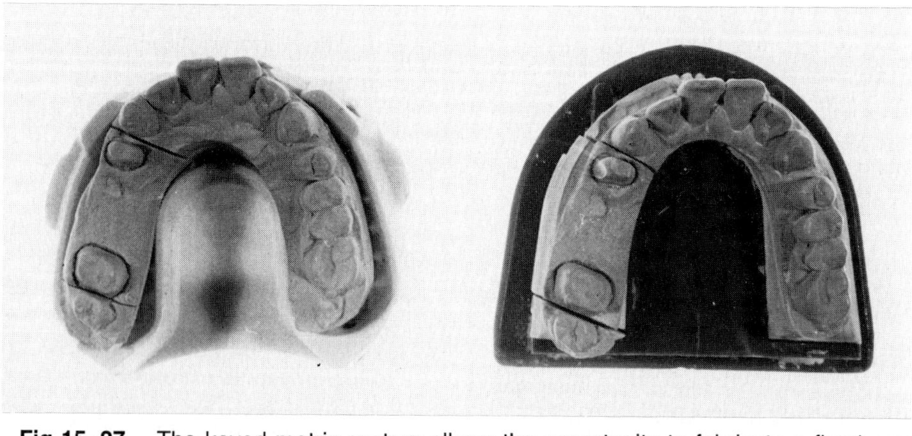

Fig 15–27.—The keyed matrix system allows the opportunity to fabricate a fixed prosthesis without sectioning the abutment dies apart and thus accurately maintain the relationship between abutments.

4. Dies are sectioned with a saw where needed. Care is taken to maintain keyed surfaces and pin holes in the cast dust and debris-free (Figs 15–6 and 15–27).

If the two pour technique is used, the trimming of the first pour to conform it to the U-shape of the tray makes it vulnerable to fracture. The added height of the tray sometimes interferes with the mounting of the working cast on an articulator. It is less convenient to remove and reseat the die because the entire unit has to be disassembled.

An advantage of the tray system is that there is no worry about dowel pins coming loose or improper saw cuts passing through the dowel pins. The relationship of a fixed prosthesis can be accurately maintained by not sectioning between the abutments. This is also possible with dowel pins (Fig 15–28).

CLINICAL AND LABORATORY CONSIDERATIONS

The Custom Guide Table

When anterior teeth are being restored, it is important to accurately reproduce the guidance controlled by them. This is only possible by making a customized incisal guide table on the articulator.[47–49] When posterior teeth are being restored, the custom guide table prevents wear and fracture of anterior teeth on the working cast and opposing cast during fabrication.

Custom Incisal Guide Table Technique

1. The custom incisal guide table is made from diagnostic casts occluding in the same relationship that the working cast will be occluded. Usually this is the intercuspal or centric occlusion relationship (Fig 15–29);

2. The pin on a semi-adjustable articulator is lubricated and embedded in a mix of autopolymerizing TMJ Fossa and Tray Acrylic.* With the cast teeth in contact, the maxillary cast is moved through all excursive movements. The incisal pin molds the acrylic;

3. The excess flash is trimmed so that when the casts are in an edge-to edge relation in protrusive or lateral excursions, the pin contacts the top edge of the custom guide table. This helps to establish the correct incisal length for the final restorations (Fig 15–30); and

4. If the anterior teeth are missing or badly broken down, a diagnostic wax-up may be done to establish anterior guidance with acrylic provisional restorations. After any necessary adjustments, an alginate impression of the provisional restoration is made, the cast is obtained from this impression, mounted in the intercuspal position, and the guide table developed (Fig 15–31).

Additional Patient Data

To fabricate a high quality esthetic restoration, the dentist may need to provide the technician with additional information about the patient. Such information might include original casts and mounted opposing cast, diagnostic wax-up, labial index, face-bow transfer, custom incisal guide table, interocclusal records, tooth color and characterization data, age, gender of the patient, and occlusal scheme.

---

*TMJ Inst. Co., Santa Ana, CA 92702.

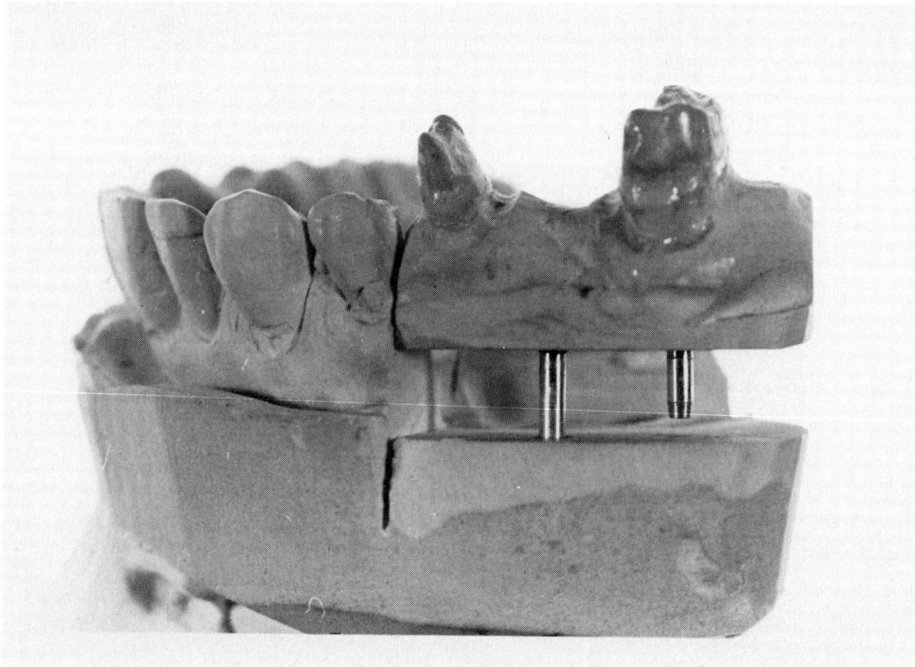

Fig 15–28.—Abutments can be maintained in the same segment using dowel pins also but they must be positioned with a paralleling aid so that they are absolutely parallel.

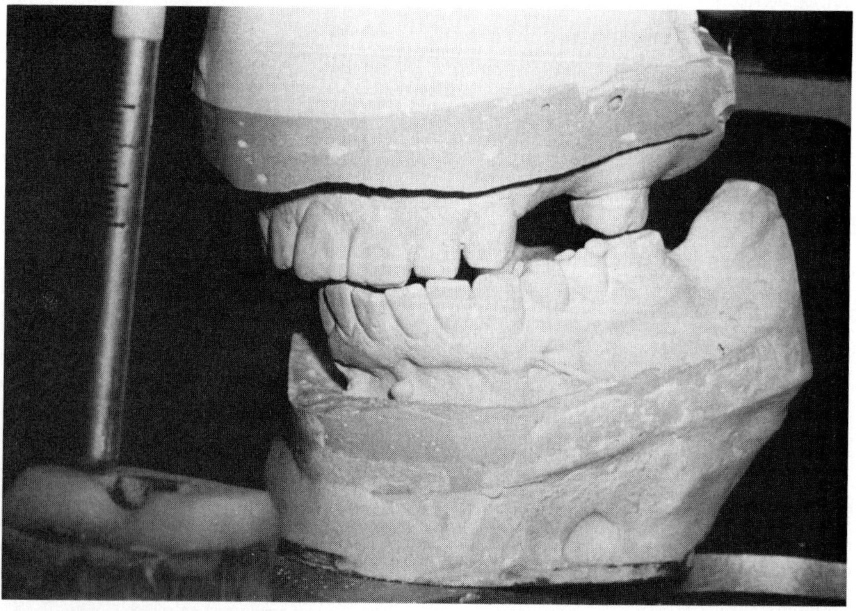

Fig 15–29.—The custom incisal guide table is developed from diagnostic casts. Note the relationship of the incisal guide pin, the custom guide table, and the incisal edges of the opposing casts.

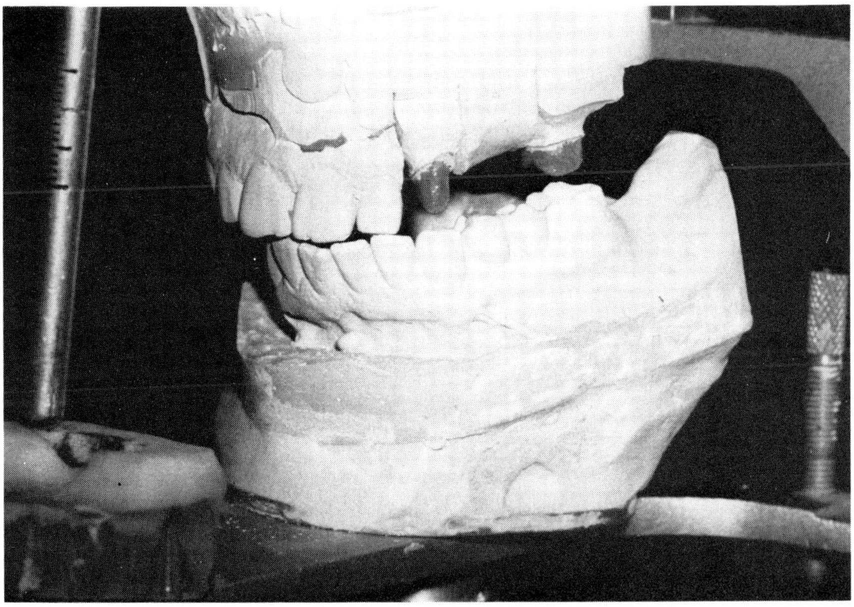

Fig 15–30.—The mounted working cast duplicates the original lateral excursions. Correct incisal length and lingual contours in the wax pattern can be easily developed.

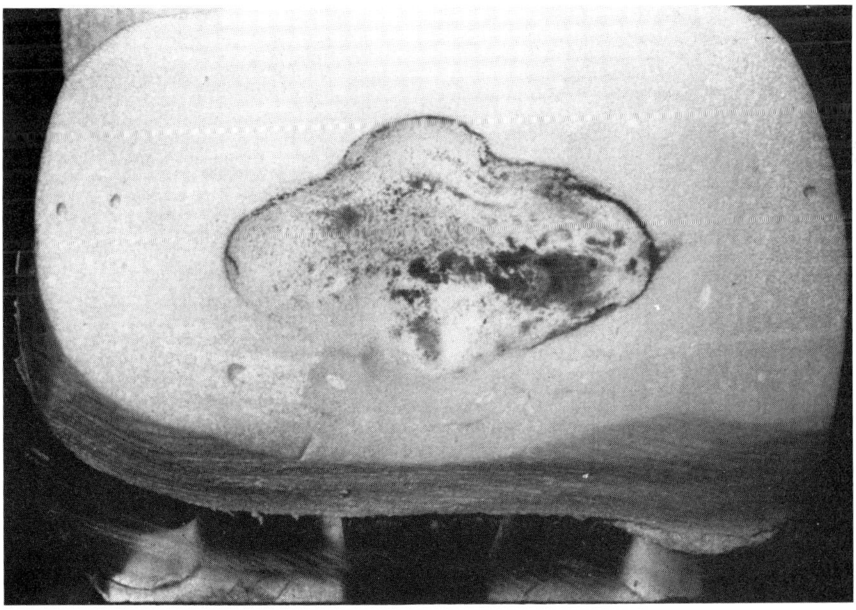

Fig 15–31.—A custom incisal guide table reproduces the patient's excursive movements as shown in this closeup of the trimmed guide table.

SUMMARY

Techniques of developing working casts and removable dies have been discussed. The final fixed restoration can only be as good as the poorest phase of its fabrication. Working casts and dies are certainly no exception. A chain is only as strong as its weakest link. Careful attention to detail and precision are of utmost importance. Accurate and complete information about the patient aids the laboratory technician in providing the best possible service for the dentist and patient.

REFERENCES

1. Phillips R.W.: *Skinner's Science of Dental Materials*, ed. 8. Philadelphia, W.B. Saunders Co., 1982.
2. Stackhouse J.A.: Electrodeposition in dentistry. A review of the literature. *J. Prosthet. Dent.* 44:259, 1980.
3. Markley M.R., Krug R.S.: Silver plating rubber base material for superior dies and casts. *J. Prosthet. Dent.* 22:103, 1959.
4. Schwartz H.B., Leupold R.J., Thompson V.P.: Linear dimensional accuracy of epoxy die resin and stone dies. *J. Prosthet. Dent.* 45:621, 1981.
5. Eames W.B., Edwards C.R., Buck W.C.: Scraping resistance of dental die materials. A comparison of brands. *Oper. Dent.* 3:66, 1978.
6. Stackhouse J.A.: Impression materials and electrodeposits. Part I: impression materials. *J. Prosthet. Dent.* 45:44, 1981.
7. Stackhouse J.A.: Impression materials and electrodeposits. Part II: electrodeposits. *J. Prosthet. Dent.* 45:146, 1981.
8. Podshadley A.G., Dilts W.E., Neiman R.: Accuracy of silver plated mercaptan rubber impression. *J. Ky. Dent. Assoc.* 25:29, 1973.
9. Gettleman L., Ryge G.: Accuracy of stone, metal and plastic die materials. *J. Calif. Dent. Assoc.* 46:28, 1970.
10. Cooney J.P.: A comparison of silver-plated and stone dies from rubber-base impressions. *J. Prosthet. Dent.* 32:262, 1974.
11. Phillips R.W., Schnell R.J.: Silver-plating rubber base material for superior dies and casts. *J. Prosthet. Dent.* 22:103, 1959.
12. Nomura G.T., Reisbick M.H., Preston J.D.: An investigation of epoxy resin dies. *J. Prosthet. Dent.* 44:45, 1980.
13. Vermilyea S.G., Huget E.F., Wiskoski J.: Evaluation of resin die materials. *J. Prosthet. Dent.* 42:304, 1979.
14. Moser J.B., Stone D.G., Willoughby G.M.: Properties and characteristics of a resin die material. *J. Prosthet. Dent.* 34:297, 1975.
15. Toreskog S., Phillips R.W., Schnell R.J.: Properties of die materials. A comparative study. *J. Prosthet. Dent.* 16:119, 1966.
16. Eames W.B., et al.: Compatibility of gypsum products with hydrocolloid impression materials. *Oper. Dent.* 3:108, 1978.
17. Eames W.B.: The casting misfit—How to cope. *J. Prosthet. Dent.* 45:283, 1981.
18. Phillips R.W.: *Skinner's Science of Dental Materials*, ed. 8. Philadelphia, W.B. Saunders Co., 1981.
19. Smith D.C., Fairhurst C.W.: Effect of hydrocolloid impression materials on the surface of the dental stone. *J. Dent. Res.* 41:1103, 1962.
20. Lorren R.A., Salter D.J., Fairhurst C.W.: The contact angles of die stone on impression materials. *J. Prosthet. Dent.* 36:176, 1976.
21. Norling B.K., Reisbick M.H.: The effect of nonionic surfactants on bubble entrapment in elastomeric impression materials. *J. Prosthet. Dent.* 42:342, 1979.
22. Shillingburg H.T., Hobo S., Whitsett L.D.: *Fundamentals of Fixed Prosthodontics*. Chicago, Quintessence Publishing Co., 1981.
23. Dilts W.E., et al.: Accuracy of a removable die-dowel pin technique. *J. Dent. Res.* 50:1249, 1971.

24. Dilts W.E., et al.: Accuracy of four removable die techniques. *J. Am. Dent. Assoc.* 83:1081, 1971.
25. Hembree J.H., Brown T.: Relative accuracy of several removable die techniques. *J. Acad. Gen. Dent.* 22:31, 1974.
26. Miranda F.J., et al.: Comparative stability of two removable die systems. *J. Prosthet. Dent.* 36:326, 1976.
27. Myers M., Hembree J.H.: Relative accuracy of four removable die systems. *J. Prosthet. Dent.* 48:163, 1982.
28. Reed G.M.: New concepts in precision dowels. *J. Am. Dent. Assoc.* 76:321, 1968.
29. Christy J.M., Pipko D.J.: A simplified method of indexing working dies. *J. Prosthet. Dent.* 19:160, 1968.
30. Stern A.J., Vernon H.M.: Development of a new tool in restorative dentistry. *J. Prosthet. Dent.* 21:536, 1969.
31. Carl W., Garlapo D.A., Brown M.H.: Modified impression procedure for removable die preparation. *Quint. Int.* 5:39, 1974.
32. Tanquist R.A., Stamps J.T., Gullat T.: Producing accurate removable dies from elastic full arch impressions. *J. Prosthet. Dent.* 48:210, 1982.
33. Troendle K.B., Troendle R.G., Cavozos E.: Positioning dowel pins for removable dies. *J. Prosthet. Dent.* 46:575, 1981.
34. Robinson F.B., Block B.: Dowel pin positioning technique for fixed partial denture working casts. *J. Prosthet. Dent.* 46:215, 1981.
35. Balshi T.J., Mingledorff E.B.: Matches, clips, needles, or pins. *J. Prosthet. Dent.* 34:467, 1975.
36. Stone T.E., Walker W.A.: A method for locating dowel pins in artificial stone casts. *J. Prosthet. Dent.* 44:345, 1980.
37. Smith C.D., Nayyar A., Koth D.L.: Fabrication of removable stone dies using cemented dowel pins. *J. Prosthet. Dent.* 41:579, 1979.
38. Tanquist R.A.: Die trimming: A guide to physiologic contour. *J. Prosthet. Dent.* 48:485, 1982.
39. Beck D.B.: Precision technique for trimming dies using a magnification device. *J. Prosthet. Dent.* 43:590, 1980.
40. Morris T.: For best periodontal health, trim dies after wax-up. *Coping* (Sterngold) 6:1, 1979.
41. Fusayama T., et al.: Cement thickness between cast restorations and preparation walls. *J. Prosthet. Dent.* 13:354, 1963.
42. Eames W.B., et al.: Techniques to improve seating of castings. *J. Am. Dent. Assoc.* 96:432, 1978.
43. Campagni W.V., Preston J.D., Reisbick M.H.: Measurement of paint-on die spacers used for casting relief. *J. Prosthet. Dent.* 47:606, 1982.
44. Fukui H., Lacy A.M., Jendersen M.D.: Effectiveness of hardening films on die stone. *J. Prosthet. Dent.* 44:57, 1980.
45. Yoder J.L., Thayer K.E.: A rubber-base impression technique for fixed partial dentures. *J. Prosthet. Dent.* 12:339, 1962.
46. Benfield J.W., Lyons G.V.: Precision dies from elastic impressions. *J. Prosthet. Dent.* 12:737, 1962.
47. Dawson P.E.: *Evaluation, Diagnosis and Treatment of Occlusal Problems.* St. Louis, C.V. Mosby Co., 1974.
48. Kaiser D.A.: Fabricating a customized incisal guide table. *J. Prosthet. Dent.* 45:568, 1981.
49. Hoyle D.E.: Fabrication of a customized anterior guide table. *J. Prosthet. Dent.* 48:490, 1982.

CHAPTER 16

Pontics and Pontic Form

KEITH E. THAYER, D.D.S.

PONTICS, THE UNITS of fixed partial dentures that replace missing natural teeth, must satisfy several needs. They must restore function, be hygienically maintainable, be biologically and esthetically acceptable, and be comfortable.[1]

Pontic design and construction is a controversial subject that is complicated by a vast number of confusing terms and empirical opinion. There is a lack of extensive research to support the opinions expressed. Our discussion of pontics will be confined to two areas, materials, and design.

MATERIALS

Three dental materials are currently in use for fabricating pontics. They are metal, porcelain, and acrylic resin. Metal may be used alone or in combination with either porcelain or acrylic resin, primarily as an esthetic veneer. Pontic fabrication is perhaps one of the few areas where material designs have become simpler rather than more complicated over the years. Previously there was a wide array of manufactured acrylic resin and porcelain facings or "pontics" available to use in conjunction with a cast backing. These included various pin facings for both anterior and posterior replacements where metal pins were a part of the facing. The popular Steele's line of facings (interchangeable facings) included flat backs, trupontics, and sanipontics. These depended on posts on the manufactured backing and slots in the facing to secure the acrylic or porcelain facing to the metal part of the pontic.

Since the developing and refining of the porcelain-fused-to-metal technique, more pontics are fabricated in this manner than all other available techniques combined. The second most common esthetic combination is the use of one of the many acrylic resins available, cured or processed to a mechanically retentive, cast pontic framework. These two combinations account for the vast majority of the esthetic veneered pontics now fabricated.

Where esthetics are not important the all metal pontic is still widely used. Originally, these were traditionally made of a dental gold alloy. As gold prices increased the search widened for a less expensive substitute. There are now many alloys available that are approximately half gold and half other metals, but provide a yellow colored metal. Where the yellow color is important these are popular. All of the nonprecious metals are silver in color and serve the same mechanical and functional requirements for pontics as the gold alloys.

In addition to the esthetic variations in the three materials, two other factors are important to consider when selecting materials. They must be resistant to wear and compatible to soft tissue.

Acrylic resin is by far the least resistant to wear. Consequently, it is seldom the material of choice for occlusal surfaces of posterior pontics. Its wear characteristics are also a factor in anterior esthetics. Unprotected functioning incisal edges may wear and deform rapidly. Toothbrush abrasion and abrasive foods or habits will wear facial surfaces over a longer period and detract from the esthetic appearance. Acrylic resin also has a tendency to gradually discolor in certain oral environments. The major advantage of acrylic resin is its resiliency and resulting resistance to fracture. Porcelain, on the other hand, is friable and subject to the same fracture as tooth enamel, but is resistant to wear and color change. These characteristics should be given careful consideration when the material is selected for a particular patient. The projected use and/or abuse of the restoration would be a major factor in material selection.

Soft tissue tolerance of the various materials is of major interest and concern. Traditionally, glazed porcelain has been supported as the most ideal and best tolerated by the soft tissue. This is usually followed in preference by gold and acrylic, respectively. More recently, numerous studies have shown no significant difference in tolerance levels of the three materials.[2–4] Perhaps equally or even more important than the material is the surface quality, contour, and area contacted by the pontic. Hence, a poorly designed or porous porcelain pontic would likely cause more gingival irritation than a well-polished and well-contoured acrylic pontic. By the same token, highly polished and well-contoured gold contacting soft tissue would be less irritating than poor quality porcelain or acrylic.

Oral hygiene maintained by the patient may be a more important factor in gingival tissue health than material, surface quality, design, and area of contact combined. According to one study,[5] when poor oral hygiene conditions existed tissue inflammation developed wherever there was contact regardless of pontic design. With good oral hygiene, healthy tissue could be maintained[6] with any pontic design, including a full saddle. However, when pontic design was changed from saddle to ridge-lap to modified ridge-lap to spheroidal, maintaining good oral hygiene became easier. This was a result of the fact that gingival embrasures were more open and there were more convex contours of pontic-tissue contact in smaller areas.

DESIGN

Pontic design involves several facets of pontic construction. These include ridge adaptation and contour, pontic connector design, and the size and shape of occlusal surfaces of pontics that must be determined, as well as contours of axial surfaces.

Ridge Adaptation and Contour

Some of the terminology applied to the surface contour of that part of the pontic opposite the edentulous ridge soft tissue include denture-base type, saddle, modified saddle, ridge-lap, modified ridge-lap, lap facing, spheroidal, modified spheroidal, egg shape, bullet shape, heart shape, sanitary, modified sanitary, and bar pontics.[1, 5–8] The differences between these are sometimes slight and may be only semantic (Table 16–1).

The denture-base type contact and the saddle (Fig 16–1) are generally not indicated. They provide no support for a fixed partial denture and are seldom, if ever,

TABLE 16–1.—Types of Pontics

TISSUE CONTACT DESCRIPTION	LOCATION OF RIDGE CONTACT	SIZE OF RIDGE CONTACT	LINGUAL FORM	EMBRASURE FORM
Denture-base type	Facial-crest-lingual	Very large	Full	Closed
Saddle	Facial-crest-lingual	Very large	Full	Slightly open
Modified saddle	Facial & crest	Large	Open to lingual of crest	Slightly open
Ridge-lap	Facially from center of crest	Medium	Open to center of crest	Slightly open
Modified ridge-lap	Facial surface only	Small	Open to facial of crest	Slightly open
Lap facing	Pinpoint facial	Very small	Open to facial surface	Slightly open
Spheroidal	Gingival crest	Very small	Convex	Slightly open
Modified spheroidal	Gingival crest	Very small	Less convex	Open
Egg-shaped	Gingival crest	Very small	Convex	Open
Bullet-shaped	Gingival crest	Very small	Flatter	Open
Heart-shaped	Gingival crest	Very small	Slight concave	Open
Sanitary	None	None	Open	No embrasure
Modified sanitary	None	None	Open	No embrasure
Bar-shaped	None	None	Open	No embrasure

a factor in esthetics, phonetics, or function. They almost certainly provide a more difficult if not impossible task for oral hygiene.

The modified saddle (Fig 16–1), ridge-lap, modified ridge-lap, and lap facing (Fig 16–2) are all comparable because they never contact soft tissue lingual to the crest of the ridge. The modified saddle and ridge-lap would usually involve a slightly larger area of tissue contact and a somewhat greater tendency to concavities in the contacting surface. The modified ridge-lap is generally flat or slightly convex in all tissue contacting areas. It is the term more often applied to posterior pontics whereas lap facing terminology applies to anterior pontics with only pin point contact on the labial aspect of the edentulous ridge. The amount of interproximal gingival embrasure opening on all of these can be varied depending on the phonetic and esthetic demands. The more open the gingival embrasures the less the area of pontic-tissue contact and the greater the ease of plaque-free oral hygiene maintenance. Because this design presents normal tooth contour appearance, it is usually

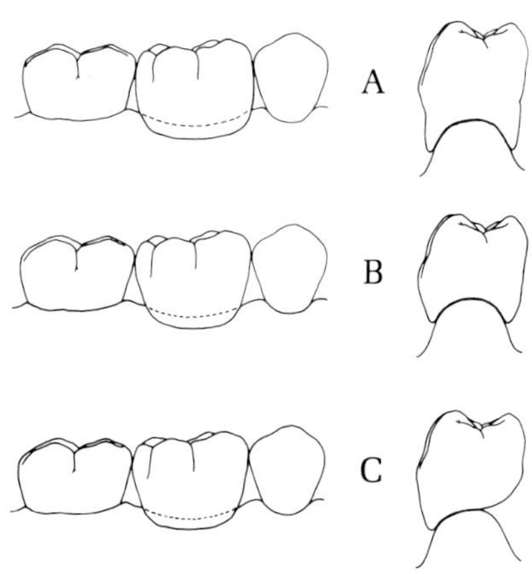

Fig 16–1.—Pontic designs: **(A)** denture-base type, **(B)** saddle, **(C)** modified saddle. All have large areas of contact of pontic to ridge both faciolingually and mesiodistally. All have definite large areas of concave contact of pontic to ridge.

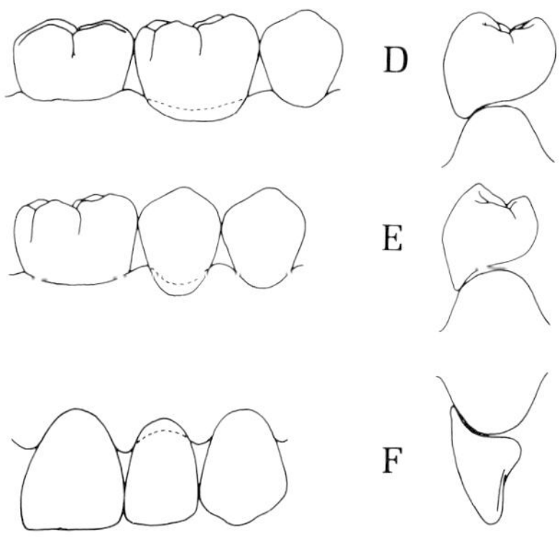

Fig 16–2.—Pontic designs: **(D)** ridge-lap, **(E)** modified ridge-lap, **(F)** lap facing. All have minimal tissue contact and only on its facial aspect of the ridge. Gingival embrasures may be esthetic but are more open. Pontic surfaces are less concave.

indicated in the maxillary arch and may sometimes be the choice for mandibular anterior replacements. Occasionally, it is used in mandibular premolars, but seldom in molars.

The spheroidal, modified spheroidal (Fig 16–3), egg shape, bullet shape, and heart shape pontics (Fig 16–4) all depend on tissue apposition at or near the crest of the ridge. They are all contraindicated whenever esthetics is a concern. They are most often used in mandibular posterior areas but are frequently the design of choice in the mandibular anterior region. Occasionally, they may be used in the maxillary posterior region. The area of tissue contact is small and the contacting surface is convex. Depending on ridge form and contour, the contact may vary in its linguofacial position. It is highly indicated when the occlusogingival pontic space is somewhat restricted. In these cases it provides the best access for oral hygiene maintenance. All of the spheroidal pontic designs are also indicated, if esthetics will allow, where there has been excessive bone loss resulting in an exaggerated occlusal gingival dimension. If the convex gingival surface of the pontic is kept at least 2 mm from the gingival crest, good gingival health and oral hygiene will be enhanced.

Positive tissue pressure is undesirable with any of the pontic designs that contact gingival tissue.[1, 6] Passive contact allows for physiologic stimulation of the gingiva in function and helps maintain its tone. If the pontic is left only a few tenths of a millimeter out of contact, the tissue will inevitably proliferate into contact unless regular stimulation, other than functional, prevents it. In the case of sanitary pontics where 2 or more mm of space is present the action of tongue, cheek, and food usually provides enough stimulation to maintain gingival health.

The sanitary, modified sanitary, and bar shaped pontics (Fig 16–5) are all designed for no contact with gingival tissue. Perhaps this is the ideal relationship for

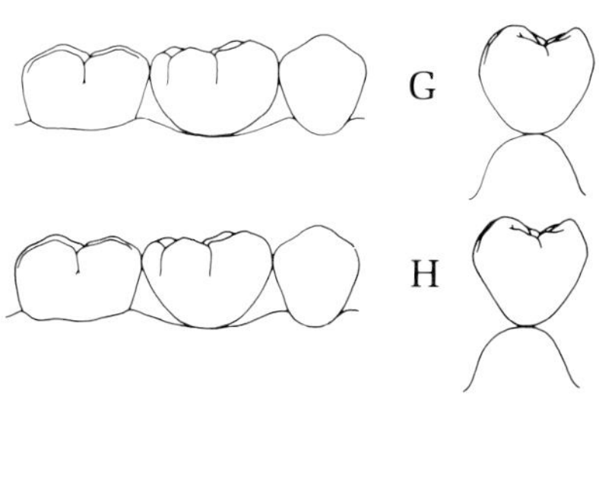

Fig 16–3.—Pontic designs: **(G)** spheroidal, **(H)** modified spheroidal. Tissue contact at crest of ridge only with no concave pontic surfaces. Modified spheroidal is slightly flattened in its gingival half of axial surfaces.

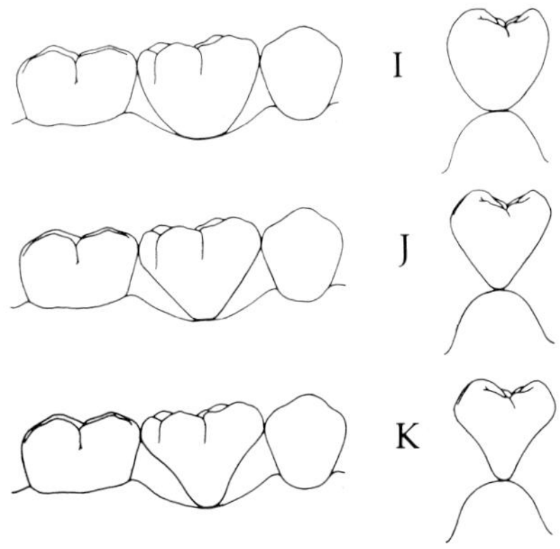

Fig 16–4.—Pontic designs: **(I)** egg-shaped, **(J)** bullet-shaped, **(K)** heart-shaped. All have small, convex tissue contact areas on crest of ridge. Gingival embrasures are open with convex, nearly flat and slightly concave axial surfaces.

tissue health. Esthetics, phonetics, and patient acceptance will seldom permit it in areas other than the mandibular posteriors. If there is not enough space between the tissue side of the pontic and the gingiva, a minimum of 2 mm, the tissue has a tendency to proliferate and eventually contact the under surface of the pontic. This surface is not contoured for tissue contact, so a more serious inflammatory result will often occur. The major difference in the design of the modified sanitary pontic[7] (Fig 16–5) is that it is concave mesiodistally and resembles an arched bridge span. It provides a strong solder joint connector with the retainers and the optimum strength with the maximum clearance from the gingiva in restricted vertical space replacements.

Regardless of pontic design, the resultant tissue health is of utmost concern. Proliferation is kept to a minimum by proper stimulation from the action of food, tongue, cheek, floss, and toothbrush. The pontic design for every patient must allow for soft tissue stimulation or exercise, if you will, by one or more of these means. If not, unhealthy gingiva will ultimately and certainly result.

Pontic Connector Design

The pontic connector design is important to the quality of the fixed partial denture. Optimum strength is required without encroachment on the gingival embra-

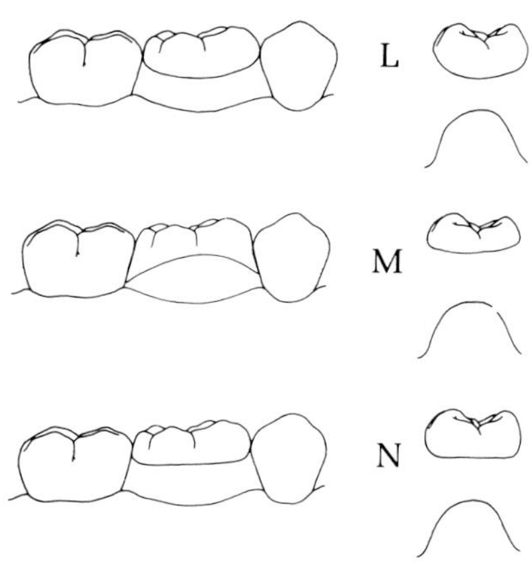

Fig 16–5.—Pontic designs: **(L)** sanitary, **(M)** modified sanitary, **(N)** bar-shaped. None of these designs have any contact with the edentulous ridge tissue.

sure with resultant irritation to the interdental gingiva. The optimum condition is provided by the modified sanitary pontic design.[7]

The connector, whether it is cast or soldered, should be well-contoured and polished so as not to invite accumulation of plaque and debris.[6] It should be as wide buccolingually and occlusogingivally as allowable without compromising gingival health. The gingival aspect should be concave mesiodistally, between the pontic and the retainer, but convex buccolingually to allow for proper cleaning and flossing.

Most pontic to retainer connectors are rigid. When the case indicates a nonrigid connector in the form of a precision or semiprecision dovetail lock design consideration should be given and care taken to satisfy the above criteria for rigid connectors. Most stress breaker connectors require more space occlusogingivally and buccolingually than do rigid connectors. Broken stress connectors are most indicated when a common path of insertion cannot be prepared on the abutment teeth. It is also indicated in some extensive restorations where cross arch splinting is desired without fabricating the entire arch in one continuous restoration. The stress-breaker may also be used for more design flexibility required by the distribution of the remaining teeth.

When multiple pontics are used in a restoration the connectors between the pontics may be developed in the same manner as the pontic to retainer connector. It is frequently necessary to create gingival embrasures between the pontics for esthetic reasons. In some posterior areas it is recommended to fuse the pontics. This results in one continuous convex area of contact to gingiva for two pontics.[9] This design is easily maintained by the patient and may enhance the strength of the connector.

Cases where there has been considerable bone loss and esthetics is a factor, present special challenges (Figs 16–6,A–C and 16–7,A–D). Fused multiple pontics that use pink porcelain to simulate gingival tissue can sometimes be helpful.[10] The fused pontics can be designed with maintainable convex surfaces. If pink porcelain is to be used a pink porcelain shade that blends with the patient's gingiva must be selected. Some labs have pink porcelain selection tabs available. A color photograph can also be helpful in pink porcelain applications.

Occlusal Surfaces and Axial Contours

Three general concepts and philosophies exist on the width of the occlusal surface.[1] One recommends the pontic be a fifth to a third narrower than the tooth being replaced. The second advocates making the pontic the same width as the tooth being replaced, whereas the last minimizes the significance of the pontic width.

Width reduction may reduce the stroke force on abutment teeth from the biomechanical aspect.[11] This is countered by the theory that proprioception exercises a control that automatically regulates occlusal forces regardless of the dimension of the opposing food tables.

Reducing the buccolingual dimension may enhance the patient's ability to clean the area.[12] In some cases, such as in premolars, narrowing may create an irregularity or depression on the lingual that in fact makes oral hygiene maintenance more difficult.

Full pontic dimension provides protection of the soft tissue and good function.

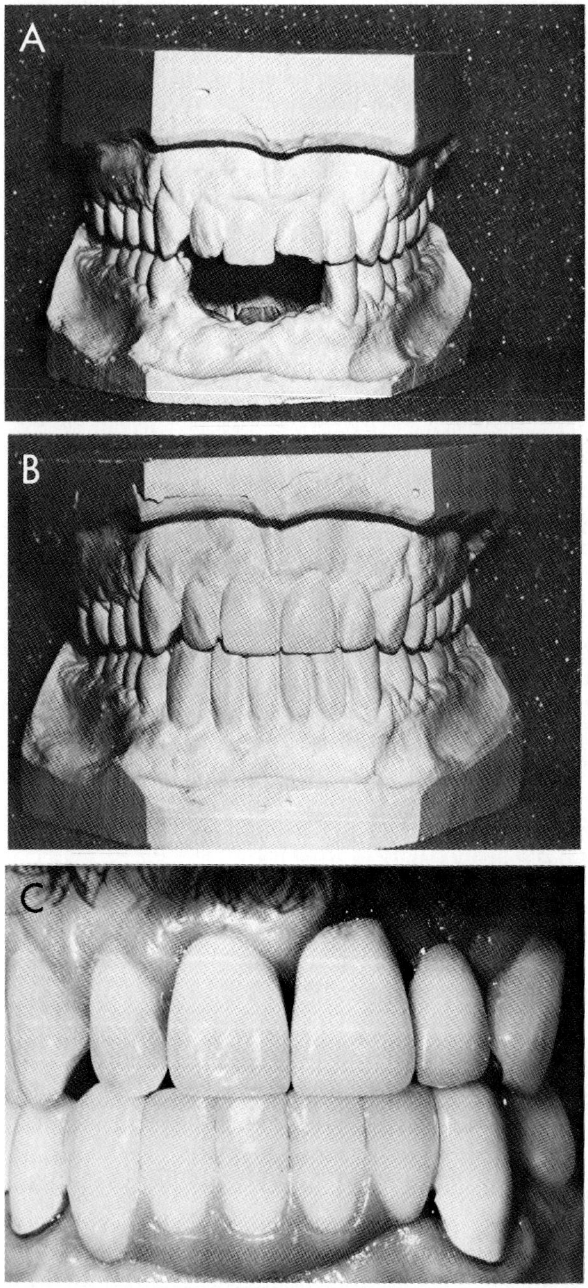

Fig 16–6.—A, study casts of patient with excessive bone loss of residual ridge. **B,** diagnostic wax-up of case for esthetic pontics. **C,** finished fixed partial denture with five pontics and pink gingival porcelain creating a fused type pontic-ridge contact. The pink porcelain controls the apparent tooth length for esthetics.

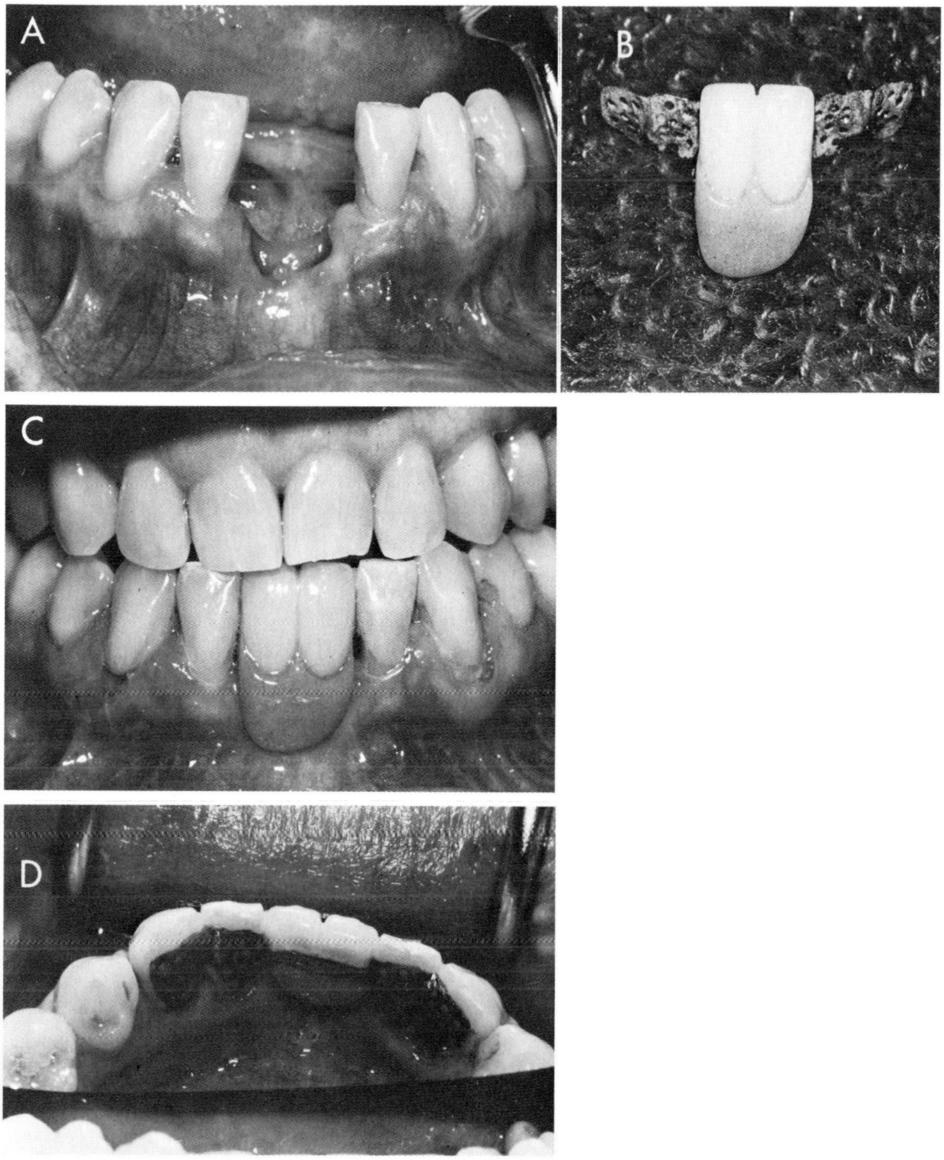

Fig 16–7.—A, missing mandibular central incisors with exaggerated bone loss and ridge defect. **B,** acid-etch fixed partial denture with pink porcelain of convex design. **C,** fixed partial denture in the mouth with controlled esthetic length of replacement pontics. **D,** lingual view of finished restoration.

Occasionally, full contour may be a factor in esthetics though the majority of width reduction is usually done from the lingual. In short pontics, occlusogingivally, full width may provide too much gingival protection and in fact promote undesirable tissue proliferation. Functional efficiency can usually be effected from good anatomy and appropriate spillways regardless of the width of the pontic.

Pontic width determination should be the result of individual determination for each restoration. The length of the span, number, and position of missing teeth, height of the edentulous space, width and contour of the residual ridge, anticipated functional load, condition of support, and numbers and location of abutment teeth should all be taken into consideration in determining pontic width.

The axial surface contours range from full anatomic to nonanatomic such as the sanitary designs and the gingival convergence seen in the various spheroidal pontics. Where esthetics require, full anatomic form is obviously important. Lingual contour both anterior and posterior should be designed to minimize food impaction and will be affected by the ridge size and form. In general, it is recommended that proximal surface contours follow normal tooth anatomy with full freedom to alter the contours where existing conditions so indicate.

Finally, the occlusal scheme that is developed in the pontic is of extreme importance. The number and location of occlusal contacts have an effect on loads transmitted to the abutment teeth. Care should be taken that there are no contacts on the inclined planes of the occlusal anatomy. These transmit undesirable horizontal loads to abutments. No balancing or nonworking contacts should exist on the pontic. If minimizing the load is important, the pontic should disclude in working and protrusive excursions as well.

RIDGE MODIFICATIONS

All of our attention has been directed to pontic materials and their shape, form, and design. One additional important consideration remains. That is the shape and condition of the edentulous ridge and tissue.[6, 8, 13] If ridge modification is contemplated, careful examination should be made. If redundant soft tissue irregularities exist because of improperly designed or maintained previous pontics, correction can often be quickly, easily, and accurately done with electrosurgery. The ideal soft tissue thickness is about 2 mm. This should be considered when electrosurgical contouring is contemplated.

If the edentulous ridge irregularities are the result of bony contours, then surgical osseous recontouring is required and recommended to provide the best possible opposing contour for our pontic. This is an often neglected or overlooked aspect of mouth preparation for fixed partial dentures. It can be quickly and easily done and can significantly enhance the success of the restoration.

SUMMARY

The attributes of the ideal pontic and the ideal ridge morphology[13] should include the following:

Ideal Pontic

1. Accurate and delicate ridge contact;
2. Minimal ridge contact. Facial aspect only for esthetic gingival pontics and ridge crest only for all spheroidal type designs;
3. Embrasure contours that promote gingival health and provide access for oral hygiene maintenance;
4. Pontic width determined in compliance with requirements for each restoration;
5. No sharp edges or angles anywhere on the pontic;

6. Axial and gingival pontic surfaces that are flat or slightly convex; and
7. Pontic materials that are carefully selected and handled. Surfaces should be free of defects and irregularities and should be highly polished or glazed.

Ideal Ridge

1. Gingiva that is firmly attached to the underlying alveolus;
2. Tissue surface that is smooth and regular, well-keratinized and healthy;
3. No subsurface bony irregularities;
4. No frenum and muscle attachments to the ridge; and
5. Ideally, a ridge with a gently concave contour mesiodistally at the crest as well as on the facial aspect of the edentulous area, and gently convex faciolingually.

REFERENCES

1. Council on dental materials and devices, pontics in fixed prosthesis—status report. Assisted by Gratton D.R. *J. Am. Dent. Assoc.* 91:613, 1975.
2. Henry P.J., Johnston J.F., Mitchel D.F.: Tissue changes beneath fixed partial dentures. *J. Prosthet. Dent.* 16:937, 1966.
3. Podshadley A.G.: Gingival response to pontics. *J. Prosthet. Dent.* 19:51, 1968.
4. Clayton J.A., Green E.: Ruffness of pontic materials and dental plaque. *J. Prosthet. Dent.* 23:407, 1970.
5. Hirshberg S.M.: The relationship of oral hygiene to embrasure and pontic design—a preliminary study. *J. Prosthet. Dent.* 27:26, 1972.
6. Crispin B.J.: Tissue response to posterior denture base-type pontics. *J. Prosthet. Dent.* 42:257, 1979.
7. Perel M.L.: A modified sanitary pontic. *J. Prosthet. Dent.* 28:589, 1972.
8. Stein R.S.: Pontic–residual ridge relationship: A research report. *J. Prosthet. Dent.* 16:251, 1966.
9. Becker C.M., Kaldahl W.B.: Current theories of crown contour, margin placement, and pontic design. *J. Prosthet. Dent.* 45:268, 1981.
10. Behrend D.A.: The design of multiple pontics. *J. Prosthet. Dent.* 46:634, 1981.
11. Beke A.L.: The biomechanics of pontic width reduction for fixed partial dentures. *J. Acad. Gen. Dent.* 22:28, 1974.
12. Howard W.W., Ueno H., Pruitt C.O.: Standards of pontic design. *J. Prosthet. Dent.* 47:493, 1982.
13. Kapin S.H., Murray J.D., Schoolnik P.R.: Pontic-ridge interrelationships in fixed prosthodontics. *Quint. Int.* 12:151, 1981.

CHAPTER 17

Finishing and Fitting of Cast Restorations

IRAJ SHAFAGH, D.M.D.

THE GOLD CASTING has rough surfaces when it is removed from the investment. Before it is placed in the mouth it must be finished, fitted, smoothed, and polished. The casting must have a smooth, highly polished surface so as to reduce accumulation of bacterial plaque that is harmful to the health of the periodontium.[1]

LABORATORY PROCEDURES

Sprue Removal

A separating disc is used to cut the sprue from the casting. Diagonal cutting pliers should not be used because the forces generated by them may distort a thin casting. The handpiece is held with a firm palm grasp while the sprue adjacent to the casting is cut. Tilting of the disc during cutting will cause the disc to bind in the cut groove. This will either break the disc or flip the casting out of the operator's hand. After the sprue is removed, the separating disc can be used to trim the remaining portions of the sprue attachment on the casting until the contour in that area is continuous with the contour of the restoration surrounding the sprue.

At this time any other rough areas of the casting should be smoothed with a coarse pumice impregnated rubber wheel. Garnet or sandpaper discs may also be used. Light pressure should be used, and the disc should be moved about quickly to avoid the formation of facets or flat spots. Then a ⅝-inch fine grit rubber wheel is used in a similar manner to further smooth the surface. The axial surface should be finished to, but not over, the margin. Wheels and discs should be rotated parallel to the margin, rather than perpendicular. Then the casting should be inspected for obvious defects. The casting may be pickled, primarily to remove surface oxides. Most pickling solutions are not designed to remove any significant amount of investment.

Fitting on Removable Die

Before contouring and smoothing, the fit of the casting should be checked by seating it on the die. It is a waste of time to finish and polish the casting before making sure that it can be seated completely, that the marginal adaptation is acceptable, and that the proximal contacts are correct.

The internal portion of the casting should be carefully inspected for any irregularities or projecting nodules or bubbles of gold. Any irregularities should be carefully removed with an appropriate size round bur. When removing nodules in the area of the line angles, a no. ½ to no. 2 round bur in the straight handpiece should be used. A no. 4 to no. 6 round bur is recommended for more assessible areas. When it is assured that there are no internal discrepancies on the casting, it is gently placed on the die and checked for complete seating and marginal adaptation. If the casting does not seat completely, its internal portion should be reinspected carefully for additional irregularities. The preparation portion of the die should also be inspected for any small surface defects. If any are found, the corresponding areas in the casting are examined and relieved.

If the casting seems to be uniformly small, the internal surface can be relieved chemically with aqua regia or electrolytically by deplating or stripping. It is extremely difficult to mechanically relieve a tight-fitting casting without substantially reducing its retention, so this procedure is not recommended routinely. When using chemical or electrolytic relief, all margins and external surfaces should be protected with either wax or fingernail polish. Stripping has its greatest effect on projections or elevations. The margin is a vulnerable portion of the casting.[2] The amount of electrolytic relief of a casting is controlled by three factors: intensity of the current, temperature of the solution, and concentration of the ions in the solution. The stripping should be done for 10 to 15 second periods, and the casting should be checked on the die after each period. If the casting does not seat after a total of two to three minutes of stripping, it is unlikely that additional relief will result in an acceptable fit.

If a casting appears to be large enough to fit the die but does not seem to seat completely, the interference should be located. There are several types of indicator pastes that can be used to locate the responsible premature areas. They vary in their effectiveness. A paste of chloroform and rouge is easily made and is as effective as any in locating internal prematurities. One of the more successful methods of locating the axial premature areas is to create a mat surface on the inside of the casting by gentle sandblasting. The casting is then seated firmly on the die, and removed and inspected for shiny or burnished areas. These areas are then carefully relieved by an appropriate sized round bur.

If, after careful selective mechanical relief or stripping, a casting does not seat completely, the casting is remade. Additional relief of the internal surface of a casting will usually result in a poor fitting casting that is clinically unacceptable.

Fitting on the Working Cast

When a casting seats completely on the removable die, it should be tried on the preparation in the working cast. Because it is necessary to have a small amount of excess contour in the casting for finish and polishing procedures, the adjacent proximal contacts on the working cast should be relieved just before adjusting the contacts on the casting. A contact that is slightly excessive can be adjusted in the mouth and is more desirable than having to add the contact with solder. The amount of overcontouring must be carefully controlled because excessive contacts are a frequent cause of incomplete seating.

The contact areas should have a satin finish. The casting is seated with finger pressure. If it does not seat completely it is removed and the proximal contact inspected for any shiny or burnished area. Coarse discs and stones should not be used for adjustment of contacts because it may result in an open or weak contact.

An abrasive rubber disc or fine sandpaper disc is preferred to remove shiny marks, and the casting is again placed on the preparation. This procedure is repeated until the casting seats completely.

Gross Occlusal Adjustment

The fabrication of fixed partial dentures requires properly mounted full arch casts that should be accurately positioned on an appropriate articulator. If the casts are mounted properly and the articulator set appropriately, the castings can be accurately adjusted. Gross occlusal prematurities can be more easily adjusted in an articulator than in the mouth because of better visibility and easier access. The gross prematurities are marked with articulating paper and relieved with a green stone until the remaining working model teeth are contacting.

At this time the grooves on the occlusal surface are smoothed with a no. 0 bud finishing bur. The cusp ridges are also smoothed and blended into the grooves on the occlusal surface with a *small*, rubber sulci disc. The axial surfaces and line angles are final checked for smoothness and proper contours. No polishing of the restoration is necessary at this time. The casting is now ready to be tried in the patient's mouth.

PATIENT PROCEDURES

The try-in procedure can be done on most patients without administering a local anesthetic. During the adjustment of the casting it is important to have the patient's tactile sense unimpaired. However, if the procedure is painful for the patient an anesthetic should be given.

The temporary restoration is removed. This should be done carefully with a spoon excavator, Backhaus towel forceps, or a straight chisel and a small mallet. Any cement left on the surface of the preparation, including the gingival sulcus, should be carefully removed. All small particles should be thoroughly washed away.

Contact Adjustment

The casting is placed on the preparation and seated with firm finger pressure. No excessive pressure should be exerted by the patient or operator on the casting. If the casting does not seat completely the most likely cause is an overcontoured proximal surface or contact area. The casting is held firmly in place and both proximal contacts tested with dental floss. Occasionally a patient will be able to tell that the restoration is wedging one or both of the adjacent teeth, particularly if local anesthesia is not used. The restoration contact should be as tight as the other tooth contacts in the mouth. If it is considerably tighter, or if the floss will not pass through the contact, the casting is removed and examined. If the casting has a satin finish on the proximal, there will be a burnished area where the tight contact occurred. Some operators blacken the proximal surface with graphite and find the offending proximal surface by a black mark on the adjacent tooth as well as by a shiny surface on the casting. Others use coating or pressure indicator pastes or rouge and chloroform.

When the overcontoured area is identified, it should be relieved and the casting reseated on the tooth. The procedure is repeated until the casting seats properly on the preparation with normal proximal contacts.

Castings with open contacts will allow food impaction and inevitably cause caries and periodontal disease. Open contacts may also cause a lack of stability in the occlusion. Such castings are corrected by soldering a contact or by remaking the casting.

Marginal Fit

The margins of the restoration should be carefully checked visually or with an explorer to make certain that there are no open margins and that the restoration is completely seated. Because radiographs are two-dimensional, the marginal fit cannot be precisely determined by this means alone. Visual and tactile examination must also be used.

If the temporary restoration is under-contoured or ill-fitted, the soft tissue may cover a subgingival shoulder preparation. Organized blood clots may form a paper-thin translucent tissue that covers the margin. In either case, the impingement of the tissue may prevent complete seating of the casting. The interfering tissue should either be removed with electrosurgery or be retracted before the insertion of the casting. It is also important to determine whether the temporary or final restoration is over- or under-contoured or if the tissue has covered the margin of the preparation.

If the casting seems too tight and does not seat uniformly, the casting may be too small. If the casting has not been previously electrolytically relieved, such relieving can be done for ten second intervals and then tried back on the tooth.

If the casting will not go into place and the proximal contacts are not too tight, there may be some minute undercut, unseen defect, or distortion preventing the seating. Water soluble indicator solutions can be used to coat the inside of the casting. The casting is replaced on the tooth and the patient is asked to seat it with occlusal force on a cotton roll or wooden stick. Areas preventing seating will appear as shiny spots on the internal surface of the casting. These spots are removed and the casting replaced. An alternative technique uses a matte finish on the inner surface of a casting that is produced by sand blasting. Shiny spots will designate areas that require relieving. If a casting persists in not seating completely and the cause cannot be quickly determined and corrected, it should be remade. If the casting fits the die but does not fit the tooth a new impression should be made.

Occlusal Adjustment

To provide a basis for comparison, the patient should be asked to close into maximum intercuspation without the new restoration. The position of the teeth adjacent to the prepared areas and the opposite side of the arch are observed for completeness of closure and occlusal contact relationships. If multiple teeth are prepared, each of the castings should be seated separately and completely adjusted before seating additional castings. After completing the adjustment of one casting, it should be removed before seating and adjusting the next casting.

Centric Adjustment

If the occlusal scheme has not been changed and the habitual or centric occlusion position is desired, the patient is asked to close in forceful intercuspation. If the mandible deflects to the side where the casting is located, the inner incline of the maxillary lingual cusp and/or the inner incline of the mandibular buccal cusp probably needs adjustment. If the mandible deflects to the side away from the casting, one of two deflective contacts requires correction. There may be a premature contact between the inner incline of the maxillary buccal cusp and the outer incline of the mandibular buccal cusp. There may also be a contact between the outer incline of the maxillary lingual cusp and the inner incline of the mandibular lingual cusp that needs adjustment.

A piece of thin marking ribbon should be cut and placed in a Miller forceps. The occlusal surface should be dried with a cotton roll or air and the ribbon held between the casting and the opposing tooth. The casting should first be adjusted in maximum intercuspation. The casting is removed from the mouth and the marks relieved only on the appropriate surfaces. Most marking ribbons tend to overmark. Because of this, marks must be analyzed carefully before grinding. Only areas that cause deflection or prevent complete closure should be removed. Care should be taken not to grind away centric contacts when adjusting mandibular side deflection and excursive interferences. A different color marking for centric and eccentric contacts is helpful in accomplishing this. The operator should also be careful not to overcorrect the casting. This can be avoided by placing a narrow strip of .0005-inch thick silver plastic shim stock over the casting and having the patient close. The shim stock should offer equal resistance from removal between restored and nonrestored teeth. If the strip holds on the casting and not the adjacent teeth, the casting is still too high. If it holds on the adjacent teeth and not on the casting, the casting is out of occlusion.

Even if habitual occlusion is desired, the dentist must avoid creating any new contact with the new restoration when the patient's mandible is in centric relation or the most retruded position. Thus the mandible should be hinged and guided into its most retruded position and closed slowly until the first tooth contact occurs. If the patient points to the tooth bearing the casting, that prematurity should be located by a different color marking ribbon and adjusted. Other markings on the casting should be retained.

Excursive Adjustment

When the occlusion has been adjusted to allow maximum intercuspation, the centric contacts are re-marked with one color of ribbon. For excursive adjustment a different color ribbon should be used. The excursive adjustment of the casting depends on the occlusal scheme desired. If the goal is a cuspid protected occlusion, contacts between the inner inclines of the maxillary buccal cusps and outer inclines of mandibular buccal cusps should be removed until the posterior teeth disclude immediately when the working side movement is made. If group function is desired, these surfaces are left in contact so that most or all posterior teeth are bearing the working side forces. In group function the most suitable posterior teeth should be contacting in working excursion.

Working side interferences on the casting are adjusted by having the patient move into a working relationship on the side of the mouth where the casting is located. Any contacts on outer inclines of maxillary lingual cusps and inner inclines of mandibular lingual cusps must be eliminated also.

Contacts on the nonworking side excursive movements are destructive interferences. These can be tested by placing the narrow strip of plastic shim stock between the casting and opposing tooth in nonworking position. The shim stock should be held tightly in the centric position, but as soon as the nonworking movement starts, the plastic stock should be easily removed from between the casting and opposing teeth. If not, the interference should be located and eliminated on the inner inclines of the maxillary lingual cusps and the inner inclines of the mandibular buccal cusp.

If anterior protected occlusion is desired, the patient should be asked to move the mandible forward. Any protrusive interferences are identified and eliminated on the distal inclines of the posterior maxillary teeth. Ideally anterior teeth should not touch in the maximum intercuspation. They should be separated by a minimum of the thickness of the .0005-inch plastic shim stock. Because anterior teeth help to disengage posterior teeth during excursive movement, the contacts that appear on them during excursive movements are considered desirable.

FINISHING

Finishing is the process of contouring and smoothing the casting by reductive grinding using successively finer abrasives until the scratches are no longer visible to the naked eye. By finishing we also burnish the margins to the prepared tooth. Because of the risk of damage to the tooth and periodontal structures, subgingival margins should be burnished on the die with a beavertail burnisher. Supragingival margins can be finished on the tooth. With proper finishing procedures, margins can be adapted to the tooth to produce an opening between the margin and tooth that is less than the film thickness of the cement.[3]

The casting is placed on the preparation. The patient seats it firmly by closing on a cotton roll. Minute marginal discrepancies can sometimes be corrected by using a burnisher and fine abrasives. If there is a visibly significant discrepancy, the casting should be repeated. Using a coarse abrasive moves or drags gold, forming a soft granular lip that can be easily broken or deformed during subsequent manipulation.[4]

Any dull burnisher can be used to press the margins against the tooth surface while the casting is held in place with another instrument or by the patient's occlusion. Burnishing on the tooth alone will not significantly reduce the surface roughness.[5] Use of a white polishing stone will reduce the roughness at the margin. The white polishing stone, lubricated with petrolatum, is used for finishing after the burnishing.

The white stone should always rotate from casting to tooth surface under heavy pressure and at low speed. Slight amounts of gold and enamel are cut. The procedure should be continued until the margin is smooth and no open margin is felt with an explorer. The final smoothing can be achieved using a rubber wheel impregnated with abrasive and/or medium and fine cuttle discs that tend to create less heat than rubber wheels. All discs and abrasive wheels should be continuously moved over the surface to avoid creating flat spots or facets. The casting can be carefully finished to the margins by orienting the disc parallel to the margin rather than at right angles to it and by never allowing the disc to extend over the margin.

To prevent any damage to the margins, the casting can be removed with a Backhaus towel forceps. A removal knob can be made an integral part of the restoration when the wax pattern is fabricated. When the casting has been removed for the last time, the knob is ground off and the area is polished.

POLISHING

Polishing refers to placing the high shine on the surface of the casting to provide a smooth surface that will be less susceptible to plaque collection. In a polished casting the scratches are no longer visible to the naked eye. All the axial surfaces are polished with tripoli on a soft mandrel bristle brush. With another soft bristle brush, used only for rouge, the axial surfaces should be polished to the subgingival margins without rounding them. Supragingival margins that are finished and polished in the mouth should not be repolished.

The grooves can be smoothed with a small finishing bur and the ridges can be smoothed with a small sulcus disc, taking care not to destroy the occlusal contacts so carefully developed earlier. The occlusal and proximal surfaces can be sand blasted or air brushed to provide a matte finish. This dull surface will enable observation of facets or burnishing produced by occlusal contacts after the casting has been in the mouth for a short time. When sand blasting, remaining surfaces of the casting that are highly polished should be protected with masking tape.

POLISHING AFTER CEMENTATION

Polishing of the accessible margins of the casting should be done after cementation with amalgloss and a rubber cup. This can be followed by a fine cuttle disc that has been lubricated to make it flexible. The discs are always rotated from gold to tooth.

A correctly contoured, well-finished, and highly polished restoration is beautiful and comfortable. The quality of the restoration is also enhanced because good contour, finish, and polish promotes caries control and periodontal health.

ARMAMENTARIUM

1. Straight handpiece
2. Contra-angle handpiece
3. Separating disc on mandrel
4. Coarse pumice-impregnated rubber wheels
5. Assorted sandpaper discs
6. Fine pumice-impregnated rubber wheels
7. Sulcus disc on small head mandrel
8. No. 0 finishing bur
9. Assorted round burs
10. Articulating ribbon
11. Assorted green stones
12. Small mallet
13. Straight chisel
14. Backhaus towel forceps
15. Miller ribbon forceps
16. Gauze and cotton pellets
17. Cotton pliers

18. Wooden stick (orangewood)
19. .0005-inch silver plastic shim stock
20. Tapered white polishing stone
21. Cuttle discs on mandrel
22. Petrolatum
23. Tripoli and rouge
24. Mandrel bristle brush
25. Rubber cup on mandrel
26. Amalgloss

REFERENCES

1. Gildenhugs R.R., Stallard R.E.: Comparison of plaque accumulation on metal restorative surfaces. *Dent. Surv.* 51:56, 1975.
2. Welk D.A., Merrill O.M.: Electrochemical etching of gold castings. *Abst. Int. Assoc. Dent. Res.* 1966.
3. Christensen G.J.: Marginal fit of gold inlay castings. *J. Prosthet. Dent.* 16:297, 1966.
4. Eames W.B., Little R.M.: Movement of gold at cavosurface margins with finishing instruments. *J. Am. Dent. Assoc.* 75:147, 1967.
5. Hobo S., Matsuki H.: Accuracy of marginal fit of cast restorations. *Dent. Outlook (Japan)* 43:731, 1974.

CHAPTER 18

Cementation in Fixed Prosthodontics

KEITH E. THAYER, D.D.S.

MANY DENTISTS CONSIDER cementation to be the most important step in fixed prosthodontic treatment. Obviously, no one phase of a multi-step treatment is any more or less important than another. One may seem to be because it is chronologically closer to the completion and consequently more vivid. The same is true of an athletic contest where the final play or final minute seems so important but may have little or no more effect on the outcome than a similar period earlier in the contest. Yet, it is that closing action that is highlighted and long remembered as being most important.

As with any other step in treatment, cementation is critically important. A decision must be made as to whether temporary cementation for evaluation of the restoration is indicated. The cement to be used must be selected. The techniques and procedures used to assure complete seating and accurate fit and the actual clinical technique steps are of utmost importance relative to the quality and success of the cementation process. This chapter will examine these factors in detail.

TEMPORARY CEMENTATION

Temporary cementation of fixed restorations is an accepted and advantageous procedure. Temporary cementation of the final restoration for extended or unlimited periods, however, has little support.[1] The exception would be for unusual periodontal problem situations. There are many advantages that accrue from temporary cementation but they are not without their potential problems.

A major concern of many dentists is being unable to remove temporarily cemented restorations from the mouth easily and safely. The amount of frictional retention of the restoration is a major factor. If a powder-liquid system temporary cement is being used, the cement will not set if vaseline is substituted for the liquid. This powder-vaseline mixture will seal the tooth from the oral environment and prevent irritation and subsequent sensitivity of the tooth. It will add only slightly to the frictional retention of the restoration. Another excellent temporary cementation material is Opotow Trial* cement. This cement sets to a rubbery consistency, similar to silicone impression material, sealing the tooth from the oral environment and adding to the retention of the restoration. Because of the resi-

*Teledyne Co., Buffalo, NY 14225

liency of the material the dentist can be confident that the restoration can be removed.

The benefits of temporary cementation allow the dentist and the patient to have the opportunity to evaluate the restoration. When esthetics is important it provides an opportunity for reaction from family and friends in lights and environments other than the dental office. Occlusion can be verified in normal function. Contacts can be evaluated for food impaction and where pontics are involved, tissue response and any food collection problems can be determined. If problems arise in any of the above areas, modification and correction can be much more easily and effectively made if the restoration can be removed from the mouth. In fact, most such problems cannot be solved without removal from the mouth.

In a large percentage of cases, the fit of the restoration is improved after a brief period of temporary cementation. Restorations seat more completely and with more ease after contacts have adjusted and abutment tooth periodontal fibers have slightly realigned the teeth to the new restoration. Most importantly, if there are any subgingival margins, the gingival tissue has adapted to the environment of the new restoration and possible trapping of soft tissue between the restoration and preparation during final cementation is virtually eliminated.

After satisfactory acceptance of the restoration by both the patient and the dentist, final cementation should be done. From the psychologic standpoint, many patients are happier with their new restoration after having had the opportunity to evaluate and adjust to it knowing that if problems should exist or arise, there would be an opportunity to correct them.

PERMANENT CEMENTATION MATERIALS

Cement has been defined as "a paste that hardens into a stony substance—not adhesive."[2] The distinction should be made between cements and luting agents where adhesive qualities exist between the material and tooth structure and/or the restorative material. Some of the newer dental cements have such qualities. The distinctions between adhesive and nonadhesive cements involve chemical versus mechanical relationships between the cement and the surfaces to which it is applied.

Zinc phosphate cements, which were introduced in dentistry toward the end of the 19th century, have become the standard for dental cements used in placing cast restorations. The material has stood the test of time and has served well. Zinc phosphate cement (Table 18–1), however, is not without its disadvantages. It is irritating to vital tooth structure and has undoubtedly contributed to the death of many pulps. Obviously, this is of no concern when using on endodontically treated teeth. Solubility of the cement in the oral fluids is another concern. The accuracy of the marginal fit of the restoration to the tooth margin has a significant effect on this concern. If the marginal fit is accurate, there will be only a minute amount of cement exposed to the dissolving action of the oral fluids. Zinc phosphate cement is not adhesive, but depends on mechanical relationships for retention of the casting. Consequently surfaces that are over-tapered, short, and smooth do not lend themselves to good retention with zinc phosphate cement. With proper attention to case selection and preparation design these problems can usually be easily overcome.

TABLE 18–1.—Final Cements

CLASS	BRAND NAMES	SITUATIONS	FEATURES	PHYSICAL PROPERTIES			
				COMPRESSIVE STRENGTH	TENSILE STRENGTH	FILM THICKNESS	SOLUBILITY
Zinc phosphate	Flecks-Mizzy Zinc Cement-SSW Tenacin-Caulk Zinc Cement-Ames Elite-Interdent Superdent-Rugby Etc.	General use Long span Multiple unit Nonvital teeth Nonsensitive teeth	Reliable, time-proved, pulpal irritant, sealer or varnish may be indicated, setting time easily controlled	Good	Good	Good	Moderate
Polycarboxylate	Durelon-Premier Carboxylon-3M Poly-C-Ash Carboset-Kerr P.C.A.-S.S.W. Chemit-Bosworth Unite-Shofu Etc.	General use Single unit Short span Sensitive teeth	Nonirritating, good adhesive qualities but tooth and restoration surfaces *must* be clean Mixing time critical, must seat restoration before cement gloss disappears Sealer or varnish must *not* be used	Fair	Good	Good	Moderate
Glass ionomer	Chembond-Caulk Fugi-M.F.Patterson Etc.	General use Vital teeth High caries patient (Fl release) Dry field *must* be maintained during setting	Fl release for high caries patients, some early sensitivity No pulpal irritation, high sensitivity to early (first 10 minutes) moisture contamination	Good	Good	Good	Low

Reinforced ZOE (EBA)	Fynal-Caulk Super EBA-Bosworth Opotow Alumina-Getz Etc.	General use Single or short span Frictionally retentive restorations (long, parallel, accurate) Sensitive teeth	Non-irritating, easy and noncritical to mix, good retentive strength, low sensitivity to moisture during set	Fair	Good	Good	Moderate
Zinc silico-phosphates	Fluorothin-SSW Lucent-Caulk Etc.	Limited use Porcelain inlays and jackets High caries patients (Fl release) Nonsensitive teeth	Irritating to pulp, Fl release for high caries patients, ideal for esthetic improvement for translucent restorations High variation in film thickness	Good	Good	Fair	Low
Resin: Acrylic BIS-GMA	Grip-Caulk Enamelite-Lee Adaptic-J.& J. Concise-3M Etc. Unfilled composite or composite thinned with bonding agent.	Limited use Problem retention cases—may "salvage" old ill-fitting restorations Nonsensitive teeth	Most irritating to pulp, excess difficult to remove	Excellent	Excellent	Poor	Insoluble

More recently, a wide range of dental cements and luting agents have been developed, modified, and introduced to the profession.[3] Of those materials, the one that has gained the most widespread use is polycarboxylate cement (Table 18–1). Polycarboxylate cement has exceptional biologic compatibility and is ideal for use on vital teeth.[4] Good retention form is still required and the mixing and cementation technique is greatly altered compared with zinc phosphate cement.

Glass ionomer cements (Table 18–1) are the newest addition to the field and are growing in popularity. Perhaps their major problem is their vulnerability to aqueous attack during setting. Setting requires the maintenance of a dry field for a minimum of ten minutes. Modifications have been made to decrease the aqueous attack problem but this results in an increased viscosity of the material that is undesirable.[2] In all other respects the material seems to be desirable.

There are three other general classes of cements that are commonly available (Table 18–1). For the most part, they are modifications of dental materials not originally developed or used as final cements or luting agents. One of these is the zinc silico-phosphate cement that is a modification of the silicate cement restorative material. A second is reinforced zinc oxide and eugenol (EBA) that was developed from the zinc oxide and eugenol temporary cements. Finally, a large group of resin cements include acrylic and BIS-GMA. All of these together account for only a small percentage of the total dental restorations currently being cemented. As can be seen in Table 18–1, each does have its advantages and disadvantages that may be important to any particular patient in some special situations.[3]

CEMENTATION TECHNIQUES

When dealing with final cements many variables must be considered as having important input into the success or failure of the procedure. Film thickness of the cement is limited by the particle size of the cement powder, but powder with a particle size of 15 μ seldom results in a 15 μ film thickness of cement. A film thickness of 20 to 30 μ is generally accepted as a good standard.[3] However, such things as mixing time, temperature, humidity, liquid age, and seating time and pressure can easily increase the thickness of the cement film to from 200 to 300 μ! In addition, the length and taper of the preparation, coupled with the accuracy of the fit of the casting and the amount and consistency of freshly mixed cement that is placed in the casting, have significant effects on the seating of the restorations.

Compressive and tensile strengths have traditionally been key measures of the quality of final cements. Together, they are generally considered to describe the ability of a cement to retain a fixed prosthesis. Compressive strength tends to measure the quality of the cement to resist crushing and resultant breakdown from repeated loading, whereas tensile strength is more likely measured by the ability of the cement to adhere or attach to the surfaces of tooth and restoration. Both of these physical properties are influenced by such things as length and taper of preparation, manipulation of the material during cementation, and accuracy of the fit in addition to the cement selected and the loads the restoration is subjected to during function.

The technique and the material have a major effect on the success of our cementation procedures. A wide range of techniques, some of which appear somewhat contradictory in their results, appear in the dental literature.[5–8] Complete seating of the restoration after application of the luting agent is always a concern. Many factors influence seating. Film thickness or particle size of the cement is one factor. These properties are indicated for the various cements on the cement chart (Table 18–1). In addition, the consistency of the mix, the amount of cement applied, the degree of set of the cement at the time of seating and the geometry of the preparation and restoration all play a part and interact to affect the amount of incomplete seating of the restoration.

RESTORATION FABRICATION TECHNIQUES

Various controls are employed during the fabrication of castings in an attempt to enhance complete seating. Variation of the water-powder ratio of the investment will affect the size of the casting. An enlarged casting will seat fully and easily but it will be enlarged at the margin as well. This produces an undesirable open margin. In addition, any frictional retention is reduced. This may affect the ability of the cement to retain the restoration. Consequently, altering the investment expansion significantly is usually undesirable. Etching of internal surfaces of castings with aqua-regia is an effective method of creating space for the luting agent. With this method the margins of the castings can be protected from the acid with wax to maintain accurate adaptation of casting to tooth margin. The same results can be obtained by electrically deplating or "stripping" the internal surface of castings. Either of these processes leaves a slightly roughened surface on the metal that enhances the retentive quality of luting agents.[9] Internal surfaces of castings can also be roughened and cleaned with various sand blasting devices.

The most popular current method of providing casting relief for cement is with the use of a paint-like die spacing material that is applied to the die in one or more coats, depending on the relief desired, before adapting the wax for the pattern.[7] This technique provides a quick, easy, inexpensive, and accurate method of obtaining relief. Marginal accuracy can be maintained by not coating the margin of the die, and no expensive electrical equipment or dangerous acid is used.

In some situations grooves may be cut in the internal surface of restorations[10] from the occlusal to within a half mm of the gingival margin without affecting marginal fit. This allows for easier escape of excess cement during cementation. The grooves are cut with a round bur and extreme care must be taken not to perforate the restoration or weaken the framework in cases where a veneer is involved.

Another effective method of enhancing complete seating is with the use of a vent hole in the occlusal of the restoration. This technique, in practicality, is limited to full cast metal restorations. It carries the additional inconvenience of closing the occlusal vent hole after cementation. This can be done in a variety of ways, ranging from fabrication and cementation of a gold inlay, to closing with another dental restorative material, to inserting a threaded pin if the occlusal vent hole has been previously sized and threaded.

CEMENT SELECTION

During the period when zinc phosphate was the only cement available for final cementation of dental castings, cement selection was not a concern. With additional materials now available, a selection must be made. It is important that the chemical and physical properties of cements listed in Table 18–1 be taken into consideration when making such decisions. Further, the working and handling properties of the material must be considered. If all dental luting agents are mixed and handled in the same manner, disastrous results will occur. A definite advantage of zinc phosphate cement is that its setting time can be controlled. Smaller increments of powder and prolonged spatulation of the mix will extend the setting time. It is virtually impossible to overspatulate zinc phosphate cement. A frozen slab technique[11] for mixing has also been developed that is designed to enhance the properties of the cement. It also helps to reduce the pulpal irritation from the cement. It does, however, have some technical disadvantages.

The other dental cements have more critical powder-liquid ratio and spatulation time requirements. Major variation will result in clinically significant alteration of the physical properties of the set cement in most cases.[2] It is important to follow the mixing and handling instructions of the manufacturer for each different cement. When using the popular polycarboxylate cements it is critical that no varnish or dentinal tubule sealer be used on the tooth. Cleaning of the prepared tooth surface with flour of pumice on a rubber cup is recommended. This will remove temporary cement particles and any plaque that may have formed on prepared margins not covered by the temporary protection. Such cleaning will enhance any chemical bond between the cement and the tooth structure. It is important not to use a pumice paste with an oily base that could contaminate the tooth surface. Because this procedure removes debris and any plaque from gingival margin areas, it is now recommended before cementation with any luting material.

Dentinal tubule sealers and varnishes have been used on sensitive teeth in an attempt to reduce pulpal irritation from zinc phosphate cement. Clinically, this practice is helpful. Studies have shown that the use of sealers and varnishes slightly reduces the retentive qualities of the zinc phosphate cement to the tooth structure,[12] but it is probably not clinically significant unless other factors reducing retention are also present. When polycarboxylate cement is used the application of sealers or varnishes is definitely contraindicated as relates to cement retention and unnecessary as relates to tooth sensitivity. They will reduce the cement-tooth interface retention of polycarboxylates.

CEMENTATION PROCEDURES

The quality of the restoration is verified from all standpoints before final cementation. Whether or not a period of temporary cementation has been used, all margins are checked clinically and radiographically, when necessary. Occlusion and contacts are evaluated. Pontic form and acceptability are considered when pontics are involved. Satisfactory esthetics and phonetics are confirmed in cases where these factors are of concern.

The restoration is thoroughly polished and cleaned. This may be done with air abrasive equipment, ultrasonic cleaners, alcohol on a cotton pellet, or a combination of these. The operating area is thoroughly cleaned and isolated for maintenance of a dry field.

The selection of the cement has been made and it is mixed. The mixed cement is applied to the internal surface of the restoration in a quantity sufficient to occupy all space between the restoration and the prepared tooth. There should be enough cement so that excess appears on all margins. This assures that all spaces between restoration and tooth are filled. However, the greater the amount of excess resulting from an over-filled casting, the greater the likelihood that the restoration cannot be fully seated during the cementation process. If desired, cement may be applied to the restoration with a brush[13] or with a metal or plastic instrument small enough to direct and control its application.

All fluid has been removed from the prepared tooth surfaces and a dry field has been maintained. The restoration is then seated to place with finger pressure. Additional biting force may be applied for further seating by the patient on posterior teeth. Interposing materials such as soft or hard wood material, a rubber polishing wheel, or a cotton roll may be used. A pressure applicator with a metal pin to engage the restoration and a hard rubber surface for opposing tooth contact may also be helpful.[14] Biting force on anterior teeth is much less effective and can be harmful if a lateral or angular force is applied to the restoration. Anterior restorations may sometimes be further seated with the use of the end of an orangewood stick that is hand held as firmly as possible on the incisal edge and then lightly tapped with a mallet. This approaches a vertical vibrating action. Horizontal vibration is also proposed as an aid to seating with contradictory results.[5, 11] The technique of vibration may be a factor in its effectiveness.

When the operator feels the restoration is fully seated it is imperative that the patient close in occlusion and be asked if the restoration feels the same as it did before the cement was introduced. If it feels different to the patient and cannot be seated further, the restoration should be removed before the cement sets. Modifications can then be made in the restoration or technique to allow it to seat fully. Incompletely seated castings require occlusal adjustment and more importantly result in open margins with likely subsequent cement washout inviting both caries and periodontal irritation. The retentive qualities of the restoration are usually affected as well.

Removal of excess cement is the final and a most important step in the cementation procedure. Excess is removed at varying times or stages depending on the cement being used. Zinc phosphate excess should never be removed before it has set to the brittle stage. It is not possible to wait too long. Polycarboxylate cement excess should never be removed when the material is in the rubbery stage of set so some of the material could be stretched and pulled from any marginal defects. Ideally it should be removed in the tacky stage as soon as it can be separated from tooth and restoration with an explorer. If the material is allowed to reach its final set, it adheres tenaciously to both tooth and restoration surfaces and is extremely difficult to remove, especially from less accessible areas. If resin cements are allowed to set completely before excess removal, a serious problem results. The polymerized resin is not friable as is zinc phosphate, frequently making removal from interproximal areas impossible without cutting with a bur.

When pontics are involved in the restoration it is important that no excess cement remain in the embrasure areas of the fixed partial denture. Tying dental floss around the pontic connector areas before cementation may be helpful in removing excess in these areas.[15] A floss with a single knot tied in the center, if carefully used, may be helpful in removing loose particles of cement beneath contacts, in the interproximal sulcus, and beneath pontics.

After removal of all gross excess and rinsing with water, a strong stream of air from the syringe should be directed into the sulcus if there are any subgingival margins. The air will dry the sulcus to improve visibility in locating any excess cement remaining on the margin. Usually the air will also mechanically retract or reflect the gingiva to improve visualization of the restoration margin. Any remaining remnants of cement on subgingival margins become periodontal irritants.

Table 18–2[10] provides a condensed version of the handling properties of three

TABLE 18–2.—CEMENT HANDLING AND PROCEDURES

CEMENT	STORAGE AND DISPENSING	MIXING	PATIENT PROCEDURES
Zinc phosphate	Room temperature, keep liquid stoppered, shake powder before dispensing, use clean, dry glass slab, dispense immediately before mixing.	Follow manufacturer's instructions, add small increments of powder, spatulate each thoroughly over large areas of slab, mix at least 1½ minutes. Frozen slab technique may be used. Do not add eugenol or other reagents to reduce irritation.	Clean tooth and restoration, establish a dry field, varnish or seal sensitive teeth, seat restoration with finger pressure followed by biting pressure where possible, check to ensure complete seating before cement sets, maintain biting force at least 5 minutes, maintain dry field during seating, never remove excess before cement is brittle, carefully recheck occlusion before dismissing patient.
Polycarboxylate	May refrigerate but mix only at room temperature. Shake powder before dispensing, dispense immediately before mixing on clean glass slab or paper pad supplied by manufacturer.	Follow manufacturer's instructions, incorporate all the measured powder with all the measured liquid as quickly as possible—never spatulate more than 30 seconds, use flexible stainless steel spatula, do not seat the restoration if the cement has lost its surface gloss.	Clean tooth prep with rubber cup and pumice, clean and sandblast internal surface of restoration, establish a dry field, *never* varnish tooth, seat restoration quickly with finger pressure where possible, check to ensure complete seating before cement sets, maintain dry field and biting pressure while cement sets, never remove excess cement during rubbery stage of set—remove just before or just after this stage, fully set excess is difficult to remove—scaler recommended, check occlusion before dismissing patient.
Reinforced ZOE (EBA)	May refrigerate but mix only at room temperature. Shake powder and liquid before mixing. Dispense immediately before mixing on clean glass slab or paper pad supplied by manufacturer. Do not add zinc acetate crystals or other modifiers.	Follow manufacturer's instructions. Mix with a flexible stainless steel spatula with a stropping motion until a homogenous fluid consistency is reached. Usual mixing time about 1 minute.	Clean tooth and restoration, establish a dry field, varnish or sealant unnecessary, carefully lubricate any resin veneers without contaminating internal surfaces, seat with finger pressure followed by biting force, wipe away excess cement with gauze sponge, check to assure complete seating before cement sets, maintain biting pressure and dry field until cement sets, remove excess after initial set, orange oil is solvent for excess on hard or soft tissue, check margins carefully for excess removal, check occlusion before dismissing patient.

popular classes of cements as well as some of the important considerations of procedures that either should or should not be performed during the cementation appointment.

REFERENCES

1. Abelson J.: Cementation of cast complete crown retainers. *J. Prosthet. Dent.* 43:174, 1980.
2. Braden M., et al.: Dental materials: Literature review part II. *J. Dent.* 8:43, 1980.
3. Clinical Research Associates Newsletter, Provo, Utah, 84601; 5:2, February, 1981.
4. McLean J.W.: Polycarboxylate cements. Five years' experience in general practice. *Br. Dent. J.* 72:915, 1972.
5. Van Nortwich W.T., Gettleman L.: Effect of internal relief, vibration, and venting on the vertical seating of cemented crowns. *J. Prosthet. Dent.* 45:395, 1981.
6. Windeler A.S.: Powder enrichment effects on film thickness of zinc phosphate cement. *J. Prosthet. Dent.* 42:299, 1979.
7. Eames W.B., et al.: Techniques to improve the seating of castings. *J. Am. Dent. Assoc.* 96:432, 1978.
8. Hoard R.J., et al.: Intracoronal pressure during crown cementation. *J. Prosthet. Dent.* 40:520, 1978.
9. Oilo G., Jorgensen K.D.: The influence of surface roughness on the retentive ability of two dental luting cements. *J. Oral Rehabil.* 5:377, 1978.
10. Meyers G.E., Silvey P.G.: Do's and don'ts for three dental luting cements. Council on dental materials and devices. *J. Am. Dent. Assoc.* 97:502, 1978.
11. Newman S.M.: Frozen-slab technique for mixing zinc phosphate cement for cast restorations. *J. Prosthet. Dent.* 43:46, 1980.
12. Chan K.C., Svare C.W., Horton D.J.: The effect of varnish on dentinal bonding strength of five dental cements. *J. Prosthet. Dent.* 35:403, 1976.
13. Ishikiriama A., et al.: Influence of some factors on the fit of cemented crowns. *J. Prosthet. Dent.* 45:400, 1981.
14. De Freitas Oliveria J., et al.: Influence of pressure and vibration during cementation. *J. Prosthet. Dent.* 41:173, 1979.
15. Berman M.H.: Problems and aids in the final insertion of complete coverage restorations. *Gen. Dent.* 27:30, 1979.

CHAPTER 19

Acid-Etch Resin Bonded Cast Restorations

VINCENT D. WILLIAMS, D.D.S.

PRIOR TO THE YEAR 1972, little had been done with the acid-etch technique in fixed prosthodontics. The work of Bowen,[1] and Buonocore and associates[2] led some clinicians to look for ways of using the acid-etch process in replacing missing anterior teeth.

Ibsen[3] and Portnoy[4] reported a direct technique that used the patient's own tooth or an acrylic denture tooth as the pontic that was acid-etched to the adjacent teeth. Stolpa[5] reported an indirect technique for a three unit fixed prosthesis on a stone model, using an acrylic tooth as the pontic, attaching it to the abutments with resin.

Most clinicians felt that these were temporary restorations, yet the longevity has been adequate. Scheer and Silverstone[6] reported a longevity of up to 24 months, on 14 cases that they had treated similarly. Paul[7] and Jenkins[8] verified the feasibility of this technique with longitudinal studies of 24 and 33 months, respectively. Rakow[9] and Gorelick[10] advocated using wires to help strengthen and retain this type of prosthesis.

A variation in this technique was used by Eisenbrand,[11] who modified a porcelain pontic with two holes, acid-etching the pontic to the adjacent teeth with resin. Jordan and associates[12] used an acrylic tooth as the pontic with pins in the abutment teeth. The pontic was attached with acid-etch composite to the abutments. The retention rate was up to 36 months on 86 cases. Nathanson and Moin[13] described a fixed prosthesis using composite as the pontic and bonded to a perforated prefabricated frame. The frame was attached to the abutments with acid-etch composite.

Other clinicians began to look at ways to improve the esthetics and permanence of these prostheses. As early as 1972, Rochette[14], advocated a unique and novel approach to the missing anterior tooth. He replaced the tooth with a porcelain-fused-to-metal pontic that was attached to a cast metal framework. The metal framework had plates of metal that were attached with composite to the lingual enamel. Howe and Denehy[15] verified the success of this type of prosthesis. Kuhlke and Drennon[16] reported 20 cases, with a retention rate of up to three years using this technique of porcelain-fused-to-metal framework. Some of the most pertinent findings of a recent study by Williams and associates[17] were: (1) the 63 acid-etch fixed prostheses in the study had an average longevity rate of 2.8 years at recall, with a range from one to seven years; (2) recurrent caries did not seem to be a problem with these restorations; (3) there appeared to be no correlation of the initial periodontal condition of the patient and that at recall examination; (4) there was a low loss of attachment (15.8%) that seemed to occur within the first year of use; (5) heavy occlusion may have played a role in the loss of attachment; (6) some washout of composite in the retention holes occurred, there was no loss of attachment attributed to this; and (7) only anterior restorations were studied.

Livaditis[18] describes an acid-etch technique for posterior tooth replacements that uses a cast porcelain-fused-to-metal restoration. It is similar in design to a unilateral, tooth-supported, removable partial denture. Occlusal rests are prepared on the abutment teeth and excess enamel contours are removed on the lingual and axial surfaces of the teeth. The buccal surface is not used because of esthetics. In most cases the metal framework extends onto the buccal line angle to resist movement of the prosthesis to the lingual aspect under function. Instead of lingual clasps, perforated lingual plates of metal are used to bond the prosthesis to the retainer teeth.

The pontic is porcelain-fused-to-metal, but the prostheses are usually made with a nonprecious alloy because it is stronger and can be made thinner without a danger of flexing. The restorations are bonded to the retainer teeth using the acid-etch composite system. Because of the greater film thickness of the conventional composites, a new bonding agent, Comspan,* is suggested. It was developed especially to bond acid-etch restorations. Livaditis[18] reported on 15 of these three unit posterior fixed prostheses in service for two to four years. Thompson and Livaditis[19] reported a new method of attachment of acid-etch restorations to the retainer teeth. They used electrolytic etching of the retainer metal instead of perforations to provide a mechanical bond of the composite to the casting. More than 140 prostheses are currently being evaluated of which 40% are posterior restorations.

DESCRIPTION OF TECHNIQUE

Full mouth impressions for study casts are made for the patient that is diagnosed for an acid-etch fixed prosthesis. These are mounted in centric relation on a semi-adjustable articulator, with a face-bow transfer. Necessary intraoral records should be made to program the articulator. After the preliminary diagnosis and treatment planning appointment has been done, the acid-etch restoration can be completed in two appointments.

First Appointment

The abutment teeth are thoroughly scaled of any calculus and cleaned with pumice. The mouth is rinsed with water and the abutment teeth isolated and dried. Retraction cord is placed in the lingual crevice of the abutment teeth, if needed, to gain lingual enamel for additional retention. A full arch impression with a final impression material of the dentist's choice is made in an individualized tray. The shade is selected using the porcelain shade guide of choice. The master cast is poured with die stone and mounted with an opposing cast on a suitable articulator. Removable dies are not made on the master cast, but the lingual gingiva may be trimmed away with a sharp scalpel or chisel. The outline of the retainer margins

*L.D. Caulk Co., Milford, DW 19963.

are drawn on the lingual of the abutment teeth with a red pencil. The case is ready to be sent, along with a work authorization, to the commercial laboratory for fabrication.

Second Appointment: Perforated Design

The teeth are again pumiced. The prosthesis is tried in the mouth to check for proper fit and a definite seat. The color, tissue adaptation, and embrasure form of the pontic are evaluated. If the prosthesis is satisfactory to the clinician and patient, the interior surface is cleaned thoroughly with a Pasche air brush, pumice, or ultrasonic cleaner. This will remove foreign materials or contamination that may prevent adhesion. Care should be taken to not touch the interface surface of the casting with fingers before cementation has taken place.

The bonding of the prosthesis to the enamel of the retainer teeth should be done with strict adherence to the acid-etch technique. Using cotton rolls and high velocity suction, the retainer teeth are kept free from saliva and moisture during the bonding procedure. A rubber dam may be used if preferred. After pumicing, washing with water, and drying with oil-free air, the lingual enamel of the retainer teeth is etched with etching solution for one to two minutes. The etchant is rinsed away with water and the tooth thoroughly dried. The etched surface is carefully examined for a chalky white surface. If necessary, the tooth may be etched again. Unfilled resin is applied to the enamel and filled resin is applied to the prosthesis simultaneously. The casting is seated on the abutment teeth. The resin is allowed to protrude through the retention areas of the metal. A celluloid strip may be used on the lingual surface of the prosthesis. Occlusion should be checked at this point. Excess composite may be removed before the final set, to facilitate trimming in the contact and the embrasure areas. The prosthesis is not disturbed while the composite polymerizes. After the final set has occurred, excess composite is trimmed with 12-bladed carbide finishing burs, disks, and polishing points. Care should be exercised not to remove the composite from the counter sunk areas of the metal retainers.

Second Appointment: Etched Metal Design

If etched castings are used as the retentive method, the prosthesis is returned from the commercial laboratory unetched for a final evaluation in the patient's mouth. Proper fit, pontic color, tissue adaptation, and embrasure form of the restoration are verified on the patient. If the restoration is satisfactory to the dentist and the patient, it is returned to the laboratory for electrolytic etching of the retainers.

On return from the laboratory the etched casting prosthesis is rinsed in acetone, chloroform, and water in that order, to remove all possible contaminants. The cleansed restoration should not be tried in the mouth again to evaluate the fit nor should the etched surface be touched with the fingers as this may contaminate the micro-retention on the retainers.

The bonding procedures for the etched castings are the same as for the perforated, except that a low viscosity resin must be used. Comspan and an unfilled resin of the operators choice make an ideal attaching media. After pumicing and etching the abutment teeth as described for the perforated retainers, unfilled resin is applied to the retainer teeth and the casting. Before the unfilled resin has polymerized, Comspan, a filled resin, is mixed and applied to the retainer areas. The restoration is carried to the mouth and seated with firm pressure. Floss tied around the pontic of anterior restorations can be a valuable aid in positioning and maintaining seating pressure while the composite sets. Polymerization should be complete in 5 to 7 minutes at which time the excess composite can be removed. Final polishing can be done with twelve-bladed carbide finishing burs, disks, and polishing points. The prosthesis should not be disturbed while polymerization is taking place.

If it is inconvenient for the clinician to return the prosthesis to the commercial laboratory for electrolytic etching, an etcher with appropriate acids, and a stereomicroscope can be purchased so that this procedure can be done in the dental office. The etch of the metal is critical. Meticulous attention to detail is required so that failure of attachment does not occur. It is also imperative that the quality of the etch must be verified under the stereomicroscope.

An imporatant factor to be considered is that not all nonprecious alloys can be etched. The metal must be a two phase alloy system for electrolytic etching to occur. An example of a nonprecious, two phase alloy for etched resin bonded prostheses is Rexillium III.*

The advantages of the acid-etch resin bonded fixed prosthesis are:

1. Little or no reduction of tooth structure is necessary;
2. The procedure is kind to young or large pulps;
3. No trauma to the periodontium occurs;
4. Maximum esthetics are possible;
5. Pontic and embrasure forms are under the control of the dentist;
6. The prosthesis is easy to keep clean;
7. Minimum chair time is involved;
8. It is less expensive than a conventional fixed prosthesis;
9. It may be reattached if it loosens with no significant clinical difference in bonding strenth;[20]
10. No permanent damage to the enamel occurs, as it does remineralize after etching;[21]
11. Individual characterization is possible with the porcelain-fused-to-metal pontic; and
12. No irreversible procedures are involved.

Disadvantages of the acid-etch resin bonded fixed prosthesis are:

1. Some clinicians may not feel that these are a permanent restoration; however, the longevity appears better with each passing year. Williams and associates[17] reported a longitudinal study of seven years, with a good retention rate;
2. The added thickness of the retainers on the abutment teeth may present a problem to the periodontium, especially on posterior teeth;
3. The composite in the countersunk areas may abrade over an extended time; and
4. The unfilled resin, a polymer, absorbs water molecules, and fluids from the oral cavity.

*Jeneric Industries, Wallingford, CT 06492.

PERIODONTAL SPLINTS

The problem of the mobile dentition, in the periodontally compromised patient, has been addressed in various ways. Traditional cast splints of precious metal have been both expensive and tedious to fabricate. The application of the acid-etch technique has been valuable in many of these situations.

McEvoy[22] and Polson[23] used only the composite resin with the acid-etch technique to stabilize the periodontally involved teeth. This is an inexpensive way to treat excessive mobility of the teeth, but the longevity and esthetics are often inadequate. Schnepper[24] advocated adding minim pins in the lingual surface to increase the permanence of these splints. He considered them a semi-permanent splint. Iacono[25] used an arch wire with the acid-etch composite technique to stabilize the mobility of periodontally involved teeth after surgery.

It remained, however, for Rochette[26] to improve the longevity and esthetics of these periodontal splints by using a cast metal framework and attaching this to the involved teeth with the acid-etch technique. These splints are esthetic and have a long life expectancy.

The advantages of this technique in perio-prostheses are:

1. Economical;
2. Esthetic;
3. Minimum chair time;
4. No alteration of the enamel or pulps;
5. Splint is easy to maintain;
6. Can be reattached if the splint becomes loose;
7. If a single tooth is lost the root may be resected, and the crown of the tooth allowed to remain as a pontic or the whole tooth may be removed and an acrylic pontic attached in its place; and
8. Does not change the shape of the gingival embrasure.

ACID-ETCH APPLICATION IN OCCLUSAL TREATMENT

Another use is the building of acid-etch lingual ramps on maxillary canines to effect a canine disclusion. This may be indicated if the patient has abraded the natural canines, has group function, occlusion, and if the clinician feels that the patient would function better in a canine protected occlusion.

A 30-year-old man presented at the dental clinic with pain in his jaws, and grinding and clenching of his teeth. His health history was essentially negative. Oral examination disclosed muscles of mastication sore to palpation and extensive wear facets on the maxillary canines (Fig 19–1). Diagnostic casts showed a discrepancy between centric occlusion and centric relation, with an anterior slide of 1.5 mm. An occlusal equilibration was done on the casts and subsequently on the patient. At this point it was deemed necessary to provide for a more favorable occlusion in excursive movements (Fig 19–2). Traditionally this has been done with full veneer crowns, three-quarter crowns, or pinlays. For this patient it was decided to use acid-etch castings attached to the lingual surface of the maxillary canines. These were made of nonprecious metal and attached to the enamel with a composite resin. Three years posttreatment the patient is comfortable and the canine risers remain firmly attached to the enamel (Fig 19–3A,B).[27]

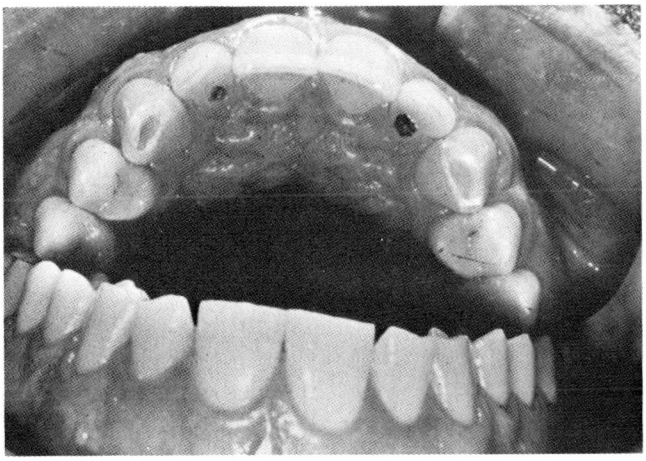

Fig 19–1.—Severe wear facets on maxillary canines of patient with history of grinding and clenching.

LABORATORY FABRICATION

The work authorization to the dental technician should specify:

1. The retainers and pontics cast in one piece;
2. Porcelain-fused-to-metal pontic;
3. The shade for the pontic;
4. Retainer margins pencil outlined on the master cast; and
5. The retention design desired: (a) perforations—number and size, (b) etched casting retainers.

The retainer designs (Fig 19–4) showed that all designs are stronger than the anterior forces of occlusion measured in human beings.[28] No retainer design failed below 75 pounds. Numerous studies[29–31] have shown that most humans cannot gen-

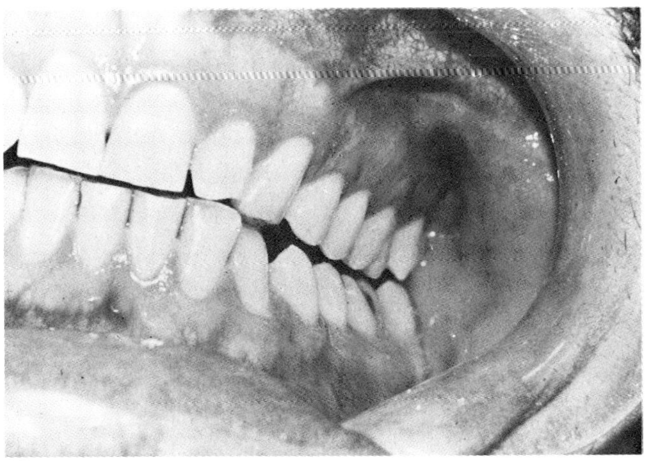

Fig 19–2.—After occlusal equilibration, canine risers are cemented on the canines and are in contact with the mandibular canines to effect a disclusion in excursive movements providing canine protected occlusion.

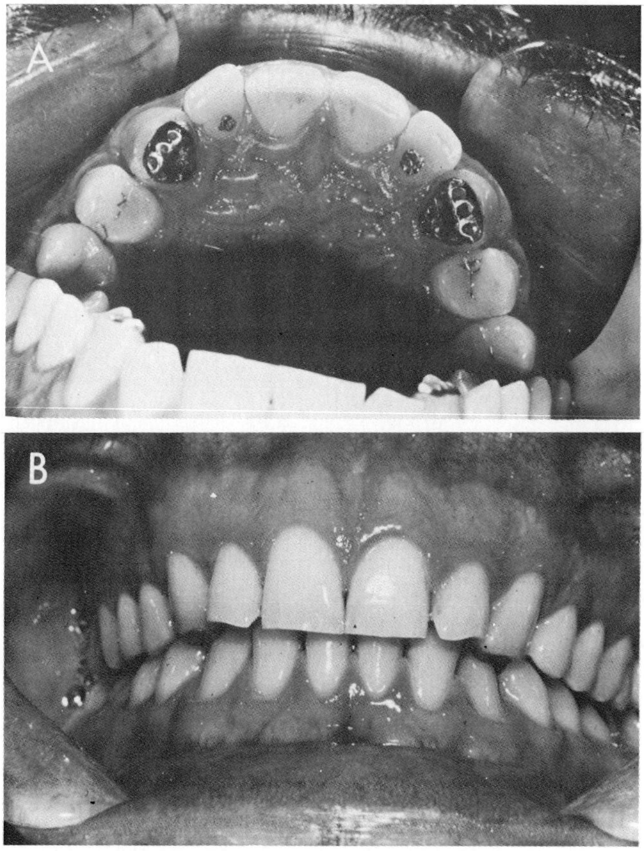

Fig 19–3.—A, palatal view of acid-etch castings in place on the canines. **B,** the dentition in centric relation occlusion with canine risers attached.

erate maximum bite forces greater than 75 pounds in the anterior portion of the dentition. Forces greater than 75 pounds were found only in the premolars and molars.

LABORATORY PROCEDURES

The vacuum pressed or duralay method may be used to fabricate an acid-etch prosthesis in the laboratory. With the vacuum pressed method the master model is first duplicated. The working model is then placed on a Dura Press* and the proper thickness plastic laminate is chosen to create a retainer thickness of 0.5 mm. The patterns may be trimmed and cut with a crown scissors to proper size and then smoothed with a green stone. If holes are used for retention, they are cut in the patterns at this time, using a no. half round bur. The retainers are returned to the master model to verify the fit and size (Fig 19–5). The pontic is developed in wax, as are the retainer margins, and the pattern is then cast as one piece in nonprecious metal. The casting is returned to the master model to verify the fit of the pros-

*Dentsply International, Inc., York, PA 17405.

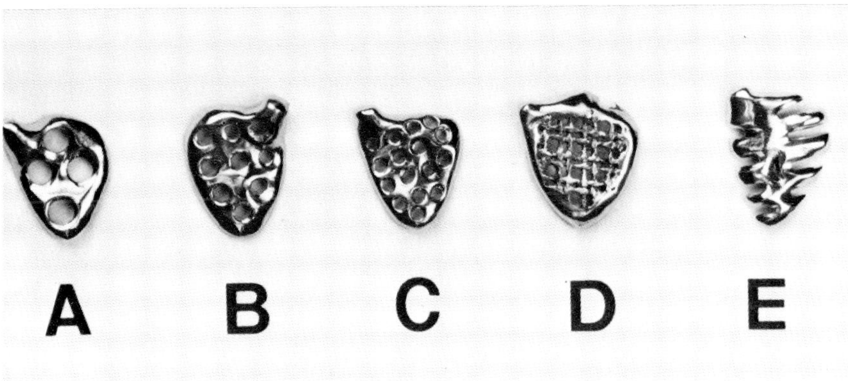

Fig 19–4.—Different retainer designs: *(A)* 4 large holes; *(B)* 9 medium holes; *(C)* 16 small holes; *(D)* meshwork retention; *(E)* slotted retainer design.

thesis. The holes are countersunk with a round carbide bur, no. 2 or four, using the high-speed handpiece (Fig 19–6).

The pontic is fabricated in the manner traditional for the porcelain-fused-to-metal technique. When the firing of the porcelain-fused-to-metal pontic is completed, the casting is polished, and the fixed prosthesis is returned to the master model. The fit of the retainers is verified and the esthetics of pontic form and embrasure areas are evaluated (Fig 19–7).

The Duralay method is the same as the previous method, with the exception of the substitution of the methyl methacrylate Duralay** for the patterns. The master model is lubricated. Using the Nealon, or bead-brush, technique with a camel's hair brush, the patterns for the retainers and pontic are fabricated (Fig 19–8). The patterns are thinned to 0.5 mm on the retainer teeth, and the holes are cut to the appropriate size. The preferred bur size is a half round, using up to 16 holes per retainer. The margins are finalized in wax, and the pattern is invested and cast in

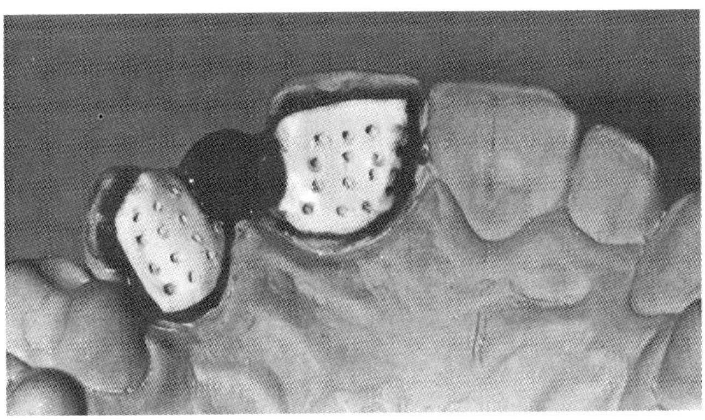

Fig 19–5.—Vacuum pressed patterns with the pontic and margins refined in wax. Patterns ready to be cast in one piece.

**Reliance Manufacturing Co., Worth, IL 60482.

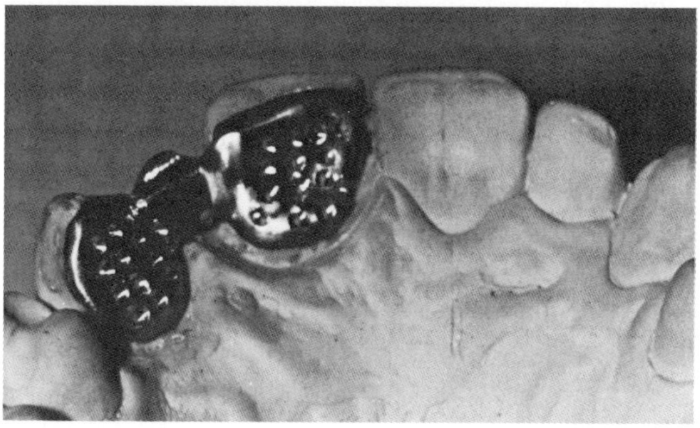

Fig 19–6.—Completed porcelain-fused-to-metal framework cast in nonprecious metal. Note that the holes are countersunk for retention.

nonprecious metal. The holes are countersunk as described previously. The addition of porcelain is the same as described in the previous method.[32]

Indications and Contraindications

This restoration may be used advantageously in:

1. Patients with a missing tooth, adjacent to intact teeth;
2. A fixed prosthesis where esthetics is of primary concern;
3. A transitional fixed prosthesis, until the pulps of the permanent teeth will withstand preparations for a conventional prosthesis;
4. Anterior periodontal splinting procedures for excessive mobility; and
5. Lingual ramps on maxillary canines to create canine disclusion.

The contraindications for the acid-etch technique are:

1. Inadequate horizontal overlap for the thickness of the metal retainer for a fixed prosthesis on the maxillary arch;
2. Short teeth with inadequate lingual enamel for attachment of the retainer;
3. Previous restorations or large areas of caries or fracture that would compromise the retention of the retainers;

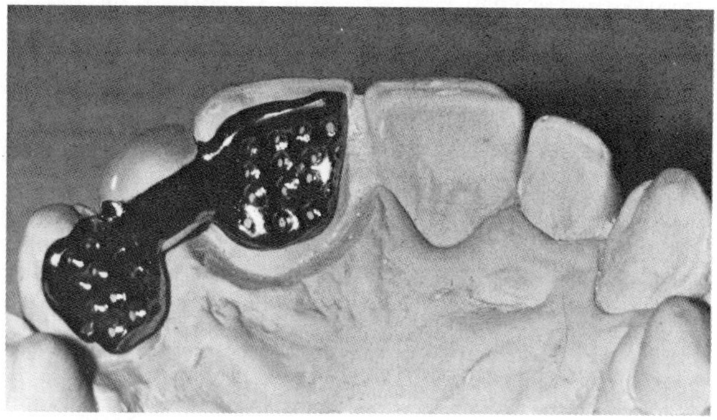

Fig 19–7.—Completed acid-etch fixed partial denture after the addition of the porcelain to the pontic.

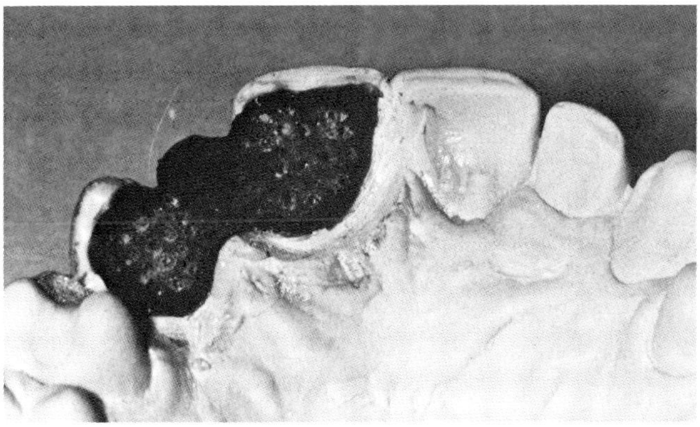

Fig 19–8.—Duralay resin pattern ready for casting in one piece.

4. Heavy anterior occlusion in excursive movements on the pontics that may compromise the prognosis of an acid-etch restoration;
5. Deep vertical overlap with centric stops in the gingival third of the teeth that would limit the area of available enamel for retentive purposes; and
6. A patient with known nickel sensitivity. Most nonprecious alloys contain nickel. A nickel free alloy, preferably nonprecious, could be used.

CASE REPORTS

A 16-year-old woman had an esthetic problem with her maxillary anterior teeth (Fig 19–9). The maxillary right peg lateral had been removed earlier, and the maxillary left lateral had been crowned with a stainless steel crown. Orthodontics had been done to close the diastema between the maxillary central incisors. Her medical history was noncontributory. The occlusion had a prematurity on the left maxillary premolar with an anterior slide of 2 mm.

Because of the indications and contraindications listed previously, it was decided

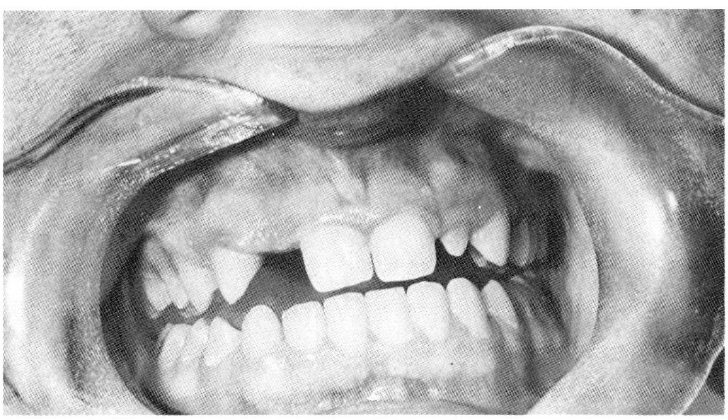

Fig 19–9.—Esthetic problem in treating 16-year-old woman. Right maxillary lateral space was excessive mesiodistally and the left maxillary lateral was a peg-lateral. Electrosurgery was used to increase the length of the clinical crown of the left lateral incisor and to equalize the height of the gingival margins.

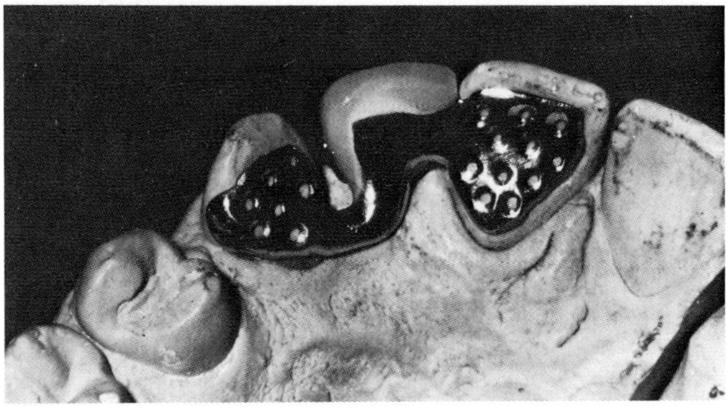

Fig 19–10.—Palatal view of acid-etch prosthesis replacing the maxillary right lateral incisor. Note the palatal strap used to decrease the width of the pontic and provide a slight diastema distal to the lateral incisor.

to proceed with an acid-etch fixed prosthesis from canine to central incisor. A palatal strap was used to duplicate the diastemas distal to the maxillary lateral incisors (Fig 19–10). The maxillary left lateral incisor was restored with a porcelain-fused-to-metal crown (Fig 19–11). This prosthesis has been in place for four years.

Periodontally involved mandibular anterior teeth may require splinting for support. Where no pontics are involved, a rubber dam is helpful for isolating the area and maintaining a better environment for etching the teeth and attaching the splint (Fig 19–12). The splint does not encroach on embrasure form and provides an esthetic result (Fig 19–13,A,B) for this 20-year-old patient with unusual tooth mobility and alarming bone loss around mandibular central and lateral incisors.

An 18-year-old woman had congenitally missing maxillary lateral incisors (Fig 19–14). Her medical and dental history were essentially negative, except for some minor orthodontics to align the anterior teeth and provide room for more esthetic pontics. The abutment teeth had no restorations. There was a small carious lesion near the incisal of one central incisor which was restored in composite.

Esthetic considerations, and conservation of sound tooth structure and existing

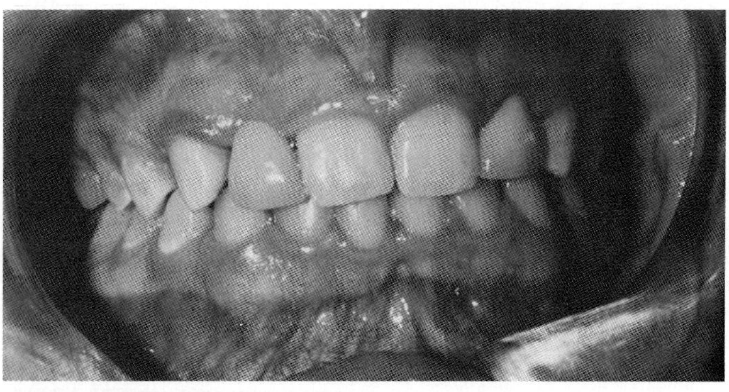

Fig 19–11.—Completed acid-etch restoration from the maxillary right canine to right central incisor. A porcelain-fused-to-metal crown was placed on the maxillary left lateral incisor. Note the position of the gingival margins following electrosurgery. This prosthesis has been in place four years.

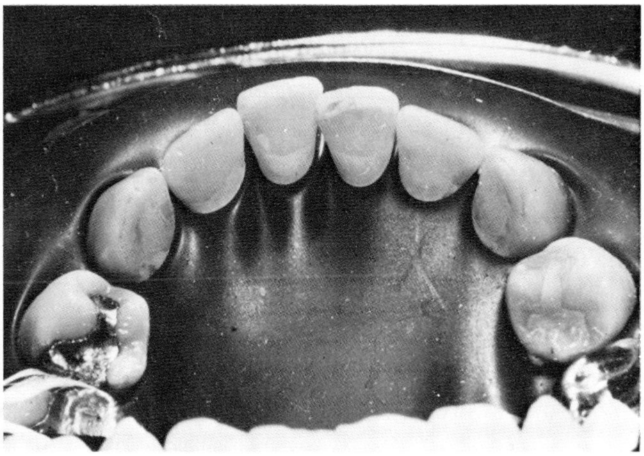

Fig 19–12.—Lingual view of teeth to be splinted in a perio-prosthesis. The mandibular incisors were mobile and needed additional support. A rubber dam is in place for the acid-etch attaching appointment.

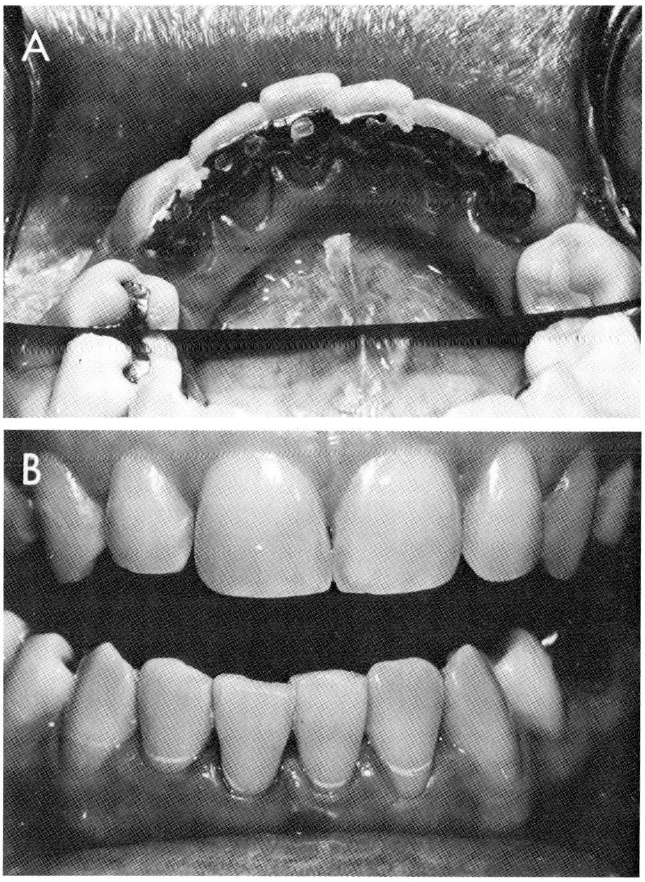

Fig 19–13.—**A,** completed acid-etch splint attached to the teeth with composite resin. This six-unit splint has been in service for three years. **B,** the splinted teeth show a good esthetic result with no encroachment on gingival embrasures. Note etched lines near gingival where etchant pooled around rubber dam. These will remineralize quickly.

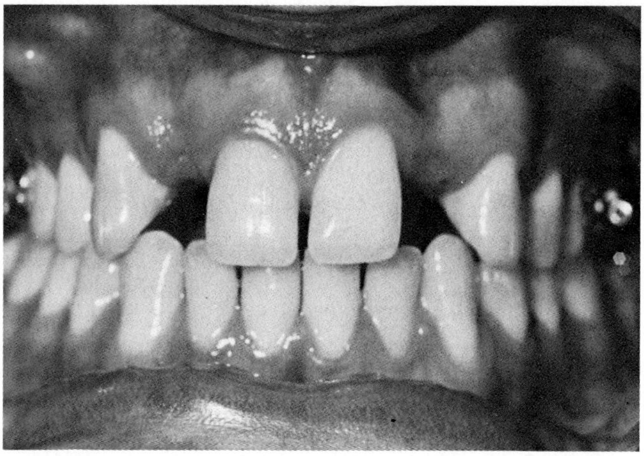

Fig 19–14.—Eighteen-year-old woman with congenitally missing maxillary lateral incisors.

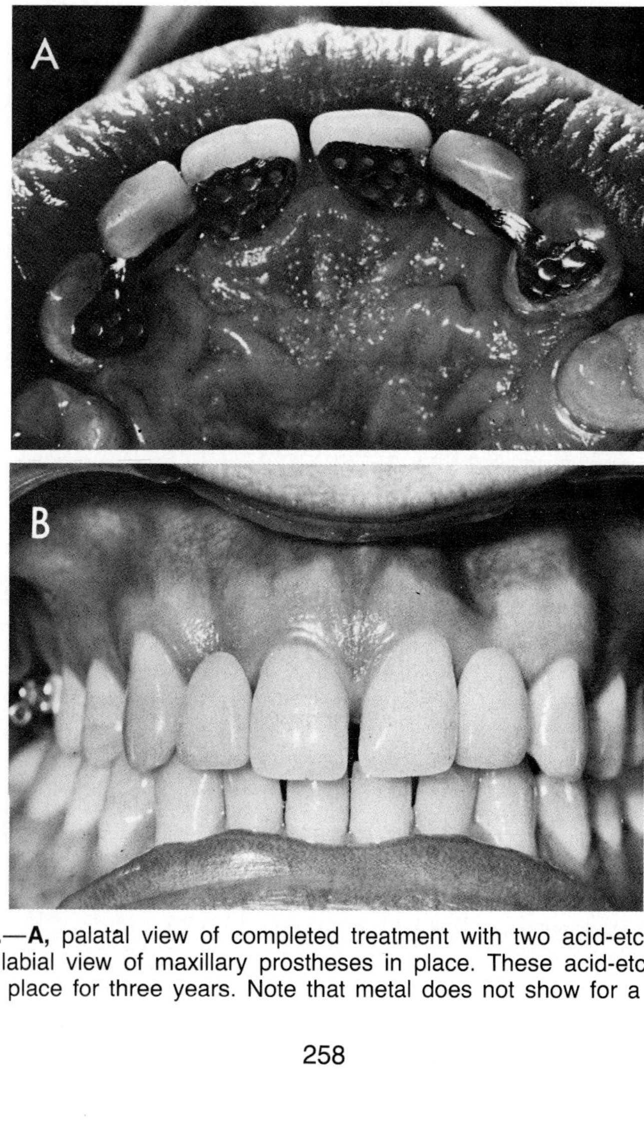

Fig 19–15.—**A,** palatal view of completed treatment with two acid-etch fixed partial dentures. **B,** labial view of maxillary prostheses in place. These acid-etch restorations have been in place for three years. Note that metal does not show for a good esthetic appearance.

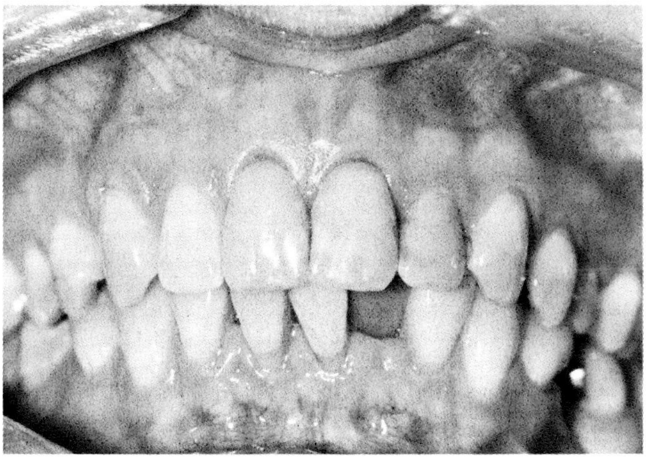

Fig 19–16.—A 42-year-old woman came after orthodontic repositioning of the six mandibular anterior teeth. A space the size of a lateral incisor remained. The mandibular incisors were slightly mobile.

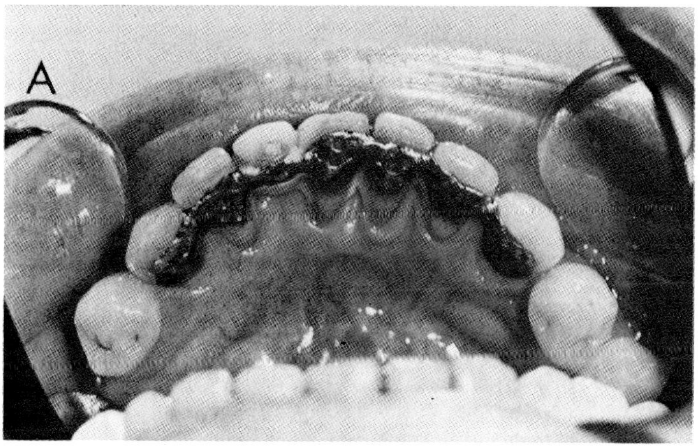

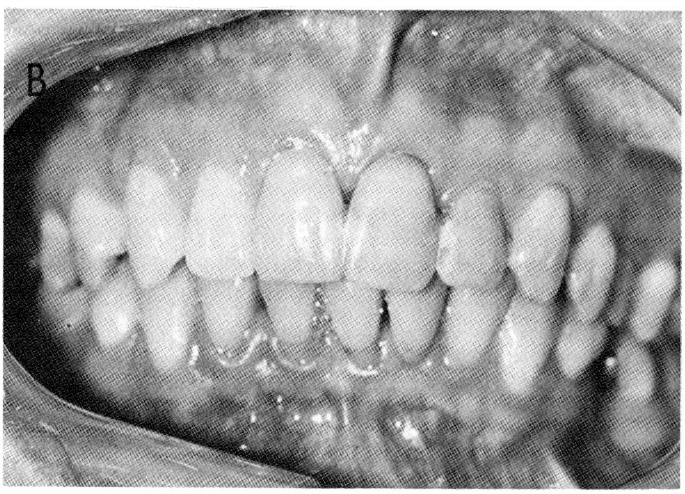

Fig 19–17.—**A,** lingual view of six unit combination acid-etch orthodontic retainer, periodontal splint, and one tooth replacement fixed partial denture. This prosthesis has been in service for seven years. **B,** labial view of the completed restoration.

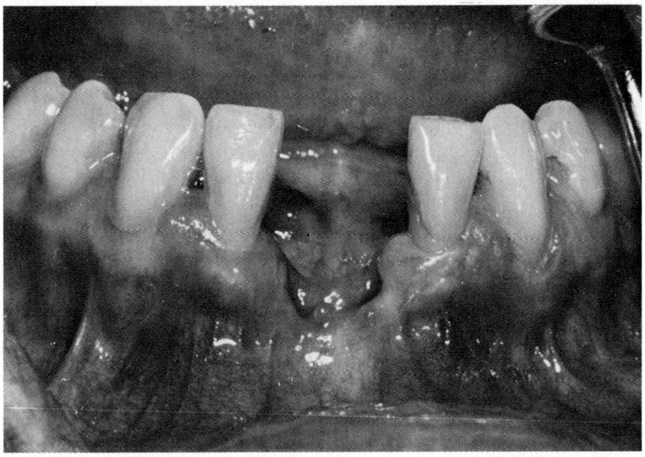

Fig 19–18.—A 57-year-old woman with a severe bony defect in the anterior portion of the mandible resulting from periodontal disease.

occlusal relationships were some of the guiding indications that led to the selection of acid-etch restorations. The final prostheses were inserted using both filled and unfilled composite resin. The two three unit prostheses from canine to central incisor bilaterally had a perforated design on the retainers and porcelain-fused-to-metal pontics (Fig 19–15,A,B). The metal used was nonprecious.

A 42-year-old woman came for fixed prosthodontic treatment for a one tooth replacement of the mandibular left lateral incisor. A one tooth space was the result of adult orthodontic treatment used to close multiple mandibular anterior interdental spacings present since childhood (Fig 19–16). Her medical history was noncontributory.

Oral examination also showed gingival recession on the two central incisors exposing the cementoenamel junction and approximately 1mm of root surface. Radiographs disclosed some bone loss and teeth had some mobility clinically. The teeth were well aligned and positioned orthodontically but the potential abutment teeth

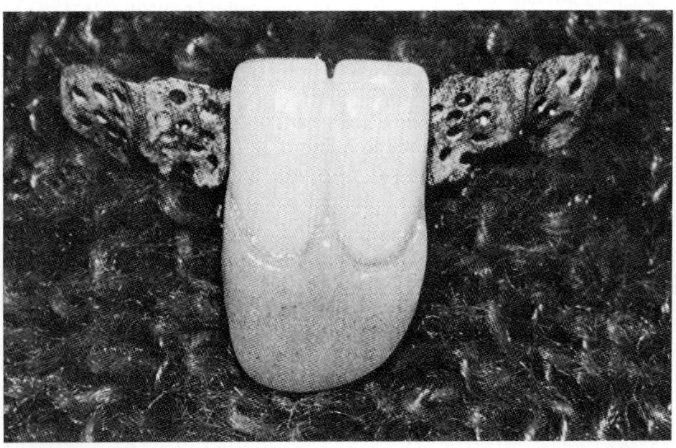

Fig 19–19.—Labial view of completed acid-etch perio-prosthesis. Note pink porcelain to simulate the gingiva.

had marked divergent inclination that would compromise the conventional preparations and require excessive tooth structure removal and over-tapering.

The use of the acid-etch application in this case resulted in a combined fixed orthodontic retainer, periodontal splint, and one tooth replacement fixed partial denture all in a single restoration (Fig 19–17,A,B). The cast metal framework of nonprecious alloy extended from canine to canine. The pontic was of porcelain-fused-to-metal design. This prosthesis has been functioning for seven years without problems.

A 57-year-old woman had "loose lower teeth." Dental examination disclosed caries, missing and mobile teeth, calculus, plaque, and Type III periodontitis. The mandibular central incisors had such severe bone loss and mobility that they required extraction. The other teeth with periodontal disease could be treated and the patient expressed a desire to save as many teeth as possible.

An esthetic problem existed if a fixed prosthesis was to be considered because of the large bony defect in the anterior area of the mandible (Fig 19–18). The mandibular lateral incisors had slight mobility. Therefore, it was decided to replace the central incisors with an acid-etch fixed partial denture splinting all six mandibular

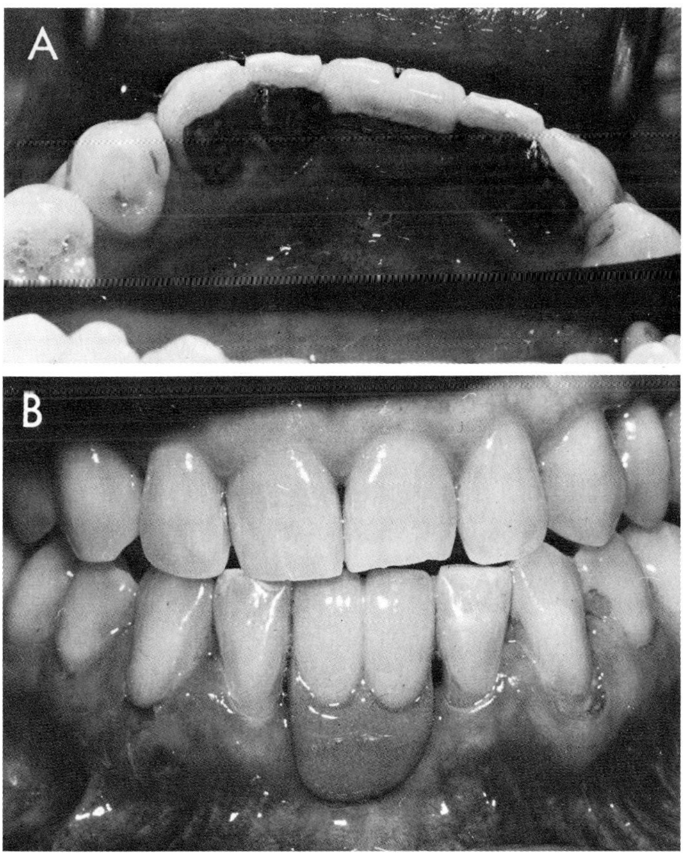

Fig 19–20.—A, lingual intra-oral view showing the completed prosthesis cemented to the teeth with composite. **B,** completed acid-etch perio-prosthesis showing improved esthetics and function. This restoration has been in service for four years.

anterior teeth from canine to canine. Esthetic considerations for the bony defect indicated that pink porcelain be used to simulate the gingiva (Fig 19–19). This restoration has now been in place for four years and is functioning well (Fig 19–20,A,B).

Acid-etch resin bonded prostheses were once considered temporary, or at best semi-permanent, restorations! After seven years of experience, it now appears that the life expectancy of these restorations compares favorably with what was previously referred to as a conventional fixed partial denture.

REFERENCES

1. Bowen R.L.: Adhesive bonding of various methods to hard tooth tissues. IV. Bonding to dentine, enamel and fluorapatite improved by use of a surface active comonomer. *J. Dent. Res.* 44:906, 1965.
2. Buonocore M.G., Matsui H., Gwinnett A.J.: Penetration of resin dentin materials into surfaces with reference to bonding. *Arch. Oral Biol.* 13:61, 1968.
3. Ibsen R.L.: Fixed prosthetics with a natural crown pontic using an adhesive composite. *J. So. Calif. Dent. Assoc.* 41:100, 1973.
4. Portnoy L.L.: Constructing a composite pontic in a single visit. *Dent. Surv.* 49:20, 1973.
5. Stolpa J.B.: An adhesive technique for small anterior fixed partial dentures. *J. Prosthet. Dent.* 34:513, 1975.
6. Scheer B., Silverstone L.M.: Replacement of missing anterior teeth by etch retained bridges. *J. Int. Assoc. Dent. Child.* 6:17 1975.
7. Paul T.J.: Replace anterior teeth without bridges or wires. *Dent. Stud.* 55:41, 1977.
8. Jenkins C.B.: Etch-retained anterior pontics. A 4-year study. *Br. Dent. J.* 144:206, 1978.
9. Rakow B.: Temporary resin bonded fixed multiple tooth prosthesis. *N.Y. State Dent.* 42:79, 1976.
10. Gorelick L.: An improved technique for fixed bonded bridgework. *J. Pedod.* 2:90, 1977.
11. Eisenbrand, G.F.: Simplified composite technique for placing porcelain pontics. *Dent. Surv.* 51:34, 1975.
12. Jordan, R.E., et al.: Temporary fixed partial dentures fabricated by means of the acid-etch resin technique: A report of 86 cases followed for up to three years. *J. Am. Dent. Assoc.* 96:994, 1978.
13. Nathanson D., Moin K.: Metal-reinforced anterior tooth replacement using acid-etch-composite resin technique. *J. Prosthet. Dent.* 43:408, 1980.
14. Rochette A.: Polymer adhesion and surface treatments. *Act. Odont.*, Paris. 98:175, 1972.
15. Howe D.F., Denehy G.E.: Anterior fixed partial dentures utilizing the acid-etch techniques and a cast metal framework. *J. Prosthet. Dent.* 37:28, 1975.
16. Kuhlke K.L., Drennon D.G.: An alternative to the anterior single tooth removable partial denture. *J. Int. Dent. Child.* 8:11, 1977.
17. Williams V.D., et al.: Acid-etch retained cast metal prostheses: A seven year retrospective study. *J.Am. Dent. Assoc.* In press.
18. Livaditis, G. J.: Cast metal resin-bonded retainers for posterior teeth. *J. Am. Dent. Assoc.* 101:926, 1980.
19. Thompson B.P., Livaditis B.J.: Etched casting acid etch composite bonded posterior bridges. *Ped. Dent.* 4:38, 1982.
20. Williams V.D., Dedmon H.W.: The retention of rebonded acid-etch retainers to enamel. *J. Prosthet. Dent.* In press.
21. Wei S.H.Y.: Electron microprobe analyses of the remineralization of enamel. *J. Dent. Res.* 49:621, 1970.
22. McEvoy S.A.: Acid-etched resin splint for temporarily stabilizing anterior teeth. *J. Dent. Child.* 41:439, 1974.
23. Polson A.M.: Temporary splinting of teeth using ultraviolet-light-polymerized bonding materials. *J. Am. Dent. Assoc.* 89:1137, 1974.
24. Schnepper H.E.: Pin-retained composites for splinting lower anterior teeth. *J. Prosthet. Dent.* 39:162, 1978.

25. Iacono V.J.: An acid etch splint for periodontally involved teeth. *N.Y. J. Dent.* 48:142, 1978.
26. Rochette A.L.: Attachment of a splint to enamel of lower anterior teeth. *J. Prosthet. Dent.* 30:418, 1973.
27. Thayer K.E., Doukoudakis A.: Acid-etch canine riser occlusal treatment. *J. Prosthet. Dent.* 46:149, 1981.
28. Williams V.D., Drennon D.G., Silverstone L.M.: The effect of retainer design on the retention of filled resin in acid-etched fixed partial dentures. *J. Prosthet. Dent.* 48:417, 1982.
29. Black G.V.: The force exerted in the closure of the jaws. *Dent. Cosmos* 37:474, 1895.
30. Howell A.H., Manly R.S.; An electronic strain gauge for measuring oral forces. *J. Dent. Res.* 27:710, 1948.
31. Anderson D.J.: Measurement of stress in mastication. *J. Dent. Res.* 35:672, 1956.
32. A special thank you to Mr. Doug Aunan, C.D.T., University of Iowa, for his technical support in preparation of this material.

CHAPTER 20

Problems and Mechanics of Shade Selection

ARTHUR N. KRACHT, D.D.S.

THERE MAY BE NO AREA of dentistry that creates more difficulties than the making of a porcelain restoration that will duplicate or replace lost tooth structure esthetically. Every color or shading system has been plagued by inadequate coordination between the shade selection process and the crown fabrication. Ideally, there should be a simple standard to effectively use for all cases but no such standard is available.

The commonly used commercial shade guides resemble denture teeth and are excellent for denture tooth selection. The resemblance is in the porcelain thickness, layering, blending, surface characteristics, and type of porcelain. They are inexpensive and available. However, if used for a veneering technique of a low fusing porcelain on a metal backing, they not only lack precision but produce unreliable results. Historically, there have been more than 125 different porcelain shade guides manufactured. New techniques and better porcelains have placed most in the obsolete category.

Clark,[1] who realized the problem, published data on the color of 6,000 anterior teeth of 1,000 patients. He duplicated the colors in ¼ inch square tabs of porcelain. The result was 361 incisal third shades or colors and 342 gingival third colors. The assumption is that the middle third color or shade is a blend of incisal and gingival shades. Clark thought that shades or colors could be assembled in a shade guide of 60 samples. Unfortunately, this shade guide and matching porcelain is not available. If it were, it might be too complicated for the average dentist to use effectively.

Culpepper[2] compared the reliability of commercial shade guides under four different kinds of lights. Perhaps because of inadequate color delineation between shade guide selectors, experienced dentists could duplicate previously selected color shades only about 22% of the time. Only 2 of 37 experienced dentists were able to select the same or "ideal" shade on successive visits. The rest of the group, on consecutive days, had a tendency to select both lighter and darker than the original shade. The problem examined by Culpepper is one that has been examined by other researchers in a variety of fields. His results are predictable.

Sproull[3] showed the disparity between the color range of natural teeth and available shade guides by a detailed spectrophotometric study on commercial shade guides and natural teeth. He converted this data to the internationally accepted

Munsell Color System. Sproull's work showed the color range needed and the results were plotted in terms of the three attributes: hue, value, and chroma.

Hue is a sensation, to which the observer is aware, of varying wave lengths of radiant energy, the color. Value is the relative quality of whiteness or blackness in a color. Low value has more black, high more white. Chroma requires a hue and denotes an increase or decrease of color saturation or purity.

This was the first study to categorize and define the physical aspects of color in dentistry. Spectrophotometric information is important to the manufacturers in developing porcelains that simulate the color curves of natural enamel. However, it does not make it any easier to communicate thoughts on what is seen, even though it does aid in explaining what we do see. The latter is important. One must be able to correctly communicate thoughts to others in the precise manner that they are seen if another person is to fabricate the restoration.

Theoretically at least, machine selection would be the most accurate.[4] One recent innovation is the shade scanner or Chromoscan.* It is a two-bridged, tri-stimulus colorimeter, consisting of a light source of fiber optic probe light that illuminates and carries reflected light from the tooth to a built-in scanner. The latter analyzes the reflected light into primary colors and displays this information in a digital read out.[5] This reading is used by the laboratory technician to select porcelain combinations. This could be a scientific step forward but, practically speaking, the instrument needs further documentation for both accuracy and effectiveness as a substitute to human eye shade selection. Research at the moment stresses laboratory support and the selection and modification of various porcelain powder color blends.

There remains a wide margin of error from one crown to the next in several areas as a result of: (1) variation in facial, gingival, and incisal preparation reductions by the dentist; (2) combinations of porcelain overlays in thickness and coloration, incisal and gingival by the technician; and (3) unreliability and arrangement of available shade guides.

We know that in a child's beautiful teeth the dentine, and the enamel, is laid down in irregular layers and that the pulp influences the color of the tooth. The aging process produces significant changes as dentin is constantly laid down pulpally. Abrasion and trauma contribute small cracks and checks that frequently stain. The influence of caries, color of adjacent restorations, and normal wear all contribute to the changing appearance of the teeth. Frequently, at age 20, the teeth may compare with Bioform shade 60 or 62, whereas at age 70 these same teeth may correspond with Bioform shade 80 or even 81.

Pilkington[6] and others experimented with "what is seen" and "what is the sequence of sight." They report the following factors to be important: light, movement, outline form, surface characteristics, and color. They proposed that tooth form and surface characteristics were more important than color. Pilkington suggests that tooth form and surface characteristics can be learned and once learned can be mechanically applied. Color is clouded by many influences, some of which are insurmountable or uncontrollable.

Gill[7] suggests using previous training in basic sciences, histology, anatomy, his-

*Sterndent Corp., Mt. Vernon, NY 10550.

topathology, and the use of several different light sources for each selection. Argue[8] suggests that teeth should be pumiced and cleaned. The tooth is then divided into incisal or occlusal aspects, and middle and gingival thirds. The locations where the middle third blends with the incisal and gingival thirds are observed and recorded. Some early authors[6, 8] suggested "looking through" the enamel and selecting the shade of the dentin. Others suggested that enamel should be considered value. Sproull[3] suggests that in reality value is simply the change in lightness or darkness of the hue and chroma of the tooth. Unfortunately, color is in the eye of the beholder. More correctly, color is what the eye sees and the brain interprets and no two people see color alike.

Color blindness[9] is an inexact term that covers all major deviations from normal color vision. The most common is dichromatism. This is a sensitivity to only two distinct colors rather than the three needed to match all colors of the spectrum. Color blindness has also been categorized as (1) protans: red; (2) deutrans: green; (3) tritans: blue; and (4) tetrans: the rare complete or total color blindness. About 8% of males are affected, mostly dichromatic, and 0.5% to 1% of females, mostly green weakness. A person with anomalous (dichromatic) color vision may make few mistakes unless they are required to make a quick choice or repeat a selection. This is because they have learned certain external clues, such as size, shape, and brightness. Examples would be—the sky is blue, tomatoes are red, buttercups are yellow.

Itten,[10] a German artist stated that 18% of the population have absolutely no color ability, 18% have a brilliant color acuity, and the remainder can be taught a reasonable amount of color acuity and make real progress in color education. Light is color and light variables are reasonably controllable. The dentist and the ceramist must use the same type, wattage, and color temperature correct light, as well as light in a full spectrum of color in both shade selection and crown fabrication. It would be ideal to select the consistently best shade under daylight, color corrected room light, color corrected spot light, and incandescent light. Starting with a common lighting environment for dentist and technician is a must! Poor dental anatomy and surface characteristics may actually be reflected as essential shade differences. The color of the backing, the opaque material, and the porcelain firing all cause shade problems.

Shade selection starts with crown preparation. If possible, the crown preparation should be made so that the technician has a standard ideal thickness of metal and porcelain. A porcelain-fused-to-metal crown preparation must be considered a radical preparation. Johnston and others[11] state that to obtain translucence the technician must have a bulk of porcelain. They suggest a 2 mm incisal reduction. Others recommend a 3 mm reduction, a minimum of 0.7 mm reduction at the gingival or shoulder, and 1 mm over the rest of the labial surface and extending proximal reduction through the contact areas. When possible, even greater labial reduction is preferred. Teeth with large pulps may require a more shallow preparation even if it means remaking the crown in future years.

Pilkington[6] and others showed that variation in color is less noticeable than tooth form. The goal is unobtrusive attractiveness by copying features of adjacent teeth faithfully to produce harmony in the dentition. Pilkington had this in mind when he said, "In dentistry, esthetics is the science of copying or harmonizing our work with nature and rendering inconspicuous our art." In a single restoration especially, the simulation of its mate is of vital importance. To aid this, the best study model is a necessity.

How deeply should the average dentist become involved in the serious elements of light, optics, and color, or in the physical, physiologic, and psychologic factors of color? Fig 20–1 is an artist's conception of the optics and physics of light. One single line is usually used for descriptive purposes. Actually the eye is bombarded by a number of light waves that range in length from 3,500 to 7,500 angstrom units (380 to 760 nanometers).

Theoretically, besides light transmission, the teeth show regular and diffused diffraction, reflection, interference, absorption, refraction, scattering, and polarization. Diffraction is defined as the spreading of light around the edges of an obstacle. Diffraction, reflection, and interference all are a part in the complex phenomenon of scattering. In general, scattering light (short waves) appear blue; whereas directly transmitted light rays lack the scattered blue and appear orange or red. This is the reason that the sun, the principal source of white light, varies from hour to hour. High in the dry, clean atmosphere the sun looks white in the deep blue sky. Early or late in the day the light rays approach at a sharper angle and a longer distance. After piercing miles of dusty or vapor-filled particles, the blue (short waves) are removed and the remaining (longer waves) appear orange and red.

Color is light, and light is one area where the dentist and technician can start on the same footing provided the difference of individual color perception is disre-

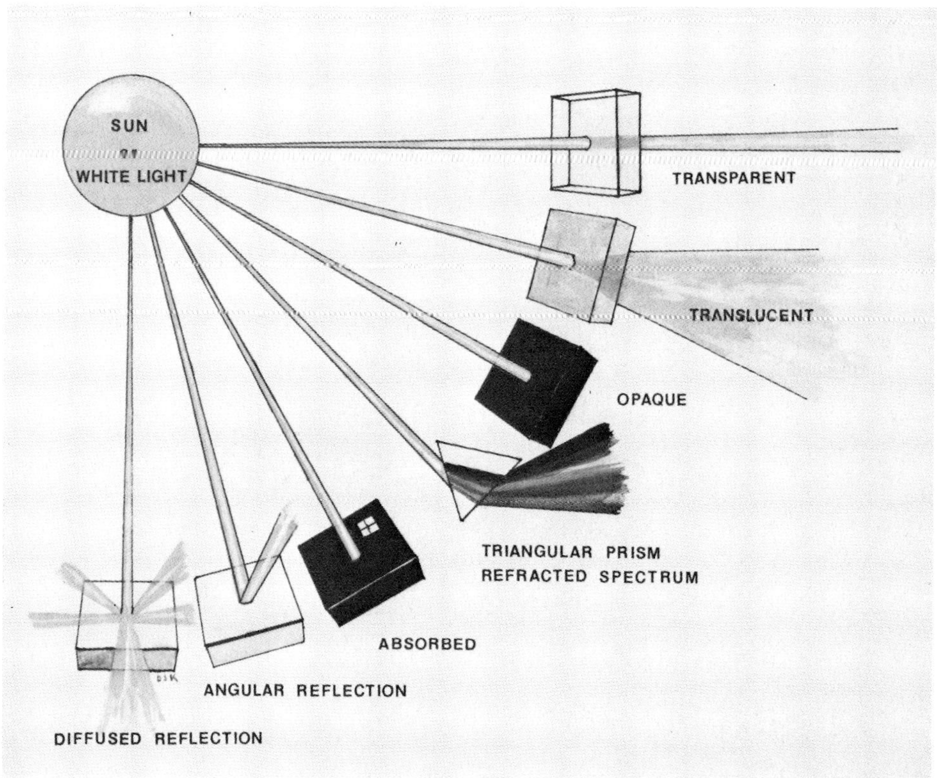

Fig 20–1.—Optics and physics of light.

garded. Both dentist and technician should have color corrected or near full spectrum white lights. The Ney Light* is one that is available. Ideal artificial light would be about 400 candlepower and Kelvin temperature of 5,500° to 8,000°. Too strong a light will wash out the color; too weak a light will not show subtle colors. The light must be comfortable to both operator and technician. It is important that the light used should neither add nor detract from the shade of the tooth.

Most dental operatories are rather subdued in color, but walls and ceilings do reflect light. Another subtle color change is the influence of lips, tongue, and gingiva on the tooth. This is, literally, borrowing from the adjacent color. Freshness or fatigue of the nervous system radically affects color decisions and even momentary fatigue of the retina can and does play unwelcome tricks when selecting a color. All of these factors should be remembered during shade selections.

Comparing sight and smell is interesting. The smell of a particular odor fatigues the olfactory cells and over a prolonged period the odor becomes less noticeable. In the eye, the fatigued cells act differently in that the effect seems to be cumulative and the result is that they send distorted signals to the brain. An example is the color of the walls in the room where the color is selected. The stimulus is there but the brain is not aware of it or simply ignores it.

It appears impossible to describe with a few words the subjective feeling of color in an objective manner. There will always be discrepancy between physical facts with psychic or psychologic facts. It is a known fact that no two people see color alike and the person best trained in color eventually will be fooled. This is similar to the conversation in which words are frequently interchanged and often incorrectly used. People understand the natural components of size, form, width, height, and length. Color is a void where people use three inept words: hue, chroma, and value.

Although not perfect, the Munsell Color Order System[12] should be accepted as the best. The reasons are that it is internationally recognized and accepted; and it is constant, simple, and flexible. There are several ways of explaining Munsell's Color Order System. It is done by sphere, tree, or wheels stacked on a common axle. A simple way to explain the differences between hue, chroma, and value is to use the analogy of the wheel. The axis represents value, the spoke represents chroma, and the rim represents hue.

HUE is simple. It is the family name of chromatic colors (red, yellow, and blue). Chroma and value are often confused, because both depend on black and white or gray.

VALUE is that quality by which we distinguish a light color from a dark one. Artists refer to it as the degree of lightness on a scale running from black to white. Black is rated zero and white ten (or 100) with gray (half black and half white) being a neutral value. Value is the axis of the wheel. The simplest way to change value is to decrease or increase the intensity of light. For this reason the term value has been substituted by brilliance and luminosity. Value can be compared with a black and white TV screen, the color was present in the original scene but you see it as brightness and darkness.

CHROMA is a subtle quality that refers to the concentration or purity of the hue. It is how we distinguish a strong from a weak color, and the richness of the

*The J.M. Ney Co., Bloomfield, CT 06002.

color such as dull, vivid, pale, weak, or strong. The degree of, or the departure from, a color sensation of black or white (gray) is the intensity of the hue or color. In a color wheel it is the spoke with the highest chroma near the rim and lowest near the axis of the wheel. Any of the above mentioned words, dull, vivid, etc., have been substituted for chroma.

Itten,[10] in his *The Art of Color* uses terms such as simultaneity and simultaneous contrast as well as harmony. Successive contrast is the basis for harmonious design because its observance establishes a precise equilibrium. To illustrate negative after-image, he states that a given hue must have a complementary hue present nearby. If the color is not there, it lacks harmony and will immediately generate a new color that is complementary to the original color. Both harmony and simultaneous contrast are closely related to retinal fatigue. Johnston[13] uses the term contrast enhancement, which is the intensifying of the difference perceived between adjacent colors or a brightness contrast. The term contrast enhancement, which is essentially borrowing color, is used interchangeably with simultaneous contrast or successive contrast.

Albers[14] explains negative after-image as the result of when the rod and cone nerve endings on the retina are tuned to receive any of the three primary colors (red, yellow, and blue). Staring at red will fatigue the red sensitive parts, so a sudden shift of sight to white results in stimulation of the yellow and blue sensory. This results in a momentary flash of green (complementary of red or red-orange). Young[15] theorized that there were three color receptors, R G B, in the forepart of the eye. In 1850, Herring theorized that there were three pairs of receptors or color coders. This led to the composite theory. In the forepart of the eye are the red, blue, and green receptors, followed by three pairs of coders, which translated all colors to the brain. One pair yellow and blue, one pair black and white, and the third pair red and green. Each pair antagonized each other, yet each pair required each other. When a green heart with a yellow border is stared at for several seconds and then the gaze is shifted to a blank white paper, a negative after-image appears as a red heart with a blue border. Herring's explanation was that there is a temporary switching of colors to the brain. If you withdraw the green and yellow stimuli, one part of the mechanism is shut down as a result of fatigue and the other part is sharply triggered. This produces a negative after-image. The literature mentions positive or true after-image that is most difficult to produce, whereas negative after-image can be easily produced by fatigue.

Harmony is another term that is explained in many ways. Is it pleasing or disagreeable? In music, is it pleasant or discordant? Harmony, technically speaking, is a balance or a symmetry of colors. Generally, complementary colors produce harmony. Itten[10] offers a suggestion that harmony, after-image, simultaneity, and simultaneous contrast are related in some way and that all are affected by retinal fatigue.

The physicist, Rainwater,[16] explains another phenomenon, successive contrast, which is closely related to after-image. When two contrasting hues are presented to the eye in rapid succession, a color effect of colors complementary to the original colors is produced. It is caused by the eyes switching back and forth rather than maintaining a fixed stare. This is quite similar to the "halo" experiment. This is demonstrated by having someone hold a colored object while you stare at it. At the end of 40 seconds they move the object towards your eye while you continue to stare. This produces a halo of complementary colors. This is said to be a result of the newly activated receptors that are not as fatigued as the original receptors were. A kaleidoscope of colors or rainbow effect results when closing your eyes after gazing at a 40 watt frosted light bulb for one or two minutes. These are some of the effects of retinal fatigue.

The effect of partial retinal fatigue is not known. For this reason it is suggested that short, quick glances not to exceed five seconds should be used when selecting shades. Some authors use terms such as "snap judgment" or "first impressions" as being the best. The color of teeth is basically yellow, and blue is its complementary color. This fact prompted the idea of shifting the eye from the tooth to a blue sheet of art paper. As blue and yellow harmonize and are in a balanced proportion, this tends to "rest" the eyes.

In 1936, Pilkington[6] mentions color fatigue and described retinal fatigue. Briefly, he stated that first impressions are best. The retina can interpret color correctly only a short time before fatigue destroys some sense of color value. He used the term "geometric metamerism." Two blocks of identical wood, but one smooth and the other rough, are both painted the same color. Under the same light the rough surface causes light to be reflected in every direction and appear darker than the smooth surface.

Preston[17] states that color is not always generated by a simple wavelength, but may result from an interaction of several wavelengths. Regardless of the type of illumination used, pairs of colored lights of the same spectral curve will always match. Pairs of colors that do not have the same spectral components may or may not match under different lighting conditions.

Practically and simply expressed, metamerism is the inability of two indentically appearing colors to continuously match each other under different lighting conditions and environments. This is a result of the difference in spectrophotometric curves. Metamerism and its effect can be lessened by choosing a shade under all lights, daylight, incandescent, and color corrected lights, as well as choosing the shade that looks best under all conditions.

An environmental factor, in addition to light, is the color of the walls of the room. If the operatory is rather subdued, color reflection from walls and surroundings can be ignored, even though they are present. Highly colored clothing should be covered with a neutral colored drape. Highly colored makeup and distracting jewelry should be removed during shade selection.

A wide variety of shade guides are helpful in shade selection. This is not necessarily to provide a wider range of colors but a variation of optical properties, other than color, from one shade tab to another. The optical properties of dentin, enamel, and porcelain are never identical. Neither are there pre-blended porcelains that can exactly duplicate a shade tab. Although the optical properties of dentin, enamel, and porcelain are so dissimilar, the actual blending of porcelain crown colors is by (1) eye, (2) instinct, and (3) chance or accident. The custom-made shade tabs are the best as they also minimize the effect of metamerism.

Some of the commercial shade guides that are currently available include: (1) Dentist's Supply Company—New Hue, Bioform, and Bioblend, (2) Vita Company—Vita Lumin Vacuum, (3) Universal Dental Company—Univac, Verident, (4) Swissdent International Company—Candular Swissdent, and (5) Meyerson Company—Meyerson's Special. All shade guide tabs with the same number have the

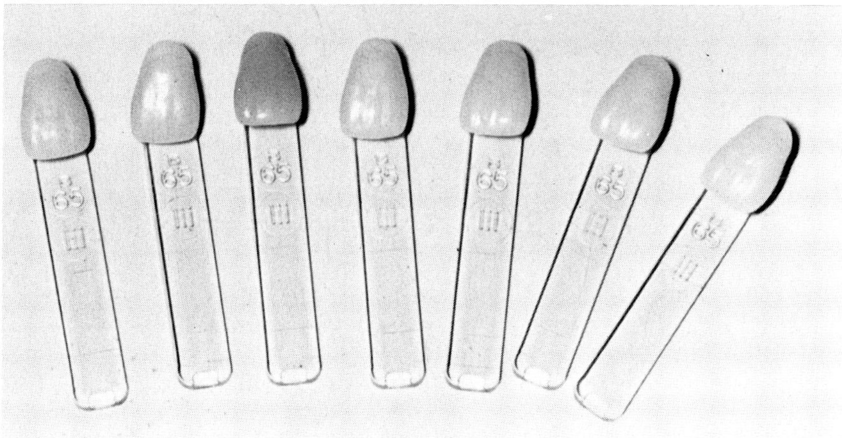

Fig 20–2.—Marked variations occur between tabs of the same shade number (65) by the same manufacturer. The tab used for selection should be sent to the laboratory technician.

same color of dentin, yet each may have a different enamel overlay. This enamel overlay gives a slightly different color reflection that is actually value (Fig 20–2). For this reason, the shade tab instead of the number should always be sent to the technician. Because the mold and position of the teeth are so important, the technician should be supplied with an accurate study cast to act as a guide to size, shape, contour, and position of the restoration. If there are major changes in size, shape, contour, or position of the restoration to be made, a diagnostic wax-up should be made and supplied to the technician.

Successful shade matching depends on several factors. First, the ability of the dentist to evaluate the color differences seen at the time the shade was selected. Second, the detection of tooth morphology as well as shade differences in the bisque bake stage so that adjustments in occlusion and other adjustments can be made. Third, a dependable shade guide. Unfortunately, no such guide exists.

There are several known reasons for color frustration in shade selection. They include: (1) lack of an accepted color system (as stated earlier, the Munsell Color System should be accepted as the best); (2) the lack of "color"training in dental graduates; (3) the failure to understand that no two people see color alike or fully understand that color is in the eye of the beholder; (4) the difficulty the majority of dentists have in selecting the same ideal shade on successive visits[2]; (5) available

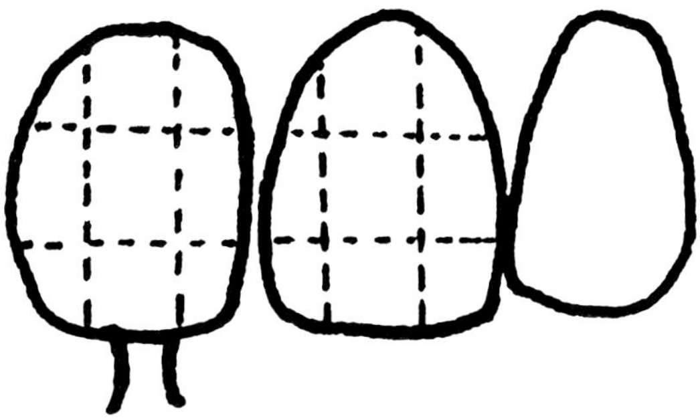

Fig 20–3.—The shade guide tab and tooth divided into nine marked areas. Marking is done with a soft lead pencil. These areas help confine the sight attention to a specific area.

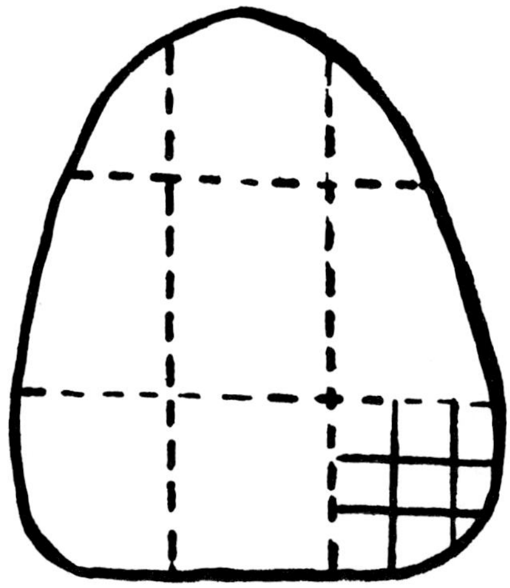

Fig 20–4.—Enlarged view with one area further subdivided with two lines each way.

porcelain denture teeth shade guides have different optical properties from natural teeth and are illogically arranged; (6) the failure of the dental student and dentist to carry a practical application of surface carving and tooth anatomy from preclinical to clinical dentistry; (7) not fully understanding after-image because of retinal fatigue and even partial retinal fatigue; and (8) failure to fully understand that color is not a characteristic of the object but is the characteristic of the reflected light from the surface of the object and its surrounding areas to the eye, which is then interpreted by the brain. Light, then, is color but involves physical, physiologic, and psychologic factors. Our goal is to evaluate the sum total of all these factors.

Sproull's[18] shade selection technique is as follows: use daylight, incandescent, spotlight, and color-corrected fluorescent ceiling lights. With a Vita shade guide, select the color family. The primary concern is to select a shade with a higher value and a weaker chroma than is desired in the finished restoration. The shade is evaluated under all lights and the one that consistently looks best is chosen. The technique of squinting is also used. Squinting switches perception from the cones to the rods. This is scotoptic vision and results in a more accurate selection of value by eliminating the confusion of hue and chroma. The ceramist delivers the restoration in the bisque bake. The dentist then modifies the form and surface characteristics and uses porcelain stains to modify the color.

The simple watching of the handpiece and the tooth will develop retinal fatigue. This alone should be ample proof that the shade pattern must be worked out and

Fig 20–5.—Shade guide tabs with ridge lap removed from one. Those that see a distinct difference of color with and without this bulk should remove this excess porcelain on all shade tabs.

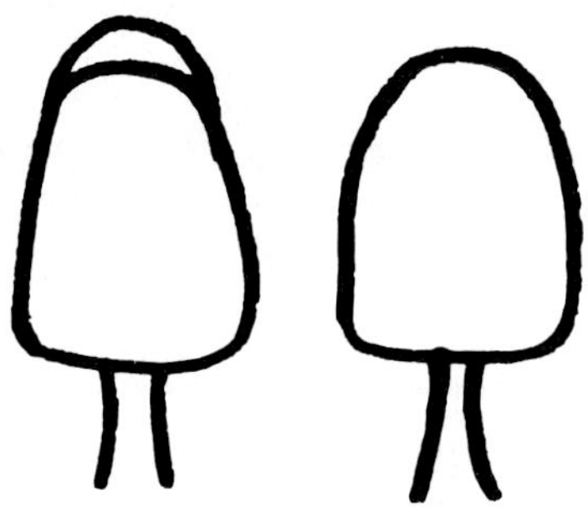

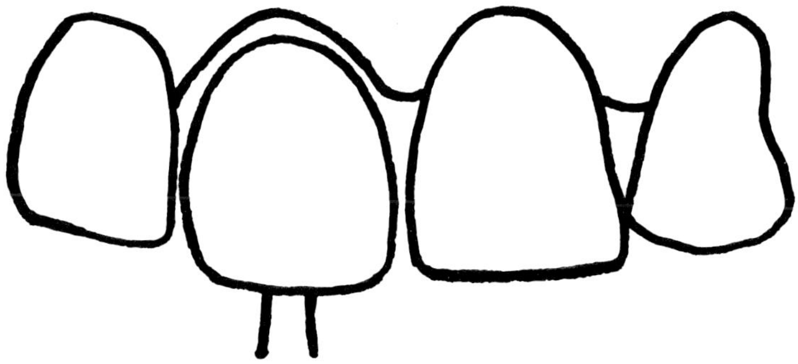

Fig 20–6.—Shade tab in edentulous space, parallel with the long axis of the tooth and the incisal of the tab towards incisal of the tooth.

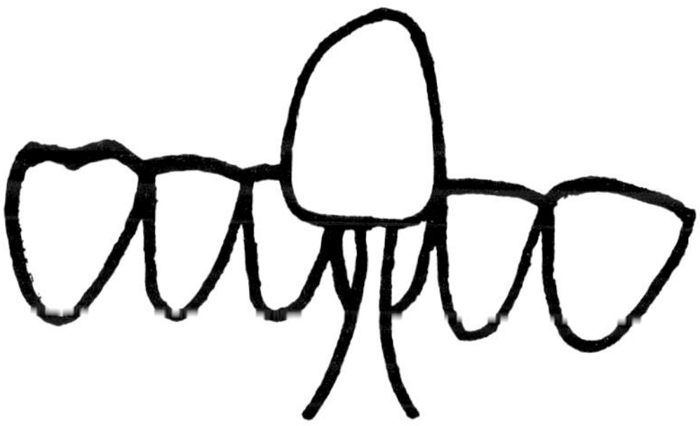

Fig 20–7.—The central shade tab is overlapping the mandibular incisors. This is an easy way to see if the shade harmonizes with the rest of the natural teeth.

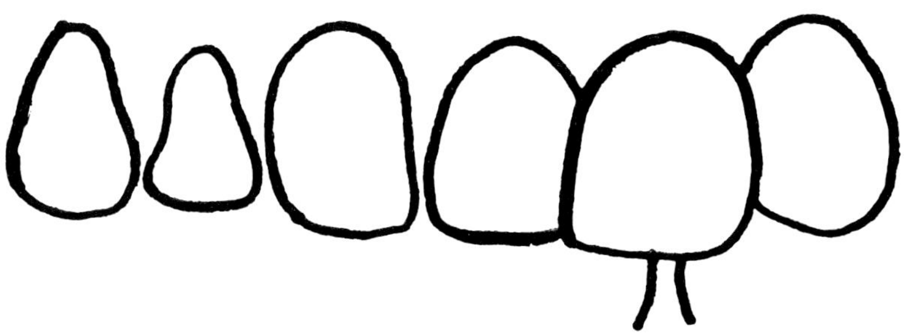

Fig 20–8.—The shade guide tab placed in the missing lateral space. In some cases, the central incisor is lighter and the canine is darker. Both shades can be recorded and the technician instructed to blend the distal half of the restoration with the canine and the mesial half with the central incisor.

properly recorded before the preparation starts. An aid to communication with the technician is a chart of the labial surface of the tooth to be restored (Fig. 20–3). A soft pencil may be used to divide the tooth into halves or draw two lines incisogingivally and two lines mesiodistally to give nine parts. Masking tape can also be used. This tends to confine the eye to one section and aids in a more accurate location of surface characteristics, grooves, translucency, stains, surface checks, and the influence of restorations in adjacent teeth (Fig. 20–4). The shade guide must be marked or covered in the same manner. The chart should list everything that will help the technician to harmonize and produce the best esthetic value of the restoration.

If the gingival area of bulk, the ridge lap area of the shade tab, is confusing, two shade tabs should be used with the gingival bulk removed from one. The two are placed adjacent to each other (Fig. 20–5). If the gingival bulk gives a sensation of a different color, grind away the gingival bulk of all tabs before use. If the bulk has been removed, the shade tab can be easily laid adjacent to the natural tooth (Fig 20–6). For overall harmony, many operators, as a second step, prefer overlapping the selected shade on the mandibular incisors (Fig 20–7).

When a lateral incisor is missing, the shade tab may be placed against the canine and the central incisor. If the central incisor is found to be NH 62 and the canine NH 65, both shade tabs should be given to the technician with instructions to blend the distal half with NH 65 and the mesial half with NH 62 (Fig 20–8). The other option is to match the central incisor only. This decision may depend on the shade of the contralateral tooth. The patient may approve, but the dentist is responsible for all shades selected.

In conclusion, teeth are composed of dentin and enamel. To fabricate a porcelain-fused-to-metal crown that will exactly simulate the appearance, texture, color, and characteristics of a natural tooth may well be impossible. The basic reasons are that

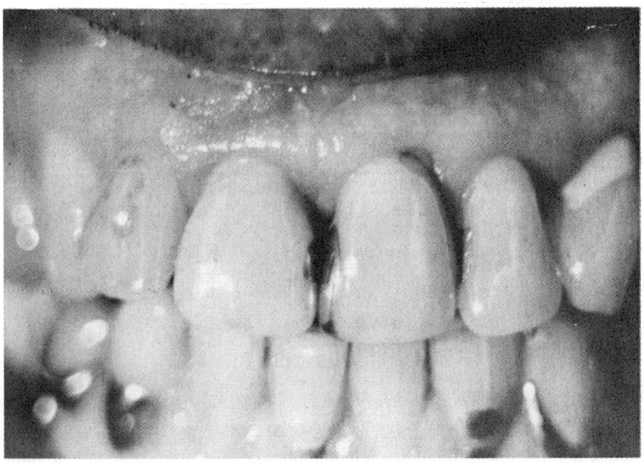

Fig 20–9.—Maxillary right central incisor restored with porcelain-fused-to-metal crown with simulated Class III mesial gold restoration. The restored crown is wider than the natural central incisor but is made to appear the same width by rounding the distal incisal angle. The labial line angle reflections of the two central incisors indicate comparable labial contour. Some brown stain on the incisal edge of this crown results in further personalization.

the enamel is usually transparent and the core of the tooth, or the dentin, is relatively opaque. Color is an agent that is physically and chemically definable as well as being an analyzable pigment. However, it requires human meaning and content through optic and cerebral perception. But excellent esthetics can be achieved (Fig. 20–9).

REFERENCES

1. Clark E.B.: Tooth color selection. *J. Am. Dent. Assoc.* 20:1065, 1933.
2. Culpepper W.D.: A comparative study of shade matching procedures. *J. Prosthet. Dent.* 24:166, 1970.
3. Sproull R.C.: Color matching, Part I. The three dimensional nature of color. *J. Prosthet. Dent.* 29:416, 1973. Color matching in dentistry, Part II. Practical application of the organization of color. *J. Prosthet. Dent.* 29:556, 1973.
4. Exposita E.: Color perception and how it affects dental shading, Sterndent Corp., Mount Vernon, NY 10550. Personal communication.
5. Selander D.: Sterngold, 60 Viaduct Road, Stamford, CT 06907. Personal communication.
6. Pilkington E.L.: Esthethics and optical illusions in dentistry. *J. Am. Dent. Assoc.* 23:641, 1936.
7. Gill J.R.: Color selection—It's distribution and interpretation. *J. Am. Dent. Assoc.* 40:539, 1950.
8. Argue, J.E.: The problem of tooth color. *J. Am. Dent. Assoc.* 24:1341, 1937.
9. Wright W.D.: *Research on Normal and Defective Color Vision.* St. Louis, C.V. Mosby Co., 1947.
10. Itten J.: *The Art of Color,* ed. 1. New York, Van Nostrand Reinhold Co., 1961, Translated from German by Ernst Van Haggen.
11. Johnston J.F., Mumford G., Dykemia R.W.: The porcelain veneered gold crown. *Dent. Clin. North Am.* 653, Nov., 1958.
12. Munsell A.H.: A Color Notation, ed. 12. Baltimore, Munsell Color, 1975.
13. Johnston J.F., Phillips R.W., Dykema R.W.: *Modern Practice in Crown and Bridge Prosthodontics,* ed. 3. Philadelphia, W.B. Saunders Co., 1971.
14. Albers J.: *Interaction of Color.* New Haven, Yale University Press, 1975.
15. Young T.: *Light and Vision.* New York, Time, Inc., Life Science Library, 1966.
16. Rainwater C.: *Light and Color.* New York, Golden Press, 1971.
17. Preston J.D., Bergen F.: *Color Science and Dental Art.* St. Louis, C.V. Mosby Co., 1980.
18. Sproull R.C.: Personal communication.

CHAPTER 21

Restoration of Endodontically Treated Teeth

MIGUEL A. PASTRANA, D.M.D.

MANY PATIENTS and dentists neglect the need for adequate restorations for teeth that have been treated endodontically.[1] Important considerations and principles involving these restorations have not been given proper attention. Improper diagnosis and treatment planning for the teeth involved, poor patient selection, and iatrogenic factors are some of the causes for failures.

It is well known that teeth that have lost their nerve and vascular supply become more brittle. This is because of the reduction in internal moisture that occurs, causing a reduction in resiliency. This renders the tooth more prone to fracture (Fig 21–1).[2, 3]

Endodontic treatment saves the tooth from extraction but only adequate restoration will reinstate it as a long-term functioning member of the mouth.[4] Before performing endodontic therapy it is necessary to carefully evaluate the tooth to assure that it can be restored adequately. The condition of the tooth must be sound enough to provide a reasonable life expectancy of useful function.

DIAGNOSIS

A careful radiographic analysis of the tooth should be done to determine: (1) extent of carious lesions; (2) extent of fractures; and (3) alevolar bone support.

If caries has caused the death of the pulp, it is important to analyze how deep the carious lesion is and if enough sound tooth structure would remain to retain and support an adequate restoration if endodontic treatment were done. It is common to encounter situations where the endodontic treatment has been possible but the construction of a restoration to protect that tooth has not been possible (Fig 21–2).

Any fractures should be carefully examined to determine if endodontic therapy is indicated (Fig 21–3,A-C). In teeth where esthetics is a factor, we have to be extremely careful to visualize what the final appearance of the area will be. If periodontal procedures that alter the level of the gingiva are needed to make the tooth restorable, the esthetic result may not be acceptable to the patient. A fracture of a maxillary central incisor, which involves the periodontal attachment on the proximal or the labial aspect, will likely require a surgical procedure that will alter its tissue level apically. This will cause an asymmetrical appearance that results in an unesthetic effect.

A third factor is unacceptable bone support for the tooth. This must be carefully

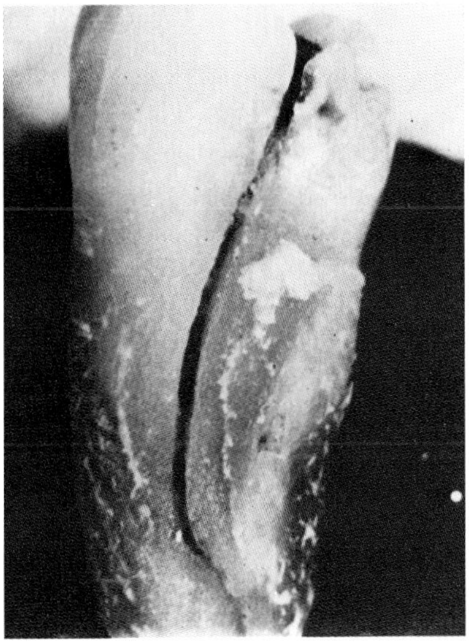

Fig 21–1.—A split tooth that had to be extracted because it was not properly protected and restored after completion of successful endodontic treatment.

studied before performing the endodontic therapy. In many instances, endodontic treatment can be successful but the tooth may not be periodontally sound enough to become an efficient functioning unit of the mouth. A healthy periodontium is extremely important in patients who are undergoing any extensive restorative treatment.[3] If there is loss of the supporting structures of the teeth the prognosis for any kind of restoration is guarded. The prognosis for the restoration can never be better than the patient's periodontal prognosis.

If any or all of the above problems are of a concern, consideration should be given to extracting the tooth and providing a fixed replacement. Such a decision must be made after considering all facets of the individual case. Certainly, it would seem advisable to extract a questionable tooth and replace it with a pontic if the adjacent teeth were also to be restored.

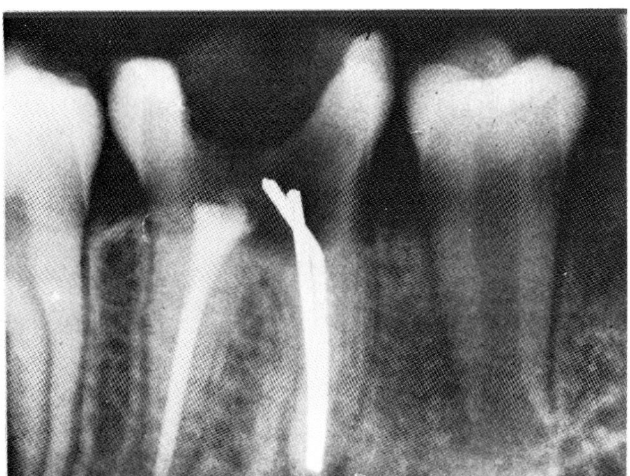

Fig 21–2.—A molar requiring extraction after successful endodontic treatment. The progression of caries through the bifurcation rendered the tooth nonrestorable.

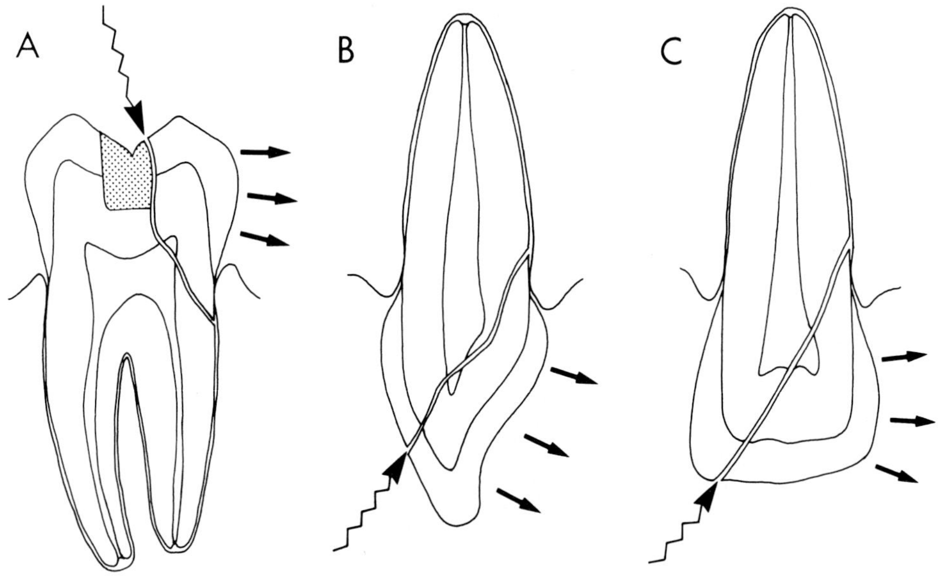

Fig 21–3.—A, a restored molar has fractured through the pulp and apically to the periodontal attachment. With proper periodontal management and endodontic treatment this tooth could be restored and returned to function. **B,** a central incisor is fractured through the pulp and apically to the periodontal attachment on the lingual aspect. With proper periodontal management and endodontic treatment this tooth can be functionally and esthetically restored. **C,** a central incisor is fractured through the pulp and apically to the periodontal attachment interproximally. Even the best periodontal management is likely to result in an altered level of the interdental papilla that might distract from the esthetics of a restoration.

The general root conformation relative to length, curvature, shape, and size must be carefully studied before determining if it is feasible to treat the tooth endodontically. Two additional factors that are frequently overlooked when evaluating patients for endodontic treatment are oral hygiene and age of the patient. A patient with poor oral hygiene is always a risk for any kind of dental restorative treatment. Restorations constructed for these patients are more likely to fail because of lack of proper care and maintenance. The patient's oral hygiene habits must be acceptable before attempting tooth reconstruction. As patients older than 55 tend to show recession of the pulpal tissues in their teeth,[5] these teeth tend to become more brittle. Endodontic therapy with these conditions will render teeth even more prone to fracture.[2] Careful analysis of the patient's occlusion is also necessary to determine if a risk is involved.

PREPLANNING ENDODONTIC THERAPY

Careful preplanning of the endodontic treatment should be done so that the canal can be filled with a material that can be easily and adequately eliminated. One of the more frustrating situations that a dentist can encounter is a tooth that needs a post, but the root canal is filled with a silver point. There is really no adequate way to prepare this canal without endangering the integrity of its walls[6] and apical seal. The best material for filling the canal is gutta-percha. This provides easy access to the canal with the reamer and safe removal to the desired depth. Removal may be done with a warm heater plugger instrument, Glidden* drills, Peeso** reamers, or pre-sized drills supplied with most preformed post kits.[5, 6] Some authors recommend the use of hot instruments for the elimination of gutta-percha because rotary instruments could alter the apical seal of the canal.[3]

Radiographs are an indispensable aid when preparing the root canal for the construction of the post.[5] Direction and depth of the preparation can be easily monitored and danger of perforation greatly reduced. Perforation of the root is not easily corrected. It requires periodontal surgery and the prognosis of that tooth may be poor.

CONSTRUCTION OF A CAST POST AND CORE

The gutta-percha should be removed from the canal at least two thirds of the root's length.[5] Another guide for minimal post length is equal to the length of the tooth's normal clinical crown. The prepared root canal should leave at least 2 to 3 mm of undisturbed gutta-percha at the apex. If these rules are violated, the life expectancy of the restoration will be shortened. Lateral forces exerted on the clinical crown will not be adequately resisted. Forces applied at the cusp tips tend to concentrate at the height of the periodontal attachment as a pressure fulcrum.[6] Long post length reduces the incidence of fracture of these restorations.[7]

The post and core should be designed to resist both lateral and rotational forces. Adequate retention should be provided to the post to prevent dislodgement from the canal (Fig 21–4 and 21–5). The core should engulf, by use of proper contrabevels, as much of the remaining tooth structure as possible.[5]

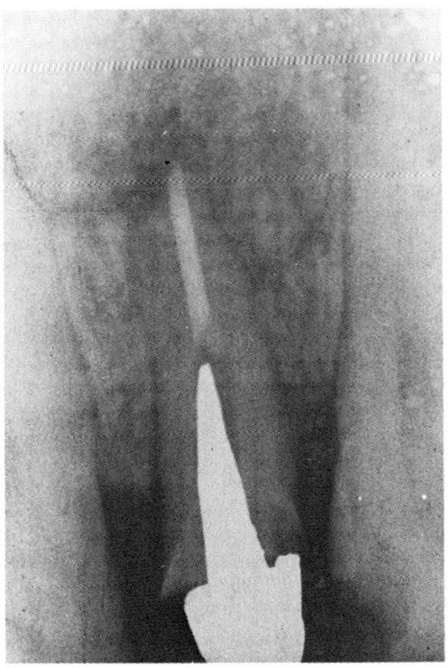

Fig 21–4.—A cast post and core that is obviously short radiographically and not well adapted to the lateral wall of the prepared canal. This greatly reduces the support and retention gained from the cast post and core.

*Premier Dental Products Co., 1710 Romano Dr., Norristown, PA 19401.
**Union Broach Co., Inc., Long Island City, NY 11101.

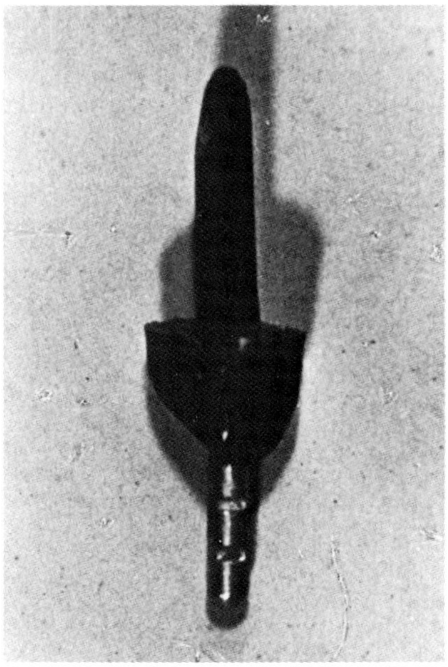

Fig 21–5.—A post and core pattern that accurately fits and fills the prepared canal will provide optimum retention.

If sound tooth structure remains in the coronal portion of the nonvital tooth, there is no need to eliminate it completely. Sound structure will serve to prevent dislodgement and rotation from lateral forces acting on the coronal portion of the tooth (Fig 21–6). In cases where all the coronal tooth structure has been lost or is removed because of weakness, an antirotational device in the form of an internal lock or an auxiliary pin may be needed to prevent rotation of the restoration.[5]

Cast posts are made from a pattern fabricated of resin or wax. The pattern is made with the aid of an old bur, a wire, plastic toothpick, or plastic dowel. Wax or resin adheres to any of these materials and is used to reproduce the form and dimension of the inner surface of the tooth. The core portion is built and shaped

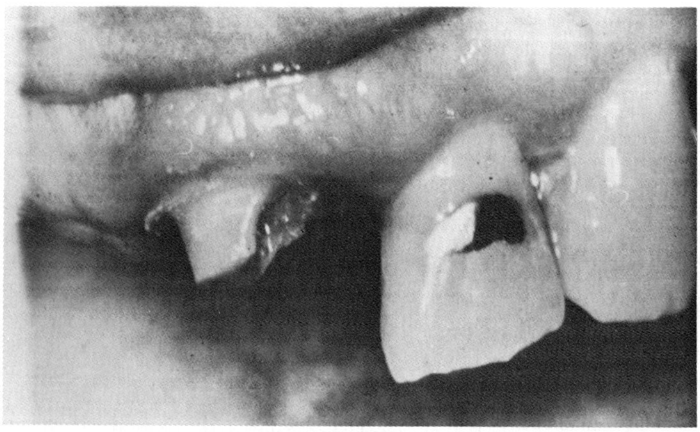

Fig 21–6.—Sound dentin is left to help support the foundation after caries has been removed and the canal prepared for the cast post and core pattern.

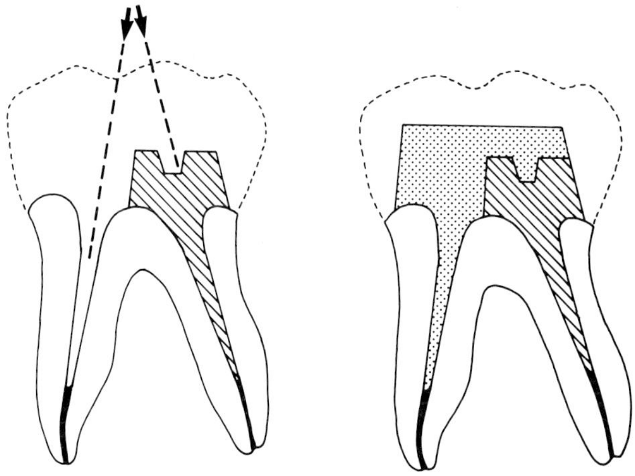

Fig 21–7.—Where maximum retention and support is needed on molar with divergent canals a two-section interlocking cast post and core is most effective.

directly in the mouth and the completed pattern is sprued, invested, and cast.

Some dentists prefer to use the indirect method for posterior teeth because of the difficult access. The cast post provides a foundation with maximum strength for restoring devitalized teeth. Retention and resistance form are the best with this conventional technique because the post is a nearly perfect copy of the internal portion of the canal. In situations where heavy masticatory forces are anticipated, this will be the method of choice for constructing the post and core.

The use of interlocking posts (Fig 21–7) also provides a good foundation for badly destroyed molars.[8] It is important to pattern the most divergent root first and to then establish the path of insertion of the other root preparations parallel to the interlocking box.

When constructing a temporary restoration for a tooth without the post in place, it is recommended that a cotton pellet or a piece of cotton applicator stick be placed in the canal to prevent cement from entering the already prepared canal. Any small particles of temporary cement in the canal will prevent the proper seating of the cast post and cause unnecessary time and effort in cleaning the canal.

Prefabricated Posts

There are a variety of prefabricated systems for restoring endodontically treated teeth on the market. Some of those are: (1) Parapost System (Whaledent Co.) (Fig 21–8,A,B); (2) Kurer Crown Anchor System[10] (Union Broach Co.) (Fig 21–9); and (3) Radix Anchor System (Star-Dental Co.) (Fig 21–10).

Most of these systems are satisfactory if the operator follows the instructions carefully and if the limitations of each system are considered. Some basic guidelines important to the selection and use of preformed posts include: (1) stainless steel is a stronger post material than gold; (2) cylindrical posts are more retentive than conical posts; (3) retention is increased by about 40% with the use of serrations on the post, as opposed to a smooth post; (4) post length should be at least two thirds the length of the root; and (5) axial forces are transmitted in line with the long axis of the tooth when cylindrical posts are used.

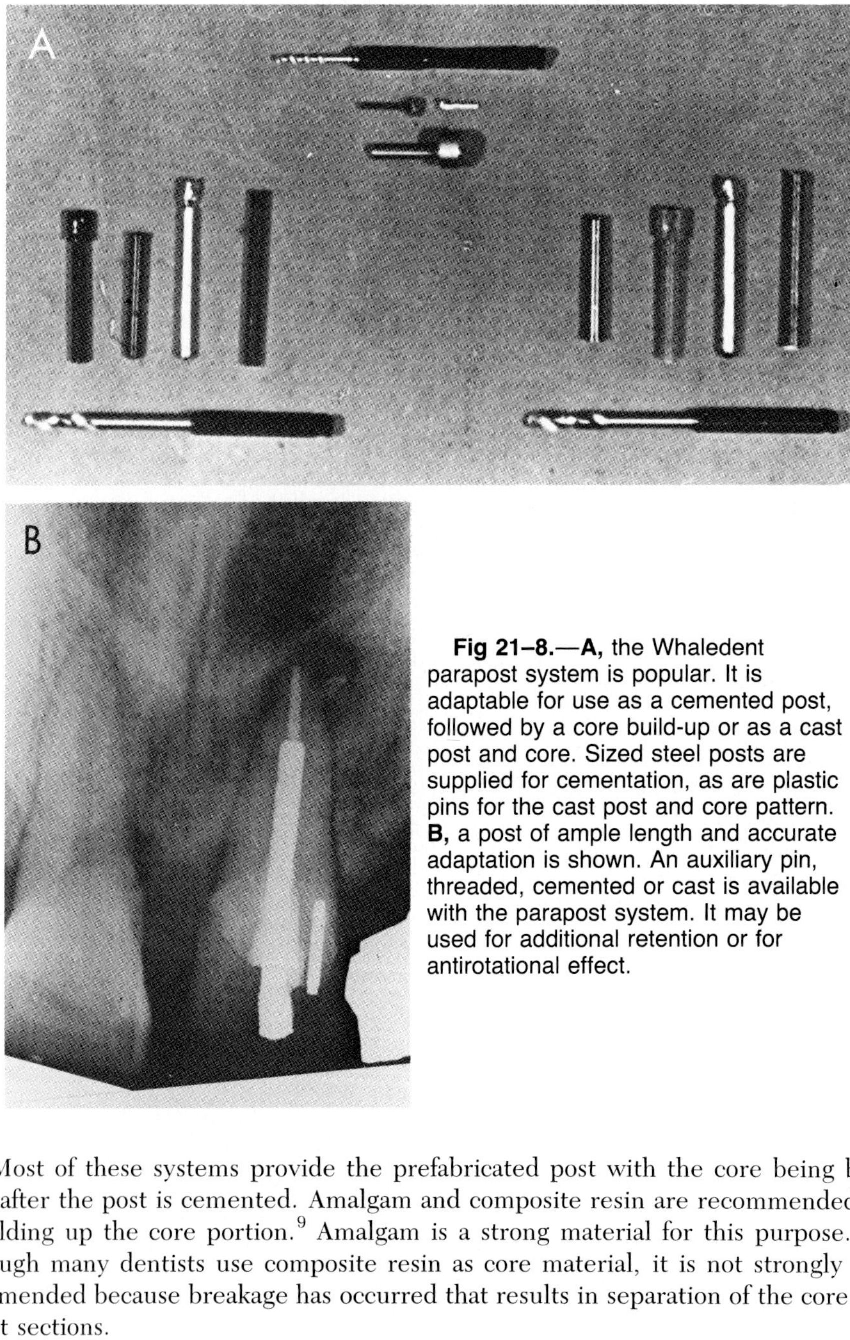

Fig 21–8.—A, the Whaledent parapost system is popular. It is adaptable for use as a cemented post, followed by a core build-up or as a cast post and core. Sized steel posts are supplied for cementation, as are plastic pins for the cast post and core pattern. **B,** a post of ample length and accurate adaptation is shown. An auxiliary pin, threaded, cemented or cast is available with the parapost system. It may be used for additional retention or for antirotational effect.

Most of these systems provide the prefabricated post with the core being built up after the post is cemented. Amalgam and composite resin are recommended for building up the core portion.[9] Amalgam is a strong material for this purpose. Although many dentists use composite resin as core material, it is not strongly recommended because breakage has occurred that results in separation of the core and post sections.

Amalgams and Composites

Anterior teeth that have been treated endodontically and that need a crown for reconstruction should have a post and core fabricated. This may be a one piece casting or one of the prefabricated posts with a coronal build-up of amalgam or

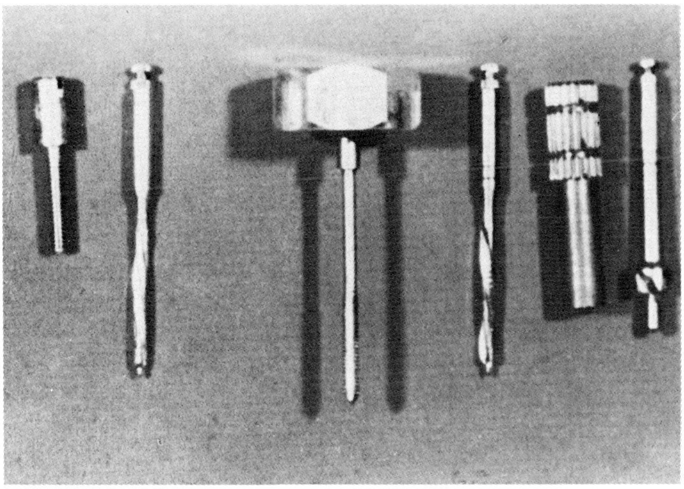

Fig 21–9.—The Kurer crown anchor system uses a threaded post with a preformed core. The prepared canal is hand threaded. The cement coated preformed post and core is turned into the threaded canal.

composite. Composite should be used only if the preparation margin for the crown extends at least 1 to 2 mm onto sound tooth structure. If this is not done, failure of the restoration may occur (Fig 21–11,A,B). During endodontic therapy, part of the internal tooth structure is eliminated. External tooth structure is eliminated when the tooth is prepared for a complete crown. A nonvital tooth tends to become brittle because of its loss of internal moisture. The combination of these factors causes the tooth to be less resistant to the lateral forces acting on it.

Posterior teeth are evaluated individually for the needs of the foundation. If sufficient tooth structure remains, a pin-retained foundation could be done before the construction of the crown.[9] If no coronal tooth structure remains, the tooth can be

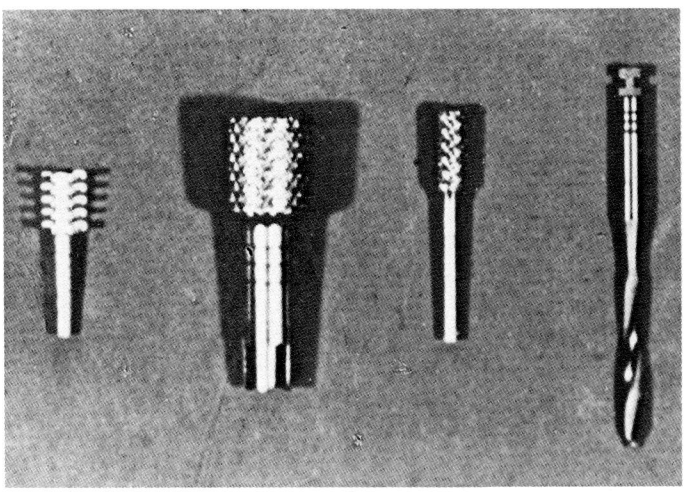

Fig 21–10.—The Radix anchor system uses a threaded post with a head designed to retain the core build-up.

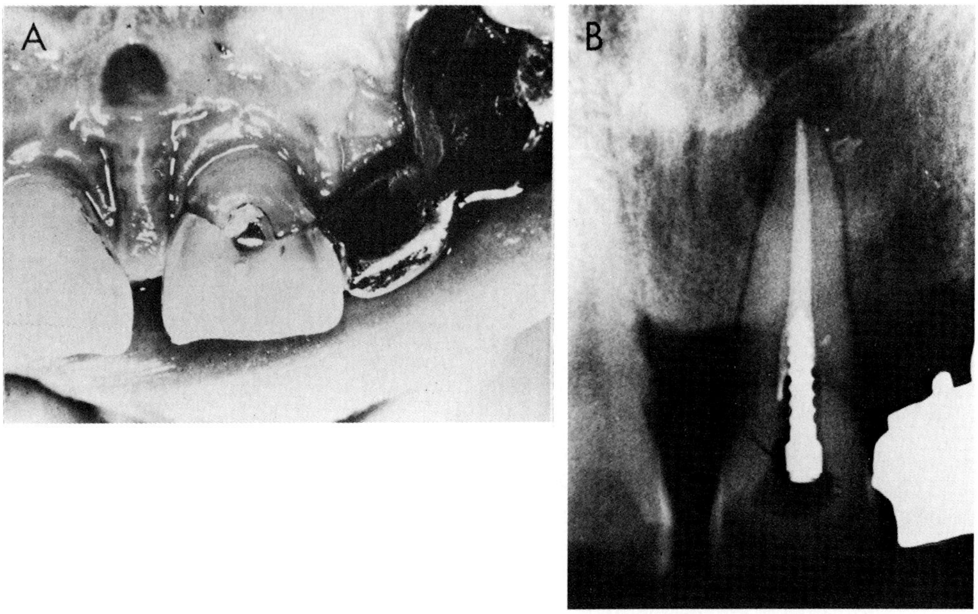

Fig 21–11.—**A,** the tooth is fractured at the level of the endodontic access opening. A preformed endodontic post is visible in the opening but failed to prevent fracture as a core was not finished and a crown was not fabricated. **B,** radiographically, the fracture is visible and the inadequate length and adaptation of the post observed. If a core had been built and a crown fabricated, the length and adaptation of the post would probably not have been adequate for long-term success.

reconstructed by the use of cast posts and cores or prefabricated posts combined with amalgam or composite build-ups, followed by the crown as the final restoration.[8] The foundation and the crown should be done separately to facilitate good marginal adaptation and provide optimum resistance to dislodgement under masticatory forces. Finishing the foundation before the crown is made eliminates problems of parallelism between the canal and the path of insertion of the crown. This provides better distribution of the forces that tend to cause fractures at the height of the periodontal membrane.

Final Restorations Indicated for Endodontic Teeth

Onlays are indicated for posterior teeth where there is a large amount of tooth structure left in good condition. The protection of the remaining cusps with this restorative procedure will permit the tooth to function properly under heavy loads. Correctly designed, they will tie the tooth together to prevent splitting. Adequate retention is attained when onlays are used as individual restorations. Any partial coverage restoration that covers and includes all of the occlusal surface is acceptable. Inlays are not acceptable because they do not protect the tooth from splitting and wedging forces.

Teeth that require a post and core or any major foundation buildup usually require full coverage restorations. These may be full cast restorations or esthetic veneer restorations. The choice depends on the preference of the patient and the location and visibility of the tooth in the mouth. Any full coverage restoration will adequately protect the nonvital tooth.

REFERENCES

1. Baraban D.J.: The restoration of pulpless teeth. *Dent. Clin. North Am.* 633, Nov, 1967.
2. Weine F.S.: *Endodontic Therapy.* St. Louis, C.V. Mosby Co. 1972.
3. Frank A.L.: Ingle J.I., (ed.) *Endodontics.* Philadelphia, Lea & Febiger, 1965.
4. Shillingburg H.T., Jr., Fisher D.W., Dewhirst R.B.: Restoration of endodontically treated posterior teeth. *J. Prosthet. Dent.* 24:401, 1970.
5. Shillingburg H.T., Jr., Hobo S., Whitsett L.D.: *Fundamentals of Fixed Prosthodontics.* Berlin, Chicago, Rio de Janeiro, & Tokyo, Buch-und Zeitschrifter-Velag "Die Quintessenz," 1976.
6. Baum L., Copper H.: *Advanced Restorative Dentistry Modern Materials and Techniques.* Philadelphia, W.B. Saunders Co., 1973.
7. Standler J.P., et al.: Analysis of stress distribution by endodontic posts, *Oral Surg.* 33:952, 1972.
8. Abdullah S.I., Bjorndal A.M.: A cast gold base for endodontically treated molar roots where divergent form precludes parallel post construction. *Dent. Dig.* 76:187, 1970.
9. Rosen H.: Operative procedures on mutilated endodontically treated teeth. *J. Prosthet. Dent.* 11:973, 1961.
10. Kurer P.F.: Retention of post crowns—a solution of the problem. *Br. Dent. J.* 123:167, 1967.

CHAPTER 22

Orthodontic Considerations in Fixed Prosthodontics

KAVITA NAKRA, D.D.S.

THE CORRECT ALIGNMENT OF the teeth is important to the prosthodontist because the functional balance of a fixed prosthesis is dependent on the position and alignment of abutment teeth. Often, this balance cannot be attained because extracted teeth are not replaced immediately, resulting in maloccclusion. The malocclusion, characterized by rotated or tipped teeth, poor contact, and elongation into opposing edentulous areas can cause problems when placing proper restorations. Often, extensive orthodontic treatment is required to make these teeth serve usefully as abutment teeth. At other times, the orthodontic treatment may be less complicated.

Orthodontic treatment for the adult patient generally involves compromise for the following reasons:[1]

1. Adult patients are less likely to accept wearing the required appliances;
2. The processes of jaw and facial growth have ceased in adult patients;
3. The tooth movement over large distances is accompanied by rebuilding and changing of bone that does not occur as easily in adults as in children;
4. Adult patients are simply not as cooperative as young children; and
5. A decision must be made between orthodontic and fixed prosthodontic treatment when a crossbite or deep overbite caused by a loss of teeth or alveolar bone has occurred.

The stability of occlusion can never be compromised for esthetics. Although esthetics is a major factor in many adult orthodontic cases, a basic decision has to be made that malocclusion itself is not to be corrected, but that minor tooth movements are to be carried out for restorative purposes.[2] This procedure is often called "minor tooth movement" to differentiate it from comprehensive orthodontics.

When abutment teeth are tipped mesially or distally in excess of 30° or when they are rotated in the same magnitude; they usually require involved orthodontic regulation. Tipping, or tipping and rotation, of such magnitude is usually a result of functional imbalances in occlusion that may be attributable to one or more extractions. When referring this kind of malocclusion to an orthodontist; the prosthodontist may expect, among other things, that the axis of the abutment teeth would be made parallel to each other. Fixed partial denture design dictates parallel axis of abutment teeth if the prosthodontist is to seat a one piece, multiple unit prosthesis. Second in importance would be to re-establish the plane of occlusion and to create the needed arch length. Last in importance would be the correction of abutment teeth rotation. Less significance is placed on orthodontic correction of minor tooth rotations, because the modern trend in prosthodontics is moving more and more to full coverage of abutment teeth.

CROSSBITES

Deep vertical and horizontal overlaps pose serious problems to the prosthodontist and are classified by Angle[1] as Class II. When maxillary and/or mandibular posterior teeth are lost, both vertical and horizontal overlap usually increase. In many cases, a poorly balanced occlusion is aggravated by the partial edentulation. In some instances, multiple posterior extractions block successful orthodontic objectives in malocclusion because vertical dimension is lost. In such cases, we should study the interocclusal distance of the teeth while the mandible is in the rest position to obtain some clues about the degree of overclosure during function. A word of caution must be inserted here concerning some of the "treatments" advocated for the correction of vertical overlap. There is a great difference between restoring vertical dimension and opening the bite to heights it never knew.

Bite planes can be used in the maxillary arch to restrain further overeruption of the anterior teeth and still permit the remaining posterior teeth to overerupt. It is difficult to achieve ideal occlusion in some Class II malocclusion cases found in the adult dentition, even though a full complement of teeth is present. A bite plane can also be used as a diagnostic splint in temporomandibular joint disturbances and mandibular displacements or in the establishment of correct vertical dimension before full mouth reconstruction. In constructing this splint, the labial wire of the bite plane may not be necessary. A mandibular diagnostic splint may be less bulky than a maxillary one. It may also create less esthetic and phonetic problems. The acrylic resin should be carried over the occlusal surfaces to the facial occlusal margins when using either maxillary or mandibular splints (Fig 22–1,A,B). To eliminate tooth guidance from premature contacts, the amount of acrylic resin on the occlusal surface should be little more than the thickness of one sheet of base plate wax. If the splint is to restore lost vertical dimension, it is made to equal the estimated

Fig 22–1.—A, B, mandibular occlusal splint in place before being occluded shows the amount of tooth coverage. Wrought wire clasps may not be necessary.

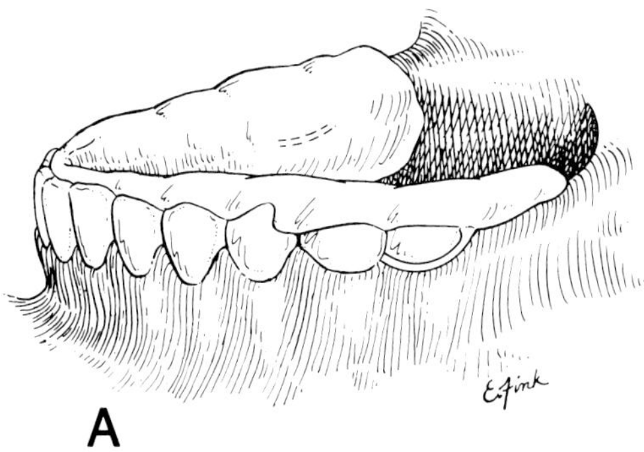
A

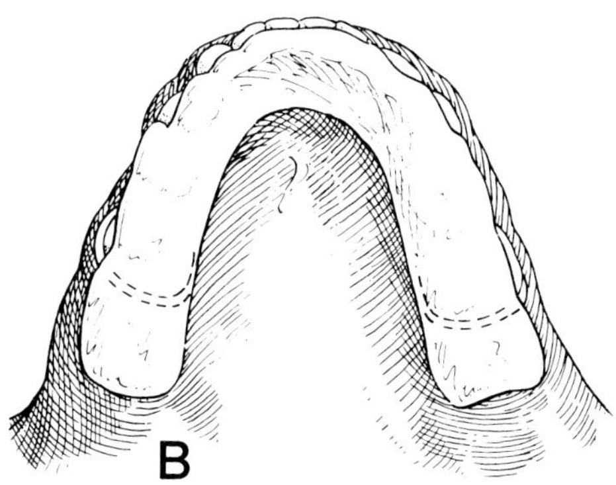
B

loss and altered later, if necessary. The diagnostic splint is occluded with the help of articulating paper or ribbon. The benefits of occlusal splints are:

1. They allow all the teeth in the opposing arch to contact the splint at the same time;
2. They allow the teeth freedom in eccentric movement;
3. With the splint in place, the mandible will be able to assume a centric relation position; and
4. The relations of the condyle, articular disc, and eminence will be more harmonious.

The occlusal surfaces of the splint may be altered by adding or removing autopolymerizing acrylic resin. These splints should be worn for a least four to six weeks with complete comfort for the patient. This will assure the prosthodontist that the vertical dimension established by the diagnostic splint can be safely duplicated in the permanent reconstruction. The diagnostic splint should be a simple, flat, plane bite plate.

MINOR TOOTH MOVEMENT

Minor tooth movement corrections can have a major effect on the results of fixed prosthodontic treatment. More ideally positioned teeth make the preparation of teeth for individual crowns and fixed partial dentures much easier. A more conservative preparation is usually possible. Frequently, better occlusion and proximal surface contacts can be attained. Esthetic appearance is often enhanced as a result of making more ideal tooth position and size, and pontic size possible.

Minor tooth movements that aid the prosthodontist in treatment include correction of anterior and posterior crossbites and closing of diastemas. Regaining pontic space may be important in fixed partial denture construction. Rotation of abutment teeth may also be helpful. These various tooth movements will be discussed individually.

Anterior Crossbite

It is important to determine whether the crossbite is a symptom of a more generalized malocclusion or purely a localized irregularity, before undertaking any corrective measures for an anterior crossbite. An effective and simple means of correcting the lingual crossbite of a maxillary incisor is to use an acrylic or cast metal inclined plane cemented to the mandibular incisors opposing the tooth in crossbite (Fig 22–2,A,B). The inclined plane should incorporate 1½ teeth on either side of the crossbite area. It should not impinge on the gingival tissue. The inclined plane should be at approximately 45° to the occlusal plane (Fig 22–3). The tooth in crossbite must be the only one contacting. The vertical dimension should not be opened more than 4 to 5 mm. The inclined plane should be smoothly polished and cemented in place with zinc phosphate cement. The correction of a malposed tooth is usually done in seven to 14 days. In no instance should the inclined plane be left cemented longer than six weeks. A prerequisite for the inclined plane is a normal or excessive vertical overlap and adequate space in the arch to bring the incisor into correct anteroposterior relationship with the mandibular incisors. If there is an end-to-end relationship, or an open bite tendency, the use of a bite plane is contraindicated.

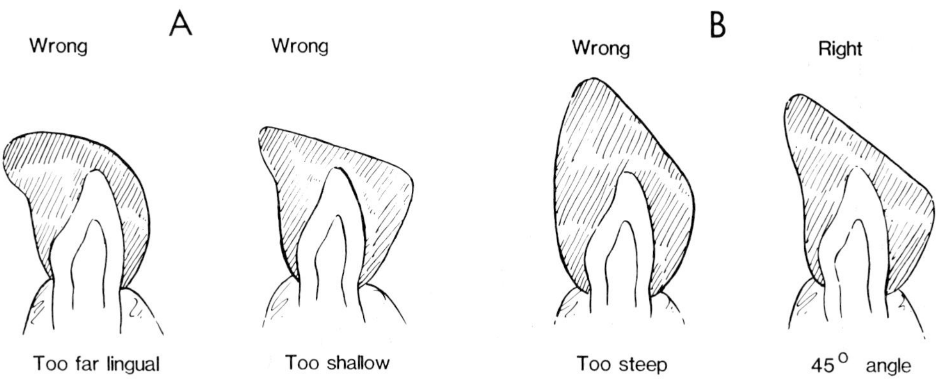

Fig 22–2.—**A,** a cross-section of acrylic guide planes in position on the mandibular teeth. The left one is too far lingual and rounded, the right at a too shallow angle. **B,** the left guide plane is at too steep an angle, whereas the right one is at the correct 45° angle.

Posterior Crossbite

Posterior crossbites usually occur whenever there is inadequate space in the arch to accommodate the teeth. Irregular eruption of teeth can also result in crossbite of a maxillary or mandibular premolar. Arch length deficiency, when seen, often requires the service of an orthodontist. One tooth alone is rarely tipped. In most cases, its antagonist in the opposite arch is out of position also. Thus, the maxillary second molar may be tipped lingually, whereas the mandibular second molar is tipped slightly buccally. In such cases both teeth must usually be moved.

Many malposed teeth are wider than the space available in the arch. Therefore, the space must be increased before the crossbite can be corrected. Crossbite correction is done by placing bands with spurs on the teeth in question and attaching elastics (Fig 22–4). There is usually sensitivity to the elastic hooks or spurs and discomfort for three to four days. It usually takes 16 to 20 weeks to eliminate second molar crossbite. If this condition is not intercepted before the eruption of third molars, crossbite correction may require removal of the third molars. Consultation

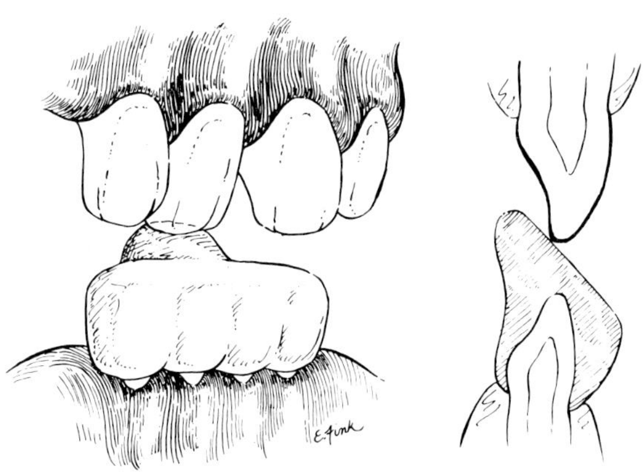

Fig 22–3.—Inclination, design, and contour of the guide plane is important. It should cover at least 1½ teeth on either side of the tooth being moved.

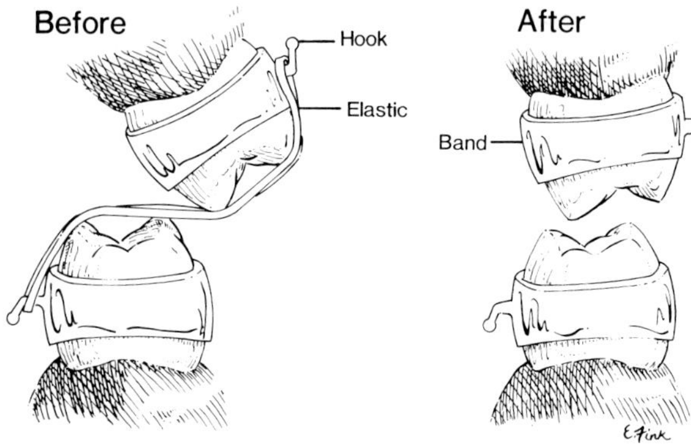

Fig 22–4.—Action of cross-bite elastics on a buccally malposed maxillary molar.

with an orthodontist on these interceptive and limited orthodontic procedures may be beneficial before instituting appliance therapy.

Diastemas

Diastemas and protruding incisors are both esthetic disabilities and dental health hazards in adults. They may also be a serious psychologic handicap. The anterior diastema stands out as a dark area between the teeth, and the patient is frequently self-conscious about it. A posterior diastema can lead to annoying and troublesome food impaction.

Diastemas may result from mesial or distal drifting of one or more teeth. Anterior teeth may migrate labially, bringing them into an arch of a larger circle. These may easily be corrected with a Hawley appliance (Fig 22–5). If diastemas of the maxillary anterior teeth exist but the tooth size, bone growth, and occlusal relationships prevent enough lingual movement to close the diastemas, more extensive orthodontic treatment is indicated.[3]

Patients with these problems may even request the removal of disfiguring incisor teeth and replacement with dentures. Because teeth can be moved in adults as well as children, numerous techniques are available to improve esthetic appearance and increase the longevity of the teeth. These orthodontic procedures should be undertaken in conjunction with conservative periodontal therapy. The patient may have to wear the appliance indefinitely as a retainer at night (Fig 22–6). An acid-etch resin bonded fixed splint retainer on the lingual may be an alternative.

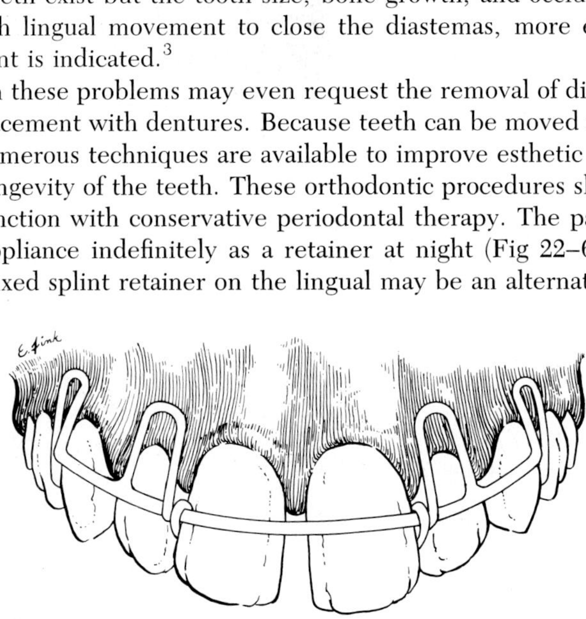

Fig 22–5.—Conventional Hawley palatal appliance with vertical loop fringe springs. Springs move central incisors together.

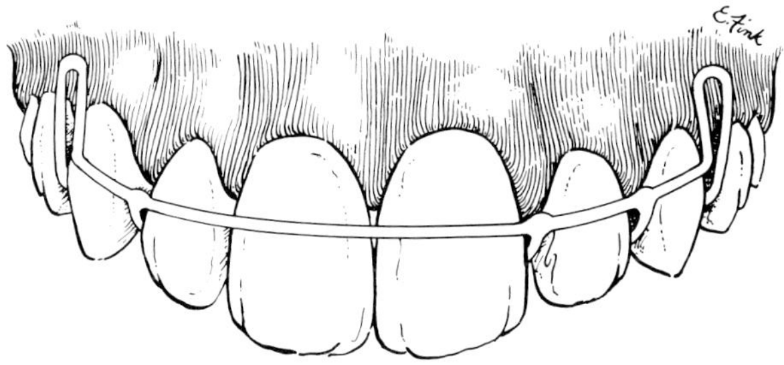

Fig 22–6.—Short spurs are adjusted to bear on distal surface of central and lateral incisors to hold them mesially.

Regaining Pontic Space

When teeth are not replaced for some time after their extraction, drifting frequently occurs and can present restorative problems. Caries with subsequent drifting of adjacent teeth into carious lesions is another common cause for loss of arch length. When the edentulous area is too narrow for a normal sized pontic to be placed in it, two options are available to the prosthodontist.[4] The first option involves excessive reduction of abutment teeth and an unesthetic narrow pontic. Another option would be to close the space by overcontouring the crowns on the adjacent teeth, making them appear undesirably wide. To have a good esthetic result, one or both of the abutment teeth may be moved to make a normal pontic space.

If the space loss is slight, a split acrylic spring-type removable space regainer may be used to re-establish the proper space (Fig 22–7). A jack screw[3] arrangement can also be built into the space regainer, with the space being opened gradually as the jack screw is opened (Fig 22–8). Then the unit is crimped on the threaded end to hold the regained space. An alternative[3] space regainer for opening a small space for premolars and first molars is the cantilever spring-and-bar space regainer (Fig

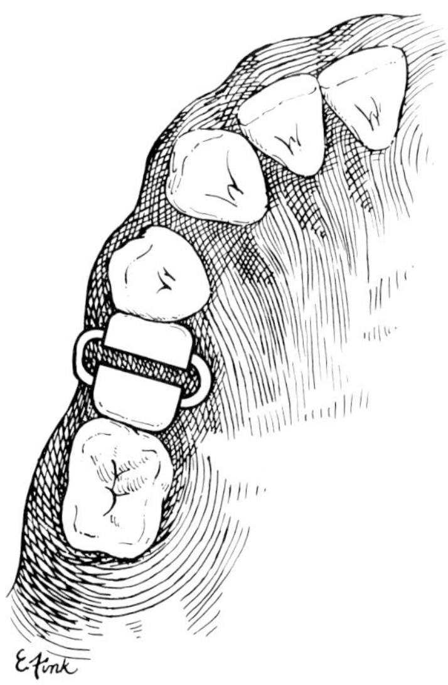

Fig 22–7.—Split acrylic spring space regainer. A compressed ellipse is formed using stainless steel wire with acrylic resin cured over it. The acrylic resin must be well adapted to the proximal surfaces of the adjacent teeth for retention. The acrylic resin is divided in the center. Pliers are used to activate the steel wire.

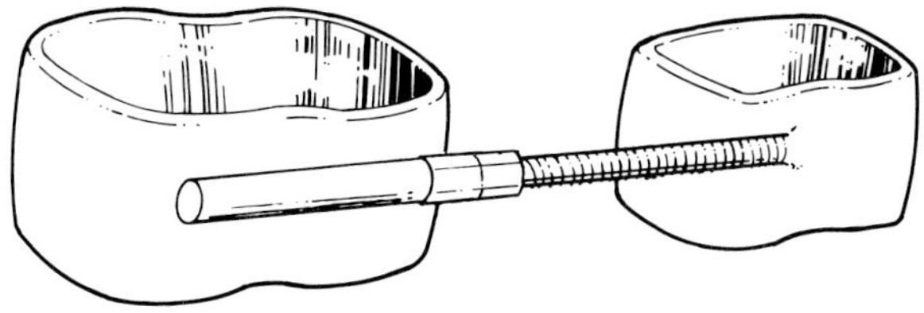

Fig 22–8.—Jackscrew space regainer moves teeth apart as screw is gradually opened. This is a fixed appliance involving banding of the abutment teeth.

22–9,A,B). This type of appliance is less resistant to displacement by the forces of occlusion than the jack screw two-unit appliance.

Rotating Abutment Teeth

Frequently, the anterior teeth that require crowns or splinting by a fixed restoration are found to be in poor alignment. If these teeth are rotated or crowded, excessive amounts of tooth structure may have to be removed, thus endangering the pulp or requiring devitalization of one or more teeth. Furthermore, the crowns constructed under such circumstances frequently have inadequate proximal contours, resulting in poor embrasures and chronic inflammation of the interproximal papilla.

Rotation is the movement of the tooth around its long axis. It is a relatively complicated tooth movement, difficult to effect and retain.[5] The production of a rotary movement requires the application of two equal and opposite pressures acting at a distance apart to produce a mechanical couple. This will produce rotation about a point somewhere between the lines of action of the two forces. It is, therefore, necessary to find, on a tooth to be rotated, two points at a suitable distance apart on which pressures in opposite directions may be applied. This requirement

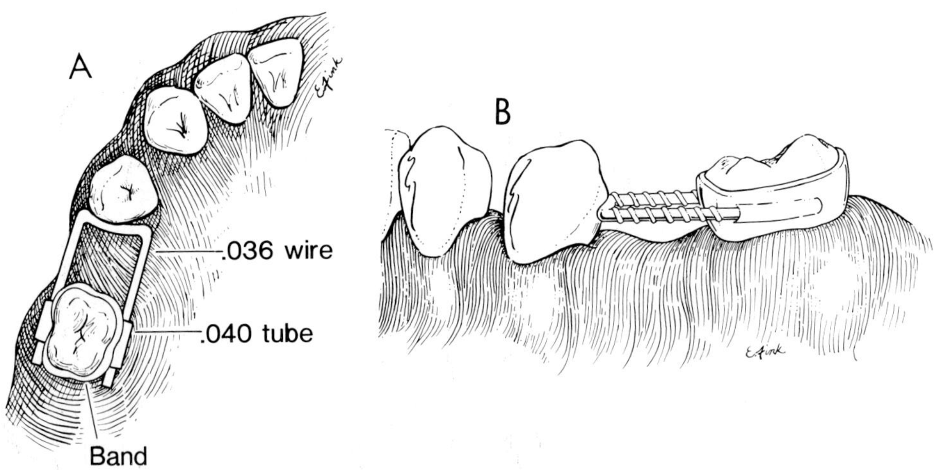

Fig 22–9.—**A,** mandibular teeth have drifted as a result of previous tooth loss. A band is placed on the molar with horizontal tubes on the buccal and lingual surfaces. A crib is fitted so that it glides freely in the tubes. **B,** coil springs are placed over the crib wires to engage both the angle of the crib wire and the tubes on the band under compression. This transmits a constant spring loaded force to the abutment teeth.

automatically eliminates the possibility of rotating certain teeth. It is important when constructing appliances for the rotation and root movement to ensure that the springs act exactly at the points intended and do not slide away to some other nearby, but unsuitable, point. For this reason, it is sometimes necessary to make springs rather stiff to ensure accuracy of application to the teeth, and to accept the short range of action inherent in such springs.

Rotation of premolars and molars usually requires a fixed appliance to ensure rotation of the tooth about the desired axis. There are, however, certain situations in which premolars and molars can be rotated with a removable appliance. A common misplacement of the maxillary first premolar is to find the lingual cusp rotated mesially and occluding buccally to the mandibular first premolar. Rotation of the maxillary first premolar, by swinging the lingual cusp distally, will produce correct occlusion. This rotation may be done by exerting firm pressure on the occlusal surface of the tooth opposite the lingual cusp. The buccal cusp rests against the mesial surface of the tooth behind and the tooth rotates about its point of contact with the second premolar. Clinically, rotations such as this take considerable time. The rotations of mandibular premolars in this way are not likely to be successful as teeth are usually almost circular in section and the formation of a mechanical couple to rotate them is difficult or impossible.

Another common tooth misplacement is the mesiolingual rotation of the maxillary first molar. This may also be rotated distally by pressure on the mesial surface opposite to the mesiobuccal cusp. Rotation takes place about the palatal root. The roots of mandibular molars are of a shape and size that is resistant to rotation. When it is necessary to rotate these teeth, it is preferable to use fixed appliances.

MANAGEMENT OF MINOR TOOTH MOVEMENT

For successful tooth movement, it is important to gain the patient's cooperation. This can be achieved by discussing the treatment plan, the benefits to be derived from the therapy, and its prognosis. The adult usually associates tooth movement with the esthetic disadvantage of wearing an appliance. In minor movement procedures, the appliance is frequently removable, and creates few social or occupational problems. In general, the adult patient who can accept a prescription for tooth movement on a realistic basis will be the most cooperative and will offer the best chance of success.

As with all other phases of dental treatment, minor tooth movement does carry some difficulties and hazards. Application of excessive force or the movement of a tooth into a traumatic position may occur. It is not unusual to see appliance pressure result in soft tissue reaction during tooth movement. Such occurrences should be detected early during the treatment and alleviated to avoid permanent damage.

PULPAL CONSIDERATIONS

The pulp size and location has a practical significance in prosthodontics. Although the pulp is not actively involved in the physiologic process of tooth movement, transient hyperemia is not unusual, even when moderate forces are applied. Extensive application of force may rapidly displace the apex of the root, causing strangulation of the circulation at the apical foramen and necrosis of the pulp.

It is true that a tooth with a vital pulp is better than one without. It is also true that pulpless teeth serve satisfactorily as fixed partial denture abutments if the root canals are carefully treated, filled, and kept under periodic surveillance. A fixed partial denture is primarily indicated for the adult patient, although it may be considered in partially edentulous arches for patients of every age. For children and early adolescents with missing teeth a fixed restoration is usually contraindicated because the abutment teeth are not fully erupted. The pulp is usually large and may be easily exposed or damaged during the preparation of the abutment. A fixed orthodontic appliance such as a space maintainer is often used. These space maintainers serve a temporary function and should be replaced by a permanent restoration when the patient has reached a more mature age.

ALTERNATIVES TO UPRIGHTING MOLARS

Crown Root Relations

Molars frequently drift mesially and tilt into an endentulous space. This makes it impossible to parallel the abutment teeth so that a fixed partial denture can be constructed. Numerous prosthetic procedures can be used to overcome this problem. A telescope coping may be constructed for the tipped tooth, making it parallel to the other abutment. This will allow the construction of a fixed restoration. A replacement using two-surface inlays or half crowns for one or both abutments may be used but these do not have the retention potential of a full coverage abutment and will frequently loosen. A semi-precision attachment stress breaker may be used.[6] This results in an uneven loading of the abutments that may be undesirable. A posterior cantilever bridge usually overloads the abutment teeth dangerously, even when multiple abutments are used.

All of these methods have inherent disadvantages. Therefore, the recommended procedure is to tip the abutment tooth back to a more normal axial position and then construct a fixed partial denture. This provides the best treatment prognosis with minimal additional effort.

Occlusal Considerations

It is important that a good functional occlusion be established so that each tooth, or group of teeth, can best withstand the stresses of mastication. The success of an extensive fixed prosthesis often depends on the tooth position and the type of occlusion present. When teeth that are to be restored are in a poor relationship, the restoration may have to follow the same general occlusal outline pattern and trauma will continue. If the teeth can be brought into a normal interdigitating relationship, it will help in the construction of a restoration with a harmonious occlusion and normal conservative tooth preparation.

Premature occlusal contacts can be treated by selective grinding to eliminate discrepancies between centric relation and centric occlusion. In some cases, however, the mandibular shift can be eliminated by moving the prematurely contacting tooth or teeth into a more harmonious alignment. This repositioning may be achieved by depression, extrusion, or movement in a horizontal direction. This may also provide better spacing for pontics and enhance the prognosis.

Even if the final fixed partial denture is good mechanically, problems will arise if it has not been inserted in harmony and balance with the remainder of the mouth structure. Although the orthodontic aid is only one phase of the reconstruction process, it sometimes may permit a result that is almost impossible to obtain in any other way.

REFERENCES

1. Moyers R.E.: *Handbook of Orthodontics*, ed. 3. Chicago, Year Book Medical Publishers, 1973.
2. Goldstein M.C.: Orthodontics in crown and bridge and periodontal therapy. *Dent. Clin. North Am.* 449, July, 1964.
3. Graber T.M.: *Orthodontics Principles and Practice*, ed. 3. Philadelphia, W.B. Saunders Co., 1972.
4. Norton L.A., Parker W.T.: Management of repositioned teeth in preparation for fixed partial dentures. *J. Am. Dent. Assoc.* 81:916, 1970.
5. Jarabsk J.R.: Orthodontic treatment preparatory to fixed denture partial prosthesis. *Dent. Clin. North Am.* 31, March, 1959.
6. Tylman S.D.: *Theory and Practice of Crown and Bridge Prosthesis*, ed. 7. St. Louis, C.V. Mosby Co., 1978.

CHAPTER 23

Periodontal Considerations in Fixed Prosthodontics

ROBERT J. CONNOR, D.D.S., and RONALD J. PETERSON, D.D.S

THE BASIC PRINCIPLES for root resection and endodontic techniques are well documented. The principles for restoring these partially resected teeth have not been as closely detailed. The purpose of this chapter is to outline the principles used in restoring partially resected teeth and to present examples that demonstrate the restoration of a variety of partially resected molars.

HISTORICAL BACKGROUND

Root resection has been used as a treatment for furcations in multi-rooted teeth for many years. The basic theory of root resection is to strategically extract a diseased root to improve the prognosis of the rest of the tooth. Black[1] attempted the technique in the late 19th century. Early attempts at root resection often failed because of endodontic complications. The technique was therefore abandoned for several decades.

Root resection entered its second period of popularity in the early 1960s. Amsterdam and others[2] presented several successfully treated cases in the literature. Amsterdam demonstrated the use of "hopeless" teeth as fixed bridge abutments. He eliminated the advanced furcation invasions present on his selected abutment teeth via root resection. The noncleanable, furcated teeth were thereby converted to cleanable abutments that Amsterdam felt presented a good long-term prognosis. The 1960s yielded numerous articles that expanded the proposed indications for root resection and many root resections were done during this time. A summary of published indications for root resection is contained in the following list:

1. Severe vertical bone loss involving one root of a mandibular molar and one or two buccal roots or a palatal root of a maxillary molar.[3]
2. Inadequate interradicular space that renders a Class I or II furcation involvement nonmaintainable;[3]
3. Bone loss in the furcation that is not treatable or maintainable;[4]
4. Decay in the furcation that is not treatable;[5]
5. An abutment tooth within a fixed partial denture or splint with a root or roots whose prognosis is hopeless;[3]
6. Multi-rooted teeth with an individual root fracture;[4]
7. A nontreatable mucogingival problem, such as a severe dehiscence;[4] and
8. Endodontic complications including a nontreatable root, a root with a broken instrument, a perforation, or an isolated area of root resorption.[4]

Many practitioners feel that root resection has been abused and that the indications for root resection are much more restrictive than those listed above. Recent studies by Ross and Thompson[6, 7] and Hirshfeld and Wasserman[8] have shown that many molars with furcation invasions can comfortably function for years without extensive surgical treatment if proper maintenance schedules are followed. It must be pointed out that these studies did not correlate success rates or predictability of molar retention with severity of the furcation invasion at the initiation of therapy. Likewise, the predictability for successful retention of a molar with advanced furcation invasions is not well documented when nonsurgical therapy is the only treatment.

Many factors are involved in determining whether a tooth with a severe furcation invasion can become a successful abutment tooth. Root resection can only be used when the retained tooth segment has enough bony support alone to allow proper function. The retained tooth segment's shape must permit optimal plaque control procedures in all sulcular areas. Therefore, when considering root resection, the therapist must decide if plaque control procedures will be facilitated by the surgery and if the retained tooth segment will have enough bony support to properly function. If a patient has lost a mandibular first molar, a fixed partial denture extending from the mandibular second premolar to the ipsilateral second molar is the restoration of choice. If the second molar has adequate bone support but has a through-and-through furcation and a narrow interradicular space, the therapist must decide if the proposed restoration would have a predictably better prognosis using the second molar with the furcation invasion as an abutment, or if a single hemisected root could support the fixed partial denture and offer better plaque control accessibility to the patient and the therapist.

Nyman and Lindhe[9, 11] have shown that selectively retained roots can serve as abutments for extensive fixed prostheses when optimal plaque control is maintained. These abutments have shown no progressive attachment loss after over five years of service. Evidently the functional adaptability of the periodontium is much greater than was previously presumed.

Nyman and Lindhe's studies tell us that partially resected teeth can be successfully used as abutment teeth if they are properly selected, correctly treated, and well maintained. If the therapist properly evaluates a patient using the above parameters and then determines root resection to be the treatment of choice for a selected tooth, he or she should feel confident in the tooth's ability to function on a long-term basis. Conversely, improperly selected teeth and an uncooperative patient will probably cause failure despite the best treatment.

BASIC PRINCIPLES FOR ROOT RESECTION

Maxillary Molars

Root resection of a maxillary molar is usually done during routine periodontal surgery of the involved quadrant. A full thickness mucoperiosteal flap is elevated and the root and furcation anatomy is identified. Adequate bone is removed to allow removal of the selected root. The removed bone must not compromise the support of adjacent teeth or remaining roots of the tooth being resected. The root is then sectioned with a diamond or fissured bur and carefully removed. After root removal, any root stump and remaining crown surface is smoothed to eliminate rough edges or furcation overhangs and to produce adequate embrasure space for hygienic maintenance after surgery. Routine osteoplasty is completed and the flaps are sutured in place.

When the sutures, and dressing, if used, are removed, the patient is instructed in personalized plaque control (P.P.C.)[11] for the resected tooth. Plaque control in these areas can be difficult for patients and must be reviewed at every available opportunity.

Mandibular Molars

Hemisection and root separation of mandibular molars does not always require an extensive surgical procedure. Teeth with Type III furcation involvements and acceptable crevice depths around the remainder of the tooth can sometimes be sectioned without elevating a soft tissue flap. The same is true with cariously involved furcations or previously treated through-and-through furcations. If surgery is required, a sequence of events similar to the previously described maxillary molar surgery is followed.

ENDODONTIC CONSIDERATIONS

Most authors agree the ideal sequence for root resection therapy includes diagnosis, endodontic therapy, periodontic therapy, and restoration of the remaining tooth segment, in that order. However, it is not always possible to handle root resection therapy in this sequence. The decision to resect a root is sometimes made at the time of periodontal surgery. When this occurs, endodontic therapy should be completed as soon as possible after root resection.[12]

Endodontic Fill Techniques

The preferred endodontic treatment sequence is to complete conventional endodontics to the apex, remove a portion of the coronal gutta percha in the involved root, and then place an amalgam filling in the canal. Some authors have advocated incomplete or sectional endodontic fill of the root or roots to be removed. However this practice is to be discouraged and a complete conventional fill should be done for all roots if possible.

Occasionally, dramatic bony healing will occur after pre-root resection endodontic therapy. This bone fill may be unexpected and is attributed to the difficulties in establishing the etiology of a bony lesion. It is now well documented that molars contain numerous accessory canals in the furcation areas.[12] The endodontic literature is replete with articles on diagnostic difficulties with partially nonvital multirooted teeth.[13, 14] The potential for misdiagnosis of an endodontic lesion as a periodontal lesion certainly exists. If the therapist elects to remove an involved root, the endodontics will probably have been completed before surgery. If the bony lesion was of endodontic origin and the cause of the problem is corrected by the endodontic treatment, the furcation may have adequate bony fill and negate the necessity to remove the root. If the involved root was not conventionally filled to the apex and contains only a sectional amalgam fill, it will be impossible to complete a conventional endodontic fill at a later date. The clinician is then faced with a potential endodontic problem that can be resolved only by placing a retrograde endodontic filling in the root. If the preferred treatment sequence is followed and if bony healing does occur after endodontic treatment, no further endodontic problems should arise. If, on the other hand, no bony healing takes place, the root can be resected as previously planned.

Periodontal Considerations in Crown Preparation Design

The relation between restorative dentistry and periodontics is interdependent. Restorative dentistry is only as good as its foundation—the periodontium. The reverse is equally true. Restorative dentistry is the basis of healthy periodontal tissues.

Faulty dentistry is a prime contributor to the causes of periodontal disease. There are basic considerations that must be adhered to when constructing any restoration to protect the supporting structures. These include proximal contact, axial contour, occlusion, margins, and polish. Protection of gingival tissues from injury from food impaction is directly related to these items.

Continuous tooth to tooth contact is essential in the dental arches if proximal periodontal health is to be maintained. Contact and proximal form are particularly important for premolars and molars.[15] Well fitting margins of dental restorations are especially important in the proximal areas for prevention of periodontal disease.[16] Imperfections such as overextension, underextension, rough or unpolished proximal surfaces, and rough margins will result in plaque accumulation and inflammation.[17, 18] If this situation is to be avoided, any irritant or irregularity that will collect plaque and produce tissue damage must not be allowed in the design or fabrication of the restoration.

The following objectives must be met with any restoration to ensure optimum occlusal function: (1) equilibration of the occlusion and articulation of the teeth to harmonize with the oral musculature and temporomandibular joint; (2) alignment of occlusal forces with the direction of the long axis of teeth; (3) establishment of a static relation between cusps and opposing fossae; (4) controlled distribution of forces in eccentric positions to the location and number of teeth best able to withstand the load; (5) reduction of steepness of cuspal inclines; and (6) non-interference with the rest position of the mandible.

Sound tooth enamel is the best biologic, physiologic, and esthetic environment for healthy gingival tissue. Therefore, when conditions permit, margins of restorations should be kept away from the gingival tissues. Gingivitis occurs more frequently around teeth with subgingival margins. Subgingival margins are extremely difficult to maintain free of plaque; they accumulate more soft deposits and develop gingivitis more easily. Whenever possible restoration margins should be placed supragingivally.

The relationship of tooth contours to the surrounding gingiva is of extreme importance. The correct external morphology of all restorations is important, but is particularly critical when full coverage restorations are involved. Perel[19] has shown that cast restorations should not be designed with excessive axial contours. Overcontouring to protect the gingival crevice from food impaction or trauma encourages the accumulation of plaque and microbial matter in areas that are difficult for the patient to clean.

RESTORING PARTIALLY RESECTED MULTI-ROOTED TEETH

Buccal Roots of Maxillary Molars

After all diagnostic tests are completed and the decision to remove a buccal root of a maxillary molar has been made, conventional endodontics is completed. At the surgical appointment mucoperiosteal flaps are reflected, the root is sectioned and removed, and osseous surgery is done. The tooth is then carefully reshaped and smoothed to eliminate any rough edges and furcation remnants. The occlusion is adjusted to eliminate any lateral loading and the surgical site is allowed to heal for at least six weeks. Most teeth do not require splinting during the healing phase although the occlusion must be carefully monitored to ensure that undesirable forces are not present. If crevice depths, tissue contours, and functional occlusion of the entire dentition are acceptable at this time, the tooth is ready for restoration.

The preparation of the tooth should incorporate the basic principles of good restorative dentistry. An adequate foundation, frequently including a post and core, is completed. Margins should be distinct and away from tissue if possible. Care must be taken to include the new curvatures and fluting from the eliminated furcation into the preparation. All margins must be placed on sound tooth structure.

The contour of the new crown must be carefully designed for the resected tooth. Contact with adjacent teeth must be established, but an adequate embrasure space must remain to allow plaque control. The occlusion must be carefully refined to eliminate excessive traumatic forces that may cause tooth mobility.[20] The occlusal table is frequently reduced in width compared with the original tooth anatomy. The new crown is often somewhat unconventional in appearance because of the absence of tooth cusps and root structure. The design of the crown should never be bulky or contain noncleanable concavities. The utmost concern during crown design must be the patient's ability to clean and maintain the new fixed prosthesis.

CASE REPORTS

Mesiobuccal root removal

This patient, referred by a general dentist, had Class IV periodontal disease and several hopelessly involved second molars. The nontreatable teeth were removed. Her maxillary first molars each contained through-and-through Type III furcation invasions (Fig 23–1). The prognosis for each maxillary first molar was questionable. As the existing furcations were not treatable or maintainable, root resection was selected as a means of furcation elimination. The decision regarding which root to remove was made at the time of surgery. In this instance, vital root amputation with subsequent endodontic therapy was used.

When flaps were reflected, bony topography and furcation anatomy favored removal of the mesiobuccal root of the maxillary right first molar and the distobuccal root of the maxillary left first molar. In each instance, the removed root had Type III furcations between it and the adjacent roots. The retained roots had interradicular bone present and furcation invasions were not severe. The root amputations were completed along with appropriate periodontal therapy in the involved quad-

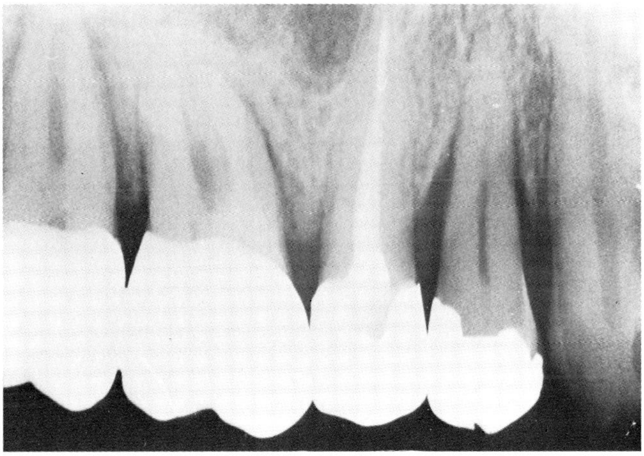

Fig 23–1.—Preoperative radiograph of maxillary right quadrant. Note the severe periodontal bone loss around the molars and the first premolar.

rants. Pulp extirpation was completed within five days after root resection. Routine endodontic therapy with gutta-percha fill was done and the surgical areas were allowed to heal for several months. Other restorative dental therapy was completed during the healing period.

After healing, tooth mobility was reduced, crevice depths were no greater than 3 mm, and the patient had excellent personal plaque control procedures (Fig 23–2). The prognosis of the teeth appeared to be greatly improved. Final restoration of the dentition was started. The maxillary molar was prepared for full coverage in compliance with the principles previously presented. In addition, the maxillary right premolars were prepared for porcelain-fused-to-metal crowns (Fig 23–3).

After final cementation of the crowns (Figs 23–4 and 23–5), the patient was instructed in proper oral hygiene techniques for all the interproximal areas and new

Fig 23–2.—Appearance of the maxillary right first molar six weeks after mesiobuccal root resection.

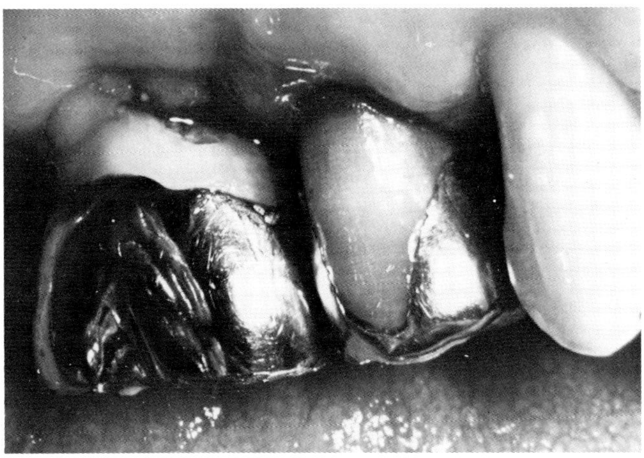

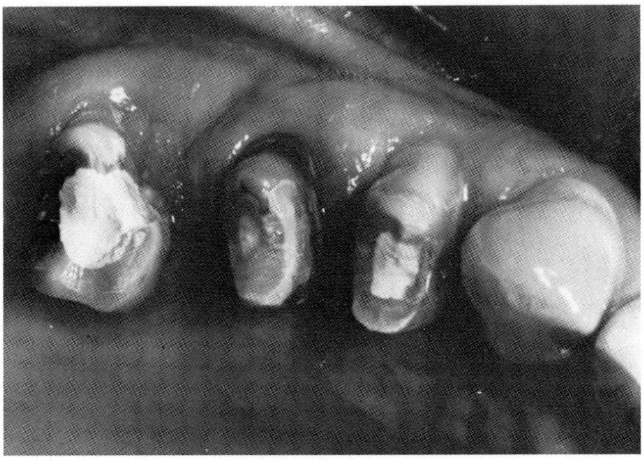

Fig 23–3.—Preparation of the maxillary right first molar for a full cast gold crown and the maxillary right premolars for porcelain-fused-to-metal crowns.

curvatures present in the restorations. Perio-Aid* toothpick holders and Proxabrush** interproximal brushes work well for plaque removal in embrasures and furcations.

Distobuccal root removal

The contralateral arch of the patient described above contained a hopeless second molar that was extracted (Fig 23–6). The distobuccal root of the first molar was the most severely involved. Type III involvement was present on both the buccal and distal furcations, being completely devoid of bone. The mesial furcation contained

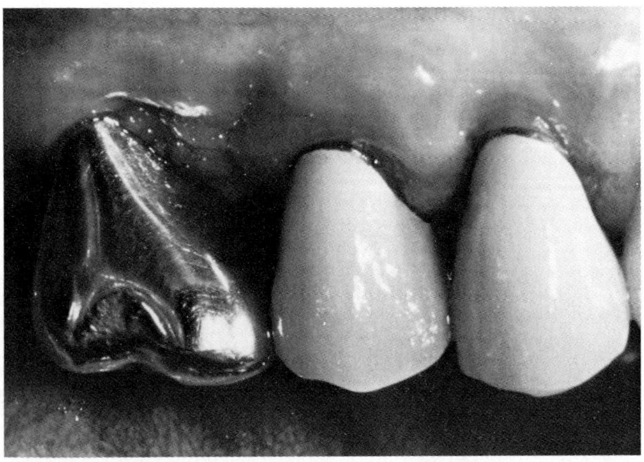

Fig 23–4.—Appearance of crowns after cementation shows adequate embrasure spaces to allow for good plaque control procedures.

*Marquis Dental Mfg., 15370 N. Smith Rd., Aurora, CO 80011.
**John O. Butler Co., 540 N. Lake Shore Dr., Chicago, IL 60611.

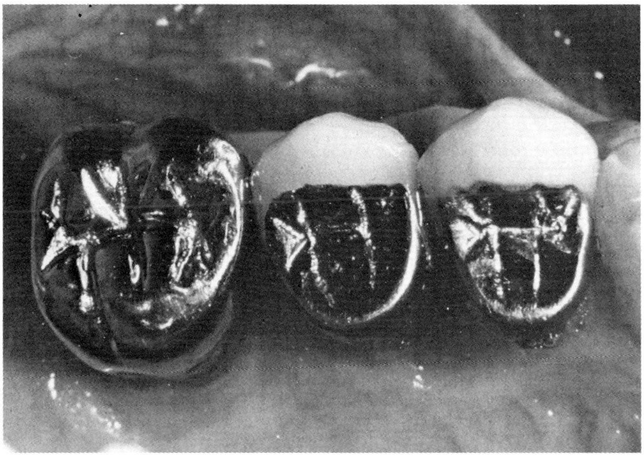

Fig 23–5.—Occlusal view of cemented crowns demonstrates proper occlusal anatomy and contact relationships.

intact bone and was only slightly probeable. The distobuccal root was selectively resected and the mesial furcation received only minor osteoplasty.

After routine endodontic treatment and complete soft tissue healing, the periodontal support appeared healthy (Fig 23–7). Final restoration was begun. Preparation design included the severe curvature created by the root resection (Figs 23–8 and 23–9). The completed crown was cemented, the occlusion adjusted, and the patient instructed in proper oral hygiene techniques (Figs 23–10 and 23–11).

Palatal Roots of Maxillary Molars

Removal of a palatal root is a far less common procedure than is removal of a buccal root, but there are instances where it is the treatment of choice. Endodontic and periodontic procedures are similar to the previously described sequence.

The crown placed after root resection must be significantly reduced in its buc-

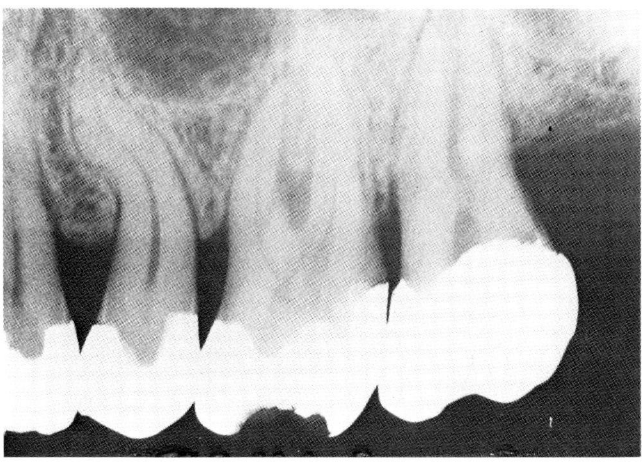

Fig 23–6.—Preoperative radiograph of the maxillary left quadrant. Note severe periodontal bone loss in molar furcations.

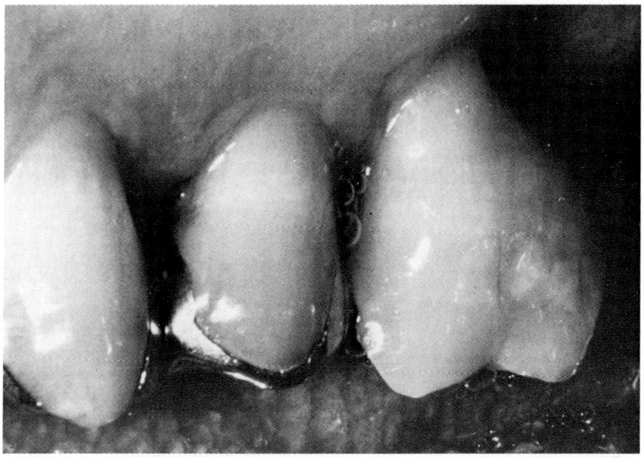

Fig 23–7.—Appearance of the maxillary left first molar after distobuccal root resection healing.

colingual dimension. If the lingual cusps were reconstructed to their original position, the crown contour would be bulky and the gingival area would be extremely difficult for the patient to clean. Further, the lingual cusp contact could act as a cantilever to torque the tooth, causing tooth mobility or orthodontic movement. The design of the crown should incorporate good centric stops in relation to the buccal cusps of the mandibular molars. No eccentric contacts should be permitted.

Improper Restoration of a Partially Resected Maxillary Molar

This patient had a maxillary molar with severe internal palatal root resorption that had perforated the root in several locations. The palatal furcations were severely involved, but the buccal furcation was sound. The patient wished to retain the tooth. Palatal root resection was performed in an attempt to save the tooth. After routine endodontics and periodontal healing, the patient was returned to the

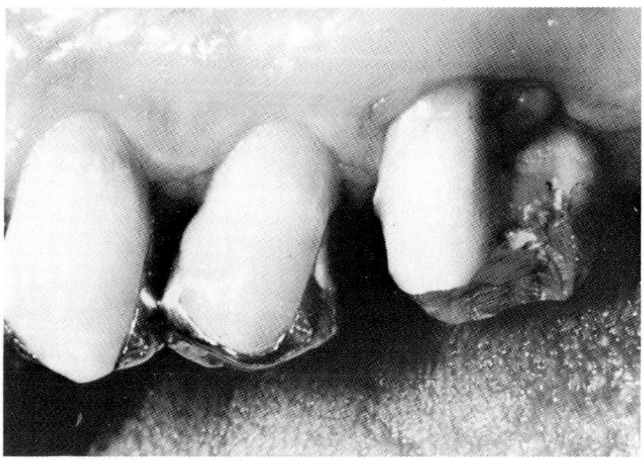

Fig 23–8.—Preparation of the maxillary molar for full cast gold crown. The small papilla of soft tissue in the root resection site was removed after tooth prepartion.

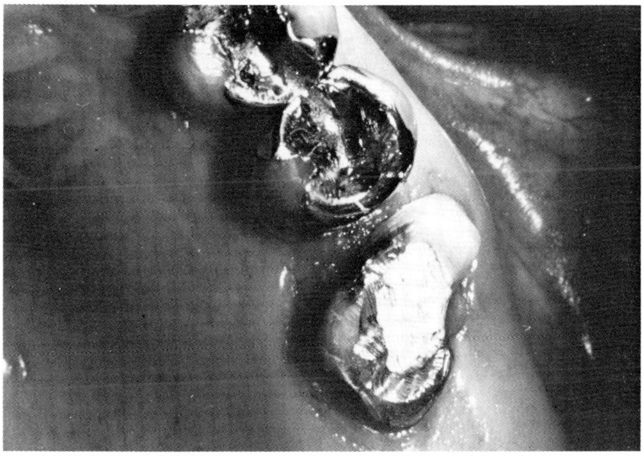

Fig 23–9.—Occlusal view of the preparation of the maxillary molar. The severe distobuccal concavity is required to establish a preparation margin where the root was resected.

general dentist for restoration of the tooth. The tooth was not adequately reduced in the buccolingual dimension and a severe tooth undercut was left on the palatal surface, which the patient could not clean. When the patient was seen at the six month recall appointment the pulp canal orifice, which had been restored with amalgam, was decayed (Fig 23–12). Proper restoration design would have covered the palatal orifice and allowed easier access for cleaning the tooth margins.

Hemisection of a Mandibular Molar

Occasionally a mandibular molar will have a severe bony defect involving only one of its roots. If maintenance of this tooth is desirable or necessary, the affected root can be removed and the sound root maintained. The periodontally sound root

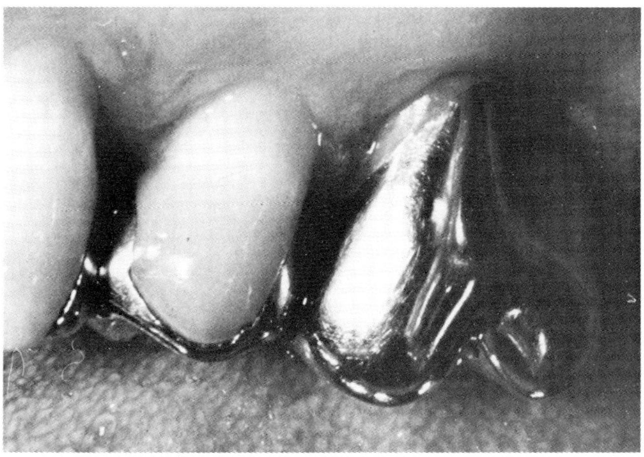

Fig 23–10.—Appearance of the cemented crown shows readily accessible crown margin for optimum oral hygiene maintenance.

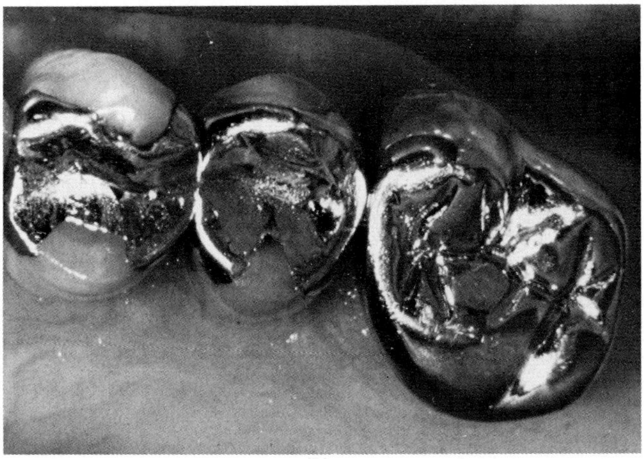

Fig 23–11.—Occlusal view of cemented crown demonstrates slightly altered occlusal anatomy and proper contact relationship.

may then be used as a fixed partial denture abutment or, in some cases, for a crown to restore proximal contacts.

The surgery technique for hemisection is quite simple. The tooth is sectioned in a buccolingual direction through the furcation and the affected root is removed. Flaps are reflected if osteoplasty is required.

The most prevalent mistake with this technique is failure to totally eliminate the furcation. After sectioning the tooth and removing the affected root, it is extremely important to ensure no overhang of the furcation remains. Such overhangs of tooth structure or restorative material can sometimes be difficult to detect clinically. A radiograph should be taken when the tooth is prepared to ensure that no noncleanable overhangs of tooth or foundation exist (Fig 23–13).

The patient had an intact mandibular dentition from second molar to second

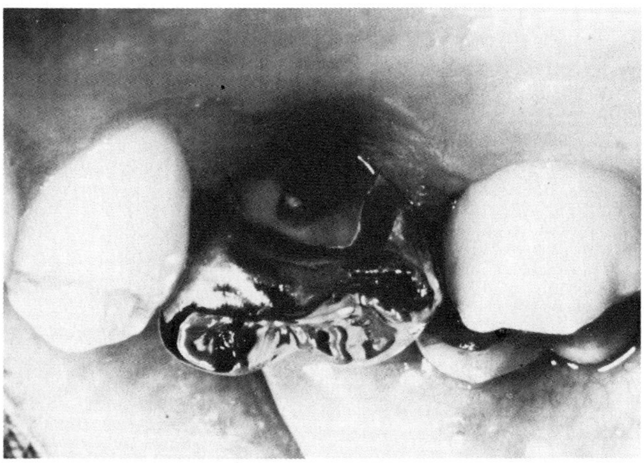

Fig 23–12.—Example of improper crown design for a tooth with a palatal root resection. The palatal aspect of the tooth was not fully covered. Caries is now present in the area of the palatal amalgam restoration.

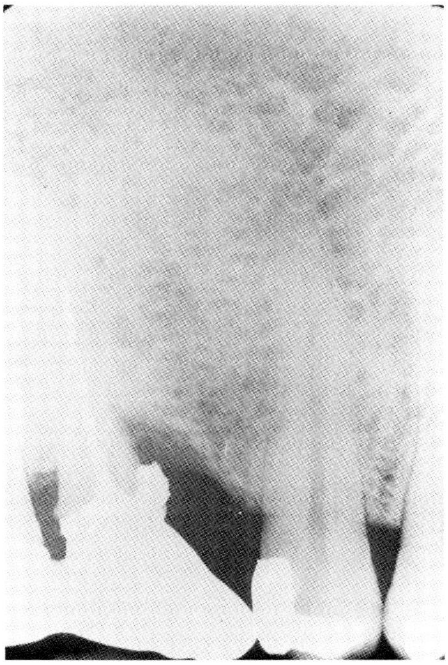

Fig 23–13.—Example of incomplete elimination of a furcation in a molar hemisection. The mesial amalgam overhang created a totally noncleanable environment that the patient had no chance to maintain.

molar, with the exception of the missing mandibular right first molar (Fig 23–14). The patient had no crevice depths greater than 4 mm except for the mandibular right second molar. This molar contained a through-and-through furcation defect, crevice depths in excess of 6 mm on the distal root, and Class II mobility. The roots of the molar were in close proximity to each other, so surgical opening of the furcation was not a treatment option. The distal root had minimal bone support and was considered a poor fixed prosthesis abutment.

Appropriate periodontal therapy and plaque control procedures were completed in all areas of the mouth. Routine endodontic therapy with gutta-percha fill was completed on the mandibular right second molar. Full thickness mucoperiosteal flaps were reflected at the time of hemisection to allow final evaluation of both roots and routine osteoplasty. The distal root was removed and minor osseous surgery was done.

Approximately six weeks later the mandibular right second premolar and the mesial root of the mandibular right second molar were prepared for a full cast gold, three unit fixed prosthesis (Figs 23–15 to 23–17). The pontic was hygienic in design, and constructed with adequate ridge clearance. Maximum embrasure space was maintained. Occlusal function was limited to the centric contacts and crowns were slightly narrowed in buccolingual width.

Root Separation of a Mandibular Molar

If both roots of a mandibular molar are periodontally sound but the furcation of that tooth is noncleanable or decayed, the clinician may elect to convert the multirooted tooth into two single-rooted teeth. This procedure should only be considered when the prognosis for both individual roots is good.

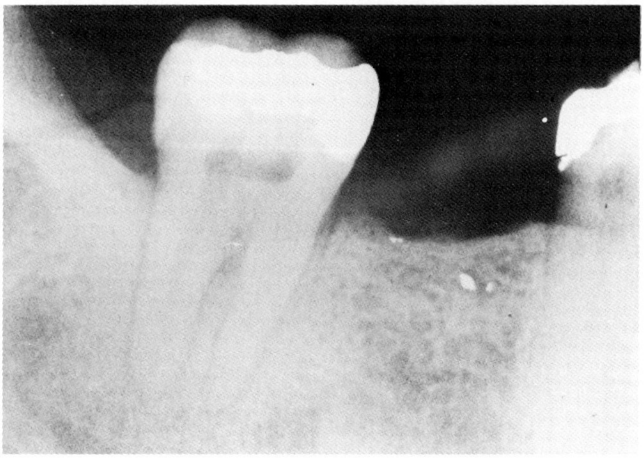

Fig 23–14.—Preoperative radiograph of the mandibular right quadrant. Deep distal pockets and furcation involvement precluded use of the entire molar as a fixed partial denture abutment.

The surgical procedure required is similar to that for hemisection, except that both root segments are maintained. The roots can often be prepared to receive crowns at the time of furcation elimination unless a flap and major osteoplasty are required. If the roots are extremely close together and there is inadequate space for fabrication of two properly contoured premolar-shaped crowns, the roots can be uprighted and separated by an orthodontic appliance to create more interradicular space.

The recommended preparation form is similar to a premolar crown preparation. The fabricated crowns should also resemble premolars. The clinician may elect to splint the crowns in the marginal ridge area if adequate space is allowed for interradicular plaque control. Splinting is not always necessary, but drifting of the distal

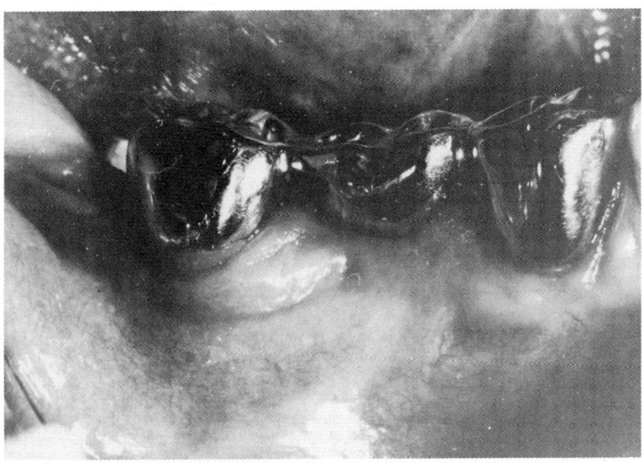

Fig 23–15.—Postoperative appearance of the three unit restoration using the mesial root of the mandibular molar as the distal abutment.

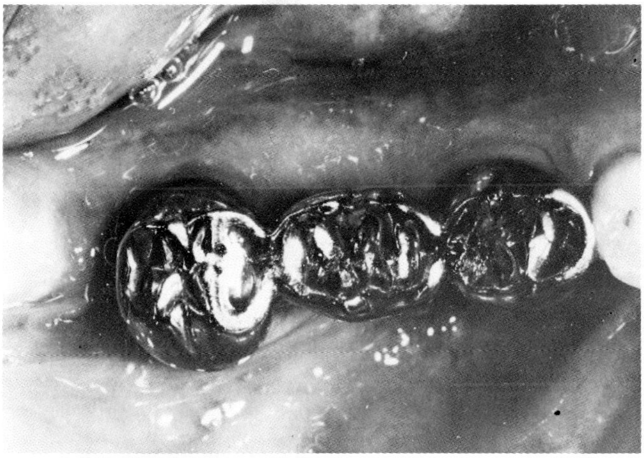

Fig 23–16.—Occlusal view of the three unit fixed partial denture. Note abutment, pontic, and connector contours.

abutment can occur if the crowns are fabricated separately and there is a distalizing component to the patient's occlusion. In either instance, the patient has the advantages of molar occlusion and a fixed restoration that is easily maintained.

Root separation of the mandibular left first molar was performed for the patient described earlier with the maxillary molar buccal root amputations. The mandibular second molar was removed. Bony support was adequate in all areas of the first molar, but it had noncleanable Class III furcation involvement (Fig 23–18). The interradicular bone could have been lowered to allow for greater patient access to the furcation, but too much supporting bone would have been sacrificed with this procedure. Root separation provided the logical method for furcation elimination.

Endodontic therapy with a gutta-percha fill was completed on the tooth. Routine periodontal surgery was done in the quadrant and osseous surgery was used to

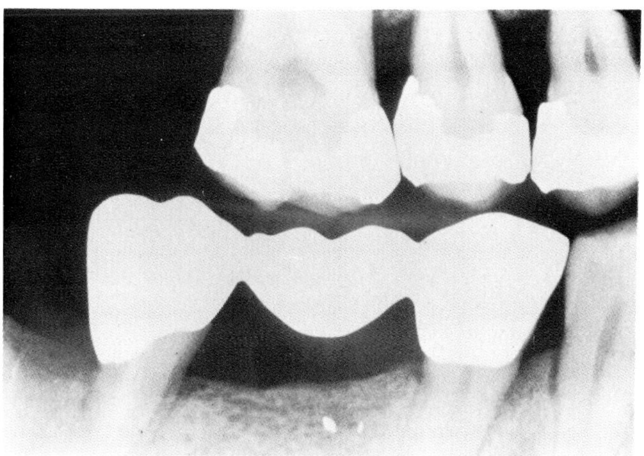

Fig 23–17.—Postoperative radiograph shows the fixed partial denture cemented in place.

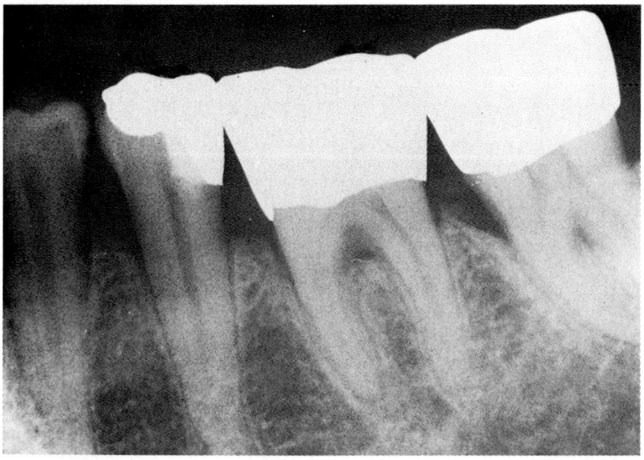

Fig 23–18.—Preoperative radiograph of the mandibular left quadrant. Note severe bone loss in the furcations of the molars.

restore positive bony architecture with minimal sacrifice of support. The tooth was then hemisected to separate the roots, and the pulp chamber was filled with restorative material. Two months after surgery both roots were stable and the decision was made to restore them as individual nonsplinted units. A large embrasure space was left between the individual crowns. The castings were cemented and the patient was instructed in oral hygiene procedures for the restorations.

When the patient was recalled six weeks later the distal crown was observed to have drifted distally and interproximal contact was lost (Figs 23–19 and 23–20). The patient was able to keep the area plaque-free and did not complain of food impaction. The occlusion was adjusted and the crown was not further altered. In this instance, splinting the crowns in the marginal ridge area would have prevented the observed drifting.

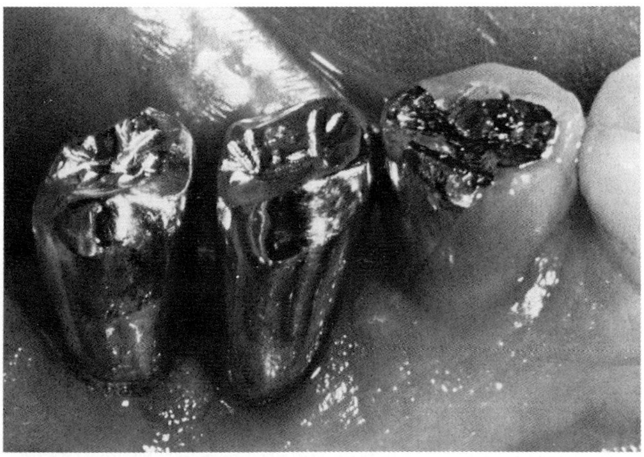

Fig 23–19.—Six week post-cementation appearance of premolar-shaped crowns on bicuspidized molar tooth. Note that the distal root has drifted distally in this lingual view.

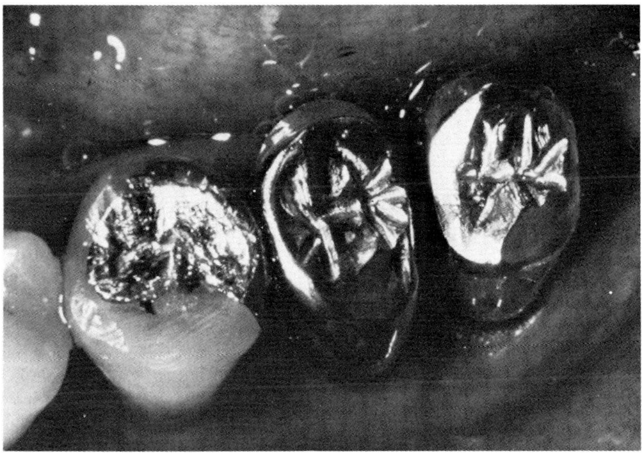

Fig 23–20.—Occlusal view of the separated molar root crowns shows their altered occlusal anatomy. The mesial root has remained in contact with the premolar, but the distal root has drifted distally.

SUMMARY

As the public becomes more aware of dentistry and willing to cooperate with the profession to save their natural dentitions, more sophisticated dental services are in greater demand. The practice of selective root resection for tooth preservation must be included as one of these services. This chapter has attempted to briefly outline some of the basic procedures involved in successful treatment of these selected teeth. The ultimate success or failure of such treatment depends on proper restoration. A partially resected tooth requires the reestablishment of near ideal occlusion and scrupulous attention to physiologic crown form and function. The patient must be willing and able to practice immaculate plaque control. It is the dentist's responsibility to provide the patient with a restoration that is able to be cleaned and to instruct the patient in proper home maintenance.

REFERENCES

1. Black G.V.: *The American System of Dentisty,* Litch W. ed. Phildelphia, Lea Brothers, 1886.
2. Amsterdam M., Rossman S.: The technique of hemisection of multirooted teeth. *Alpha Omegan* 53:4, 1960.
3. Schluger S., Youdelis R., Page R.: *Periodontal Disease.* Philadelphia, Lea & Febiger, 1977.
4. Basaraba N.: Root amputation and tooth hemisection. *Dent. Clin. North Am.* 13:121, 1969.
5. Abrams L., Trachtenberg L.: Hemisection-technique and restoration. *Dent. Clin. North Am.* 18:415, 1974.
6. Ross I.F., Thompson R.: A long term study of root retention in the treatment of maxillary molars with furcation involvement. *J. Periodontol.* 49:238, 1978.
7. Ross I.F., Thompson R.: Furcation involvement in maxillary and mandibular molars. *J. Periodontol.* 51:450, 1980.
8. Hirschfeld L., Wasserman B.: A long-term survey of tooth loss in 600 treated periodontal patients. *J. Periodontol* 49:225, 1978.
9. Nyman S., Lindhe J.: Prosthetic rehabilitation of patients with advanced periodontal disease. *J. Clin. Periodontol.* 3:135, 1976.

10. Nyman S., Lindhe J., Lundgren D.: The role of occlusion for the stability of fixed bridges in patients with reduced periodontal tissue support. *J. Clin. Periodontol.* 2:53, 1975.
11. Robinson R.E.: How patients are motivated and taught to practice effective oral hygiene *Periodont. Abstr.* 16:100, 1968.
12. Lowman J.V., Burke R.S., Pellen G.D.: Patent accessory canals; incidence in molar furcation region. *Oral Surg.* 36:580, 1973.
13. Cohen S., Burns R.: *Pathways of the Pulp.* St. Louis, C.V. Mosby Co., 1976.
14. Ingle J.I., Beveridge E.E.: *Endodontics,* ed. 2. Philadelphia, Lea & Febiger, 1976.
15. Hancock E.B., et al.: Influence of interdental contacts on periodontal status. *J. Periodontol.* 51:445, 1980.
16. Saltzberg D., et al.: Scanning electron microscope study of the junction between restorations and gingival cavosurface margins. *J. Prosthet. Dent.* 36:517, 1976.
17. Gilmore N., Sheiham A.: Overhanging dental restorations and periodontal disease. *J. Periodontol.* 42:8, 1971.
18. Parkinson C.: Excessive crown contours facilitate endemic plaque niches. *J. Prosthet. Dent.* 35:424, 1976.
19. Perel M.: Axial crown contour. *J. Prosthet. Dent.* 25:642, 1971.
20. Wentz F., Jabarak J., Orban B.: Experimental occlusal trauma imitating cuspal interferences. *J. Periodontol.* 29:117, 1958.

CHAPTER 24

Problems in Fixed Prosthodontics

ALBERT T. GOLDBERG, D.D.S.

A REALISTIC APPROACH to fixed prosthodontics is that "total" success or "total" failure is seldom achieved. Because of many complexities of treatment, a level somewhere between the two extremes will be experienced. This chapter will deal with areas in fixed prosthodontics where problems occur and errors are made. The five major problem areas are diagnosis and treatment planning, patient management and mouth hygiene, preliminary mouth procedures, tooth preparation and case fabrication, and dentist-laboratory interaction. Factors that the dentist must be aware of while treating the patient in each of the above areas will be examined and discussed.

DIAGNOSIS AND TREATMENT PLANNING

Treatment Expectations

Dentists should not overlook the treatment expectations that the patient may have when designing fixed restorations. Most patients have similar basic requirements but because of cultural, socioeconomic, and environmental differences, treatment plans must often be modified to better meet their needs and desires.

Esthetics is a prime example where differences in expectations occur. There are many differing opinions as to what is desirable and constitutes beauty. This makes it important for the dentist to talk with the patient and agree on case esthetics early in the treatment so that future misunderstandings do not occur. Although it may be possible for a dentist to modify or change the mind of a patient concerning an esthetic need, care must be taken to clearly communicate the reasons for the type of treatment contemplated. For example, if an extremely short molar located in a visible area of the mouth needs a complete crown it can be difficult to place an enamel colored veneer on all surfaces. A dentist must try to persuade the patient to accept a crown with a metal occlusal surface that would improve the retention, strength, and occlusion of the restoration.

Adequately functioning fixed restorations are another important treatment expectation to the patient. Patients have varying functional capacities resulting from habits, genetic and developmental factors, and unchangeable pre-existing mouth conditions. All of these can interrelate to complicate treatment planning and must be discussed with the patient before treatment. When constructing a posterior fixed partial denture, teeth of the opposing arch may often extrude into the edentulous space. If this condition is not corrected, an irregular occlusal plane will result and the patient's occlusal function can be disturbed (Fig 24–1).

The third and perhaps most important treatment expectation of the patient is for the dentist to increase the life expectancy of a restoration while minimizing the cost in time and money for its fabrication. With the onset of third-party payment, unstable economic conditions, and increased complexity of dental techniques and materials, the dentist must take additional care and further continuing education to help ensure the realization of this expectation. A dentist who remakes a crown supporting a clasp of a serviceable removable partial denture will need to know the latest techniques so that the partial denture can continue to function for the patient. The dentist's continuing education could be a valuable help in saving the patient time, money, and discomfort.

Medical and Dental Histories

The problems of failing to take and properly record an adequate past and present medical and dental history from a patient before treatment are well documented in the literature. An inadequate medical and dental history can lead to serious consequences during and after treatment. The moral, legal, and monetary consequences of such an oversight can be devastating to a dentist's practice.

Any chronic medical problem that makes it difficult for a patient to sit in a dental chair for a sufficient length of time to adequately complete a dental procedure must be determined before treatment is started. Severe chronic osteogenic, respiratory, and circulatory problems are but a few of the obvious situations that could make it difficult to properly complete any extensive fixed prosthodontic service.

Unstable patients with less obvious severe psychologic problems can frustrate any competent dentist. Some of these patients have related chronic drug abuse problems. Severe chronic alcohol abuse and other social drugs may contribute to the unreliability of the patient and the physical deterioration of hard and soft structure in the oral cavity.

When a patient asks about the longevity of proposed restorative treatment, it is

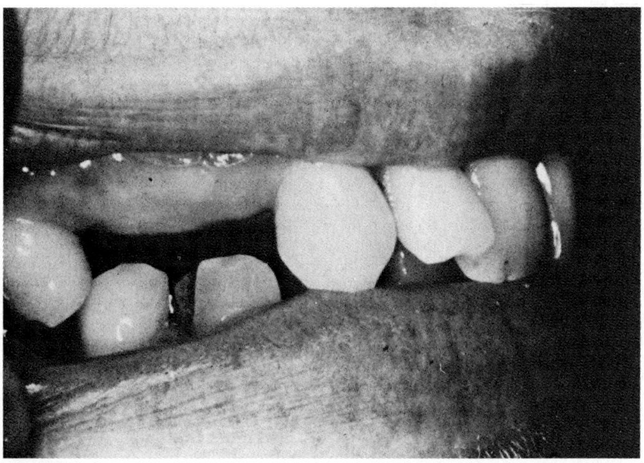

Fig 24–1.—Loss of vertical dimension and extrusion has resulted in the mandibular premolars encroaching on the maxillary pontic space.

helpful to understand the past dental history of a patient. With this knowledge, a dentist can more accurately prepare a treatment plan for the present and future. Often, a dentist is not able to secure a patient's past dental records, but must rely on the patient's knowledge of their treatment. An old, enlarged, closeup photograph can help a dentist view the past anterior esthetics and possibly the vertical dimension of a patient. The taking of some of the dental history by talking with a patient in a relaxed manner can also point out which of the patient's teeth are visible in conversation and laughter. A dentist should ask the patient's opinion about the acceptability of past treatment. This can be used by a dentist to avoid making any mistakes the patient felt were previously made.

The dental history must delve into any areas of pain in, and possibly associated with, the mouth. The most common areas are pulpal involvement, periodontal problems, and temporomandibular joint and muscle disturbance. A patient's oral hygiene practices must be inquired into because they are the foundation for treatment and can certainly affect future success.

Intraoral Records and Radiographic Examination

The preceding material dealt primarily with the extraoral nature of oral diagnosis and treatment planning. This section will deal with material that is intraoral in nature. More care is being taken to not overexpose patients to radiation, but the importance of a recent complete mouth radiographic series is still acknowledged. Radiographic information is manditory to determine if abutment teeth have adequate bone and trabeculation patterns, sufficient root length, and properly shaped roots to support fixed prostheses. Radiographs can help check the success of, or the possible need for, future endodontic treatment. The pulp size and periodontal membrane width can indicate that a tooth is under stress and whether the tooth is responding favorably to the stress. Teeth that need foundation restorations before fixed prosthodontic treatment because of the presence of caries or faulty restorations can be identified. Unerupted teeth and root tips could become a major embarrassment by creating problems after a fixed appliance is completed.

Mounted Diagnostic Casts

When diagnosing a fixed prosthodontic case, some information can be more easily and accurately obtained with mounted diagnostic casts. Difficult removable and fixed partial denture designs should be planned using the diagnostic casts to help in recognizing occlusal interferences, extruded and tipped abutments, and possible path of insertion problems (Fig 24–2). The design of pontics is made much easier by studying duplicated soft and hard tissue loss and the length of the span of missing teeth. Many preliminary procedures in fixed prosthodontics could not be done without accurate mounted diagnostic casts.

Intraoral Exam

Some information is more accurately gained from the intraoral examination than from casts. Mobile abutment teeth can present special problems for a fixed prosthodontic appliance. Sensitive teeth should be identified during the intraoral exam. Oral hygiene and the periodontal evaluation are critical and must be viewed intraorally. The shade of the teeth being treated or replaced must be finally deter-

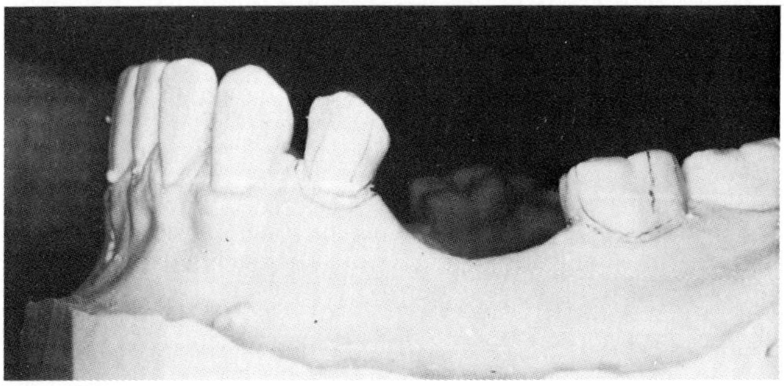

Fig 24–2.—The diagnostic cast shows a path of insertion problem caused by a severely tilted mandibular premolar abutment.

mined from the intraoral exam. Caries, old restorations, and oral habits must all be observed and charted during the intraoral examination.

PATIENT MANAGEMENT AND MOUTH HYGIENE

Before treatment is started the dentist must discuss with the patient the treatment that is included for the quoted fee and the method of payment expected. If this is not done, a patient can become so annoyed with the financial arrangements that it affects the acceptance of the restorations. The approximate number of appointments needed should be explained so that the patient is aware of complicated procedures that may take lengthy or numerous appointments. Any limitations or special problems that are anticipated must be discussed with the patient and the method for handling them explained. It is also important to begin with the oral hygiene instructions before the initiation of treatment so that a dentist can obtain an early indication of the patient's interest in maintaining a clean mouth.

During treatment a dentist should relieve the patient's stress by being reassuring about the treatment. Adequate medication should be given to make certain that the patient is comfortable. Analgesics, anesthetics, and antisialogogues are among the most common. Certain types of foods should be avoided during treatment. These are foods that are extremely hard, sticky, hot or cold, and are likely to be discoloring. The dentist should have the patient demonstrate the correct method for cleaning provisional restorations properly.

After the appliance is completed, the dentist still has a responsibility. Postcementation examination of a restoration is necessary and must be done routinely. The dentist should inquire about the comfort and satisfaction of the appliance. Radiographs should be taken periodically to check for periapical disease and recurrent caries. The soft tissue response, occlusion, and marginal integrity should be examined. Finally, the patient's oral hygiene practices must be monitored to make sure that they are doing their part to maintain the appliances properly.

PRELIMINARY MOUTH PROCEDURES

Soft Tissue Treatment

The soft tissue, especially surrounding the abutment teeth, must be healthy before the fabrication of the appliance. Extensive periodontal procedures may be indicated or less involved crown lengthening by electrosurgery may be needed in isolated areas. Whatever the need, this important aspect must not be overlooked. If the pontic is to have a natural appearance, the edentulous ridge may need to be recontoured so that the gingival surface and tooth embrasures appear natural (Fig 24–3 and 24–4).

Hard-tissue Treatment

A less obvious, yet important, preliminary procedure is prophylaxis. Prophylaxis can ensure that gingival margins are not placed on calculus, and that accurate tooth color selections can be made with clean teeth. Occlusal equilibration is another important aspect of preliminary procedures. It is much easier to correct damaging lateral interferences and prematurities in a patient before treatment, than to grind and adjust extensively in gold or porcelain material later. The reshaping of teeth should be considered. Incisal edges may need recontouring, extruded teeth reducing, and proximal contacts of adjacent teeth reshaping. This must be done before the final impression for the working and opposing cast. All of these relationships are critical to the fabrication of the appliance.

The abutment teeth must be caries free and fully restored before crown preparation (Fig 24–5). The extra time and expense involved is usually reflected in the quality and prognosis of the finished restoration. Caries in a restored tooth can easily go undetected radiographically. Visible margin caries, decalcification, or cervical erosion may not be eliminated when preparing the tooth as anticipated. There is too much time and money invested by the patient to take the unnecessary risk of not removing all old restorations and caries and replacing with a new amalgam foundation before starting the crown preparation. If exposures are encountered or the tooth determined to be nonvital, endodontic treatment is done at this time to avoid the need to open through the lingual or occlusal aspect of a new restoration.

Errors relating to the placement of the foundation are frequently associated with poor selection of pin site and direction or poor condensation of the foundation material. Lack of care results in pin holes drilled into pulps or periodontal membranes. With the aid of bite wing X rays, periodontal probing of root surfaces, and smaller diameter pins, most of these problems can be avoided. Placing pins too close to

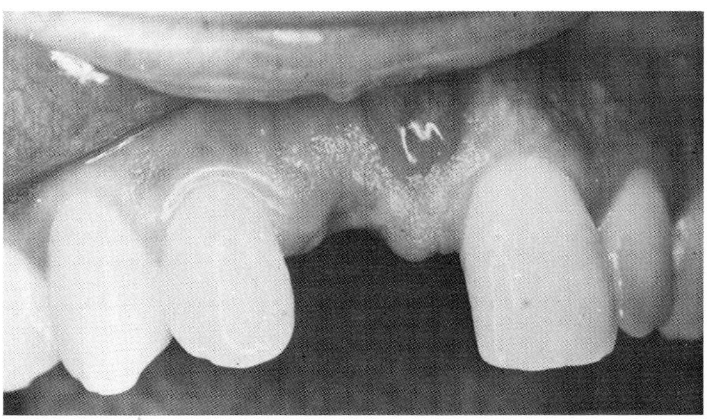

Fig 24–3.—An edentulous ridge that is uneven and has a low frenum attachment. Such conditions should be corrected before fixed prosthodontic treatment is begun.

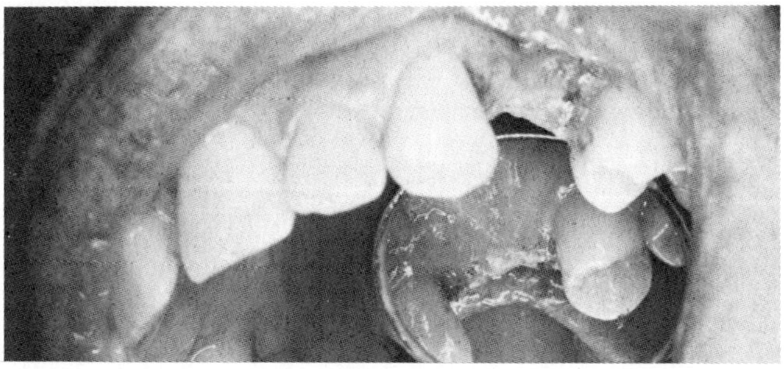

Fig 24–4.—This is a recontoured edentulous ridge immediately after electrosurgery. A much more esthetic and effective pontic can be constructed on more ideal contours.

facial surfaces thereby preventing sufficient reduction of that surface for esthetic veneers, can be a problem.

The post and core is another foundation procedure that is often omitted because of the added time, expense, and difficulty. The nonvital tooth is more brittle than a vital tooth. Often large amounts of coronal and radicular dentin are lost, leaving the crown and root weakened. If sufficient lateral forces are applied to such a tooth, fracture can easily occur. Posts should be placed when there is any doubt that fracture could occur. Posts may be cast, or selected from one of the many preformed ones available. They should be of sufficient length and diameter to retain the core and properly support the root, crown, and especially the neck of the tooth where fractures frequently occur. Care must be taken not to dislodge the apical seal or perforate the root when removing segments of endodontic filling material. Posts should not create latent internal pressure that could split already weakened nonvital roots. Posts and cores should be made separately from their overlying crowns for accuracy. A properly shaped foundation can greatly facilitate the ease with which a crown preparation can be made.

Miscellaneous Preliminary Procedures

Diagnostic wax-up of pretreatment casts is helpful or necessary for both patient and dentist to preview the completed case (Fig 24–6). Answers to esthetic consid-

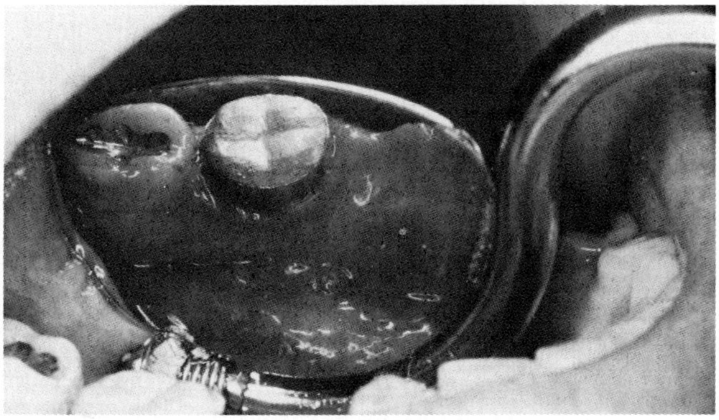

Fig 24–5.—An abutment tooth restored with an amalgam foundation before crown preparation.

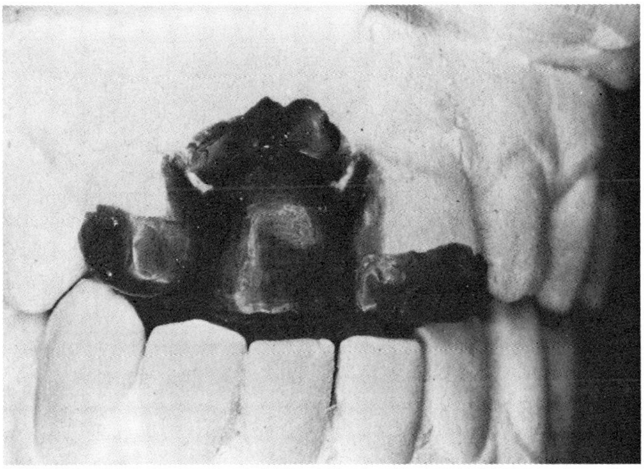

Fig 24–6.—A diagnostic cast with a diagnostic wax-up for a fixed partial denture demonstrates future tooth contours and position.

erations for the patient, and functional and technical problems of concern to the dentist, can be provided by diagnostic wax-ups.

Orthodontics repositioning is a preliminary procedure that can not only upright inclined abutments, but can improve the overall esthetics of a case. Failure to use orthodontics, when indicated, can compromise the final functional and esthetic result of many cases.

Pretreatment acrylic appliances may be needed in extensive reconstruction cases. An occlusal splint is used when the existing vertical dimension needs to be altered. A custom incisal guide table may be used when an existing acceptable anterior guidance needs to be copied accurately. A vertical dimension maintainer appliance, or index, may be used to check occlusal reduction when there are insufficient occlusal stops remaining to maintain vertical dimension during tooth preparation.

TOOTH PREPARATION AND CASE FABRICATION

Retainer Selection

Many problems encountered in tooth preparation are the result of dentist errors in retainer selection. Factors that must be taken into consideration when selecting a suitable type of retainer for a fixed appliance are esthetics, strength of the tooth and retainer, caries index, occlusion, pulp size, path of insertion, and cost for the patient. If consideration is given to satisfy these factors, errors in tooth preparation can be reduced.

Abutment Preparation

Inadequate reduction in tooth preparation has serious consequences all through the appliance fabrication and shortens the life expectancy of the restoration. Inadequate occlusal reduction will not permit development of properly shaped cusp inclines and placement of cusp tips and fossae. Bulky axial contours will enlarge the crown circumference and adversely affect the periodontal health of the tissue. Inadequate facial reduction prevents shading of veneers and pontics to blend harmoniously without over building the surface and again affecting the periodontal health. Insufficient interproximal reduction encroaches on embrasure spaces and will affect esthetics and make proper cleaning by the patient impossible.

Excessive reduction of an abutment tooth creates as severe problems as insufficient reduction. It can reduce the retention and the stability of the restoration (Fig 24–7). The tooth can be weakened and the vitality of the pulp jeopardized. It is, therefore, important that the tooth be neither over- or under-prepared. The amount of tooth structure removed should be what is necessary to allow for the selected retainer.

The path of insertion can be a problem, especially in long span appliances with pier abutments. Prostheses involving tipped or malaligned abutments, both anterior and posterior teeth involved in the same restoration, preparations with grooves, boxes, or pins, and cases involving precision and semiprecision attachments all require special attention during the preparation. In some instances, it is advantageous to make the preparations on study casts before the actual mouth preparation. The results can be surveyed to ensure that the contemplated path of insertion is possible.

Problems frequently arise regarding finishing lines. The questions that must be answered include what type of finish line is desired, where should this finish line be placed and to what depth axially and gingivally should the finish line be made? If an esthetic veneer is to be used, the axial reduction must be sufficient to provide space for the veneer, strength for fabrication procedures, and be properly designed and placed to satisfy the esthetic requirements. In addition, the finishing line should cover wear facets, eroded cervical areas, and decayed or restored parts of teeth. The placement of the finish line must strike a balance with retention and resistance needs, the patient's oral hygiene abilities, esthetic requirements, and periodontal tissue health. Often a compromise must be made when considering all

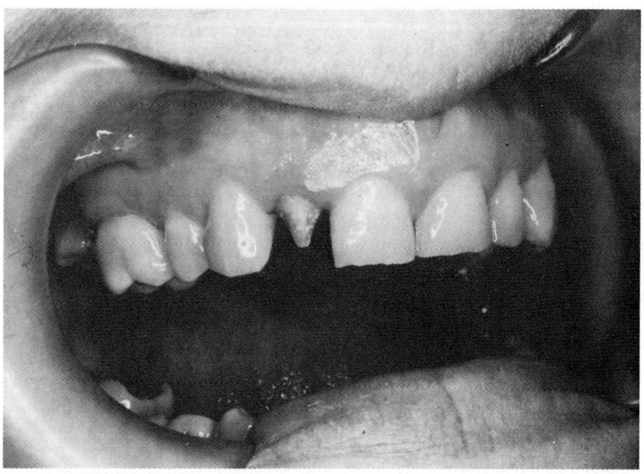

Fig 24–7.—An overprepared tooth can have its vitality impaired. This preparation would not provide adequate retention or stability for even a single crown.

of these factors together. The reasons for the dentist's decision should be explained to the patient if it involves the esthetics or prognosis of the case.

Finally, consideration for the vitality of the pulp during the preparation is paramount. Insufficient water and air coolant plus dull cutting instruments and a heavy pressure can generate excess friction and heat. This can cause transient and irreversible hyperemias of the pulp that can later lead to the death of the pulp (Fig 24–8). Prudent cutting procedures that maintain the integrity of the pulp can not be overemphasized.

Treatment Restoration

The terminology "treatment restoration" is now frequently used instead of "temporary protection." This term emphasizes the need for additional care in its fabrication but distinguishes it from the "permanent restoration." Because of the nonpermanent nature of restoration life, this term is also inaccurate. Perhaps a better choice would be "final restoration." Even though the life of the treatment restoration may be extremely short when compared with the final restoration, on occasion the treatment restoration may have to be worn for months or years because of unforseen circumstances. A poorly fabricated treatment restoration can cause severe problems for both the dentist and the patient. The following common errors should be avoided.

Overextension of the margins of the treatment restoration can cause irritation of the gingiva that will result in soft tissue damage. If underextended margins are left, the pulp can become irritated from sensitivity and the preparation margins may be damaged.

Improper cementation of the treatment restoration can cause irritation of surrounding tissue if all excess cement is not removed (Fig 24–9). If the occlusion is not accurately checked after cementation, occlusal trauma can cause the pulp to become hyperemic. If the esthetic considerations are not met, the patient can be disappointed. Soft tissue irritation can occur from overcontoured, rough, and unfin-

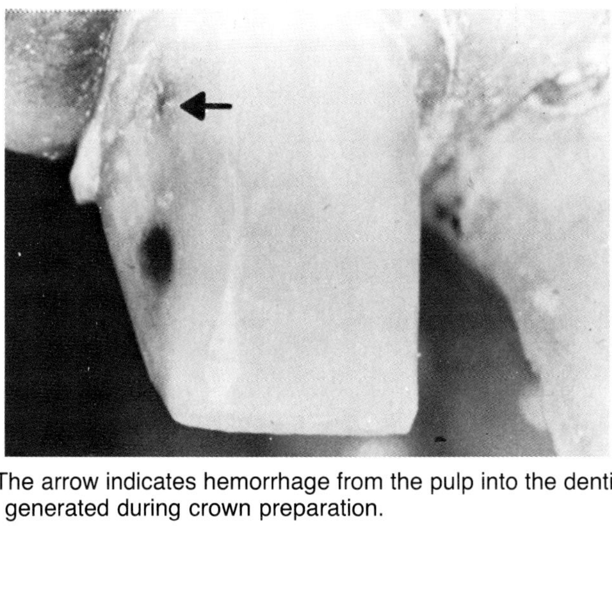

Fig 24–8.—The arrow indicates hemorrhage from the pulp into the dentin resulting from excessive heat generated during crown preparation.

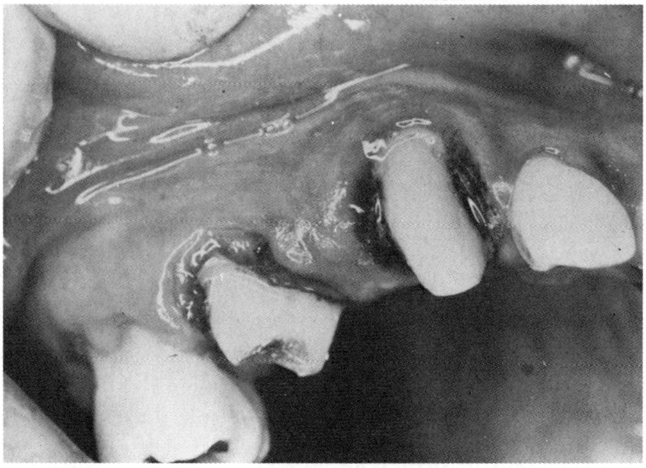

Fig 24–9.—Severely inflamed marginal gingiva resulted from failure to remove excess temporary cement from margins of treatment restoration.

ished margins. Without proper proximal and occlusal contacts teeth can shift in a short period and affect the fit of the final restoration.

Final Impression Procedures

An accurate final impression begins with an adequate impression tray. Impression trays that do not properly fit the arch and cover the area to be impressed usually lead to an inaccurate impression. Underextended trays lead to unsupported impression material and insufficient coverage of the impressed area. Overextended impression trays lead to distortion from excess stress during removal of the set impression material in the mouth. Impression material that is not adequately secured to the impression tray can be distorted when removed from the mouth.

Impression material must be placed in intimate contact with all parts of the prepared teeth. Therefore, marginal tissue should not impede the placement of the impression material on the prepared margin of abutment teeth. Whether electrosurgery or tissue retraction with mechanical or chemical agents is used, care must be taken not to injure the delicate soft tissue surrounding the teeth. If injury does occur disastrous results causing hemorrhage, recession, and periodontal pocket formation can affect the final restoration.

Some errors that occur in impression making can cause distortions that are often difficult to detect. Removing an impression before the material has reached its final set or using impression materials that are past their shelf life are some common causes of problems. Improper mixing can also lead to hidden distortions. Voids, subsurface porosities; and incomplete details are usually errors made with the hasty handling of the impression material in its flowable stage. It is important to check for the complete removal of all the impression material, as small tags of some impression materials, if left trapped in sulcular areas, can cause irritations and even periodontal abscesses. The best check of the adequacy of an impression is close examination of the dies and, ultimately, the fit of the final restoration in the mouth.

Dies and Working Casts

After an accurate impression is made, the construction of dies and mounted casts is the next critical step. The major error found in these areas is improper pouring and sectioning of the dies. The dies must be stable in their base to make accurate placement in the arch possible. Dies and casts that have voids or bubbles create difficulties in making accurate wax patterns for construction and occluding of these castings. Dies must be both trimmed and marked by the dentist to avoid over or underextension of the margins (Fig 24–10). Failure to complete this critical step leaves room for errors and adds needed time for adjustment of margins later. To reduce the time required for occlusal adjustment during casting try-in, scrupulous attention must be given to the mounting of the working cast on an adjustable articulator using accurate interocclusal records. With these few precautions observed, the construction of the castings will be made much easier.

The Final Restoration

Checking a restoration in the patient's mouth for the first time should be done in systematic and orderly manner. If the castings fit without problems on the working cast but do not seat completely on the abutment teeth in the mouth, the abutments are checked for any remaining temporary cement or debris. Next, the retainers are checked for debris or bubbles on the inside and for overextended margins. If the restoration still fails to seat, the proximal contacts should be checked for excessive contact. Pontic-alveolar ridge contacts are checked for excessive blanching of the soft tissue. If the restoration still does not completely seat, the next step is to relieve the inside of the retainers where obstruction is thought to occur. Marking materials such as chloroform and rouge are helpful in locating the offending areas. Often they are found in sharp line and point angles and along extremely long and parallel axial walls. Finally, it may be necessary to separate the abutment retainers to determine which is the offending retainer or if the alignment

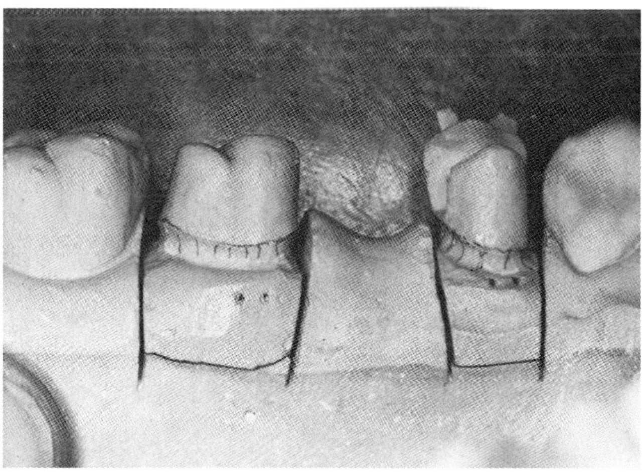

Fig 24–10.—Dies are trimmed and marked before construction of the fixed partial denture.

of the retainers is in error. A decision must be made to remake one or more retainers or to solder the parts of the appliance back together after a soldering index is made in the mouth. The decision to resolder is made only after each segment has completely seated with accurate gingival margins.

A loose fitting retainer may be no problem provided that the retainer shows no faciolingual, mesiodistal, or torqueing movement when it is fully seated. A tight fitting retainer should be relieved until it seats with finger pressure to allow complete seating during cementation. A retainer that has a hole in it or has extremely thin areas that are to be covered with facing materials must be soldered before the facing material is placed. This will minimize the problem of cracking or displacement of a facing from the internal hydraulic pressure generated on a thin area of metal and exerted on the weak facing material during cementation (Fig 24–11).

The contact of the pontic with the alveolar ridge involves two problems. Esthetic problems are solved by making the shape of the facial surface compatable with the missing tooth, adjacent teeth, and the opposing arch teeth. The pontic must appear as if it is growing out of the alveolar mucosa and be properly placed mesiodistally and faciolingually (Fig 24–12). The second problem relates to the oral hygiene of the pontic as it rests on the alveolar ridge. It is important to keep the gingival surface of the pontic convex so that plaque can be removed with floss. The contacting surface should be smooth and of glazed porcelain or highly polished metal. Contact should not extend lingually past the midpoint or crest of the alveolar ridge.

The errors made with connectors between pontics and retainers fall into three categories: placement, size and shape, and finishing errors. A connector must be placed in the contact area. Its size and shape depend on the length of the span and the area of the arch for which the appliance is fabricated. The vertical dimension of the connector has more effect on strength than the horizontal dimension. It goes without saying that short span anterior appliances have less bulky connectors and are shaped differently from long span posterior appliances. The common factor between both anterior and posterior and short and long span appliances is the need for proper finishing and polishing of the connectors, so that they have smooth, well-shaped embrasures that can be easily cleaned by the patient (Fig 24–13).

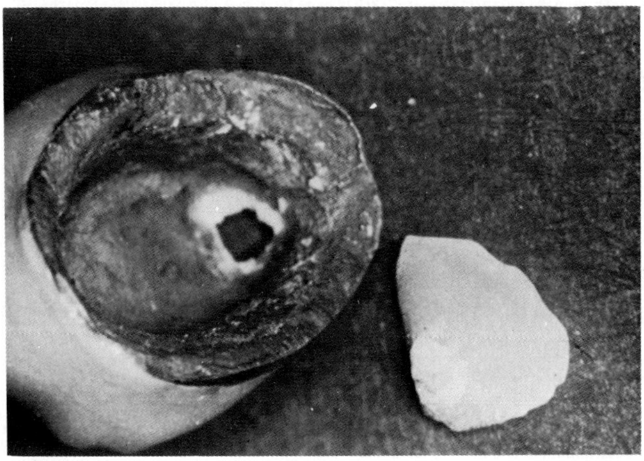

Fig 24–11.—Porcelain has fractured from the metal framework because of an unrepaired hole in the coping before the placement of the porcelain.

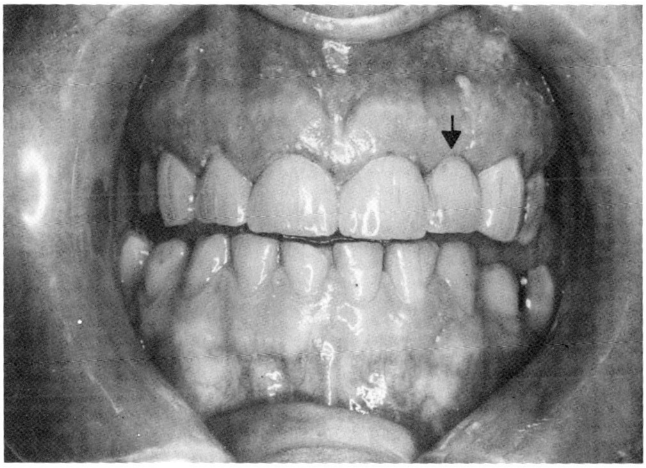

Fig 24–12.—The arrow indicates a maxillary lateral incisor pontic that appears to be growing out of the alveolar mucosa. Its contour and placement are compatible with the rest of the teeth in the mouth.

Once an appliance has been inspected for esthetics, marginal integrity, and occlusion, and is acceptable and comfortable to the patient, it is ready to be cemented. The selection of the cement is important. Errors in the mixing, seating, and removal of excess cement can destroy any previous effort by the dentist. The cementing procedure should be viewed as one of the important final steps to complete successful treatment.

DENTIST-LABORATORY INTERACTION

Dentists Needs

Dentists must use the services of dental laboratories to render the most complete treatment possible for their patients. This means that a good relationship must be

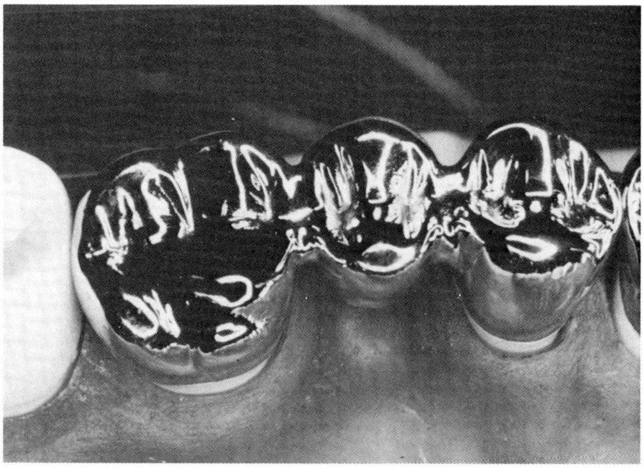

Fig 24–13.—The connector is strong, well-shaped, and polished enabling the patient to keep the appliance clean.

maintained between the laboratory and the dentist. The dentist must be able to communicate any special instructions that may be needed for treatment of a case. It is helpful if a laboratory is close and has someone available to discuss any special requests or problems that the dentist may have. Dentists need to have their laboratory work returned promptly within an agreed on time span. The work must be done precisely, neatly, and following the dentist's instructions accurately. The quality of both the work and materials should be of the highest standard. A dentist must feel secure that the dental laboratory is concerned in presenting the best possible product for the dentist and patient.

Laboratory Needs

The needs of the dental laboratory closely parallel those of the dentist. A detailed written work authorization must be sent to the laboratory that accurately describes the design, materials, customization needed, and the date the work is requested. Not only must the prescription be precise and neat, but the working casts should be properly prepared. The dies should be stable and accurate duplications of the prepared teeth with well trimmed and marked margins. The preparations should be properly tapered and with a common line of draw. Space should be adequate enough to create esthetic facings without overcontouring. Sufficient space should be present to create functional occlusion and adequate embrasures. If these few principles are followed, many of the problems that dentists have with dental laboratories, and dental laboratories have with dentists, will disappear and the quality of work of both will benefit.

SUMMARY

This chapter is designed to influence the delivery of fixed prosthodontic treatment. By effectively dealing with the above problem areas, dentists should more easily avoid errors and satisfy the restorative dental needs of their patients. This in turn will lead to a greater satisfaction for the dentist.

GENERAL REFERENCES

Horn H.R.: *Practical Considerations for Successful Crown and Bridge Therapy.* Philadelphia, W.B. Saunders Co., 1976.

Johnston J.F.: *Modern Practice in Crown and Bridge Prosthodontics,* ed. 3. Philadelphia, W.B. Saunders Co., 1971.

Kornfeld M.: *Mouth Rehabilitation, Clinical and Laboratory Procedures,* ed. 3. St. Louis, C.V. Mosby Co., 1974.

Schweitzer J. M.: *Oral Rehabilitation Problem Cases, Treatment and Evaluation, Vol. 1, 2.* St. Louis, C.V. Mosby Co., 1964.

Shillingburg H.T., Hobo S., Whitsett H.D.: *Fundamentals of Fixed Prosthodontics.* Chicago, Quintessence Books, 1976.

Tylman S.D., Malone W.F.P.: *Tylman's Theory and Practice of Fixed Prosthodontics,* ed. 7. St. Louis, C.V.Mosby Co., 1978.

CHAPTER 25

Fixed Prosthodontic Repairs

KEITH E. THAYER, D.D.S.

ALL FIXED PROSTHESES are subject to damage that will require repair or remake. When repairs are possible and feasible, they certainly should be considered. Both patient and dentist should be aware, however, that repairs may not carry as long a life expectancy as the original or as a remake. Their cost, in time and money, is usually considerably less than that of a remake. Some repairs are undertaken on an emergency or short-term basis, whereas others are projected as a long-term solution. Most repairs should have a contingency plan in case of failure. Usually that contingency plan would be a remake of the restoration. The decision to repair over remake is frequently affected by the size or the complexity of the restoration being repaired. If the restoration is an individual unit the cost of remake might be little different from that of repair and the final result and prognosis of a remake might be much better.

CAUSES OF FAILURE

Failures result from a wide variety of causes. These include recurrent caries on margins of crowns and abutment retainers, cement failure from wash out or breakdown, preparation fractures, acrylic veneer wear or loss, porcelain fracture, solder joint or major connector fractures, and periodontal involvement. Clinical examples and problem solving options of each will be discussed.

Caries

Recurrent caries on restoration margins may be repaired with amalgam, or composite if esthetics requires, if they are accessible and the restoration is functioning adequately in all other respects. If the caries is in a nonaccessible area, usually interproximal, the only option may be to remove and remake the restoration. It is imperative that enough of the gingival portion of the restoration and of the restored tooth is removed so a visual and tactily check for complete caries removal can be made before placing a repair restoration. After the cavity preparation is completed, the restoration should be carefully checked for any loosening or dislodging of the crown or retainer that resulted from the caries removal. If careful attention is paid to detail of the repair, the prognosis should be quite good.

Cement Failure

Cement failure may or may not be associated with recurrent caries. A troublesome problem is created when cement failure occurs on one or more units of a multiple abutment restoration, but one or more units remain cemented. If the remaining cemented units can be removed intact, the restoration may be successfully recemented in many cases. There are a wide variety of removal techniques that can be used. Tapping on the cemented unit with a reverse action crown remover may be successful if the preparations are relatively short and tapered or if some breakdown of the cement has already started to take place. Before attempting removal in this manner the patient should be apprised of the possible consequences of fractures of prepared tooth structure. The degree of force applied should be determined relative to the retentive qualities of the preparation and the type and extent of any foundation material present, if these factors are known. If the restoration cannot be removed with a crown remover the addition of the use of an Amurol* sugarless fruit drop or a Richwil** crown remover interposed between the restoration and the opposing teeth allows the patient to exert a constant negative load on the restoration in a completely vertical direction instead of the torquing action from the crown remover. The supplemented action of the crown remover or tapping with a chisel and mallet, combined with the unseating load exerted by the patient may be enough to break the cement joint (Figs 25–1 and 25–2). The Amurol or Richwil technique alone is effective and highly successful in removing highly retentive restorations that are being tried in, fitted, and occluded. It eliminates any marginal damage that could occur if a metal instrument were used on the restoration margin instead.

Numerous modification techniques can be used with the crown remover, including the tying of ligature wire around contacts or the application of a grappling hook type appliance in an attempt to help increase the amount or improve the direction of unseating forces.

If the restoration is not removed intact, a variety of crown removal kits are available such as the Golden West crown remover.*** This uses a sized hole cut in the

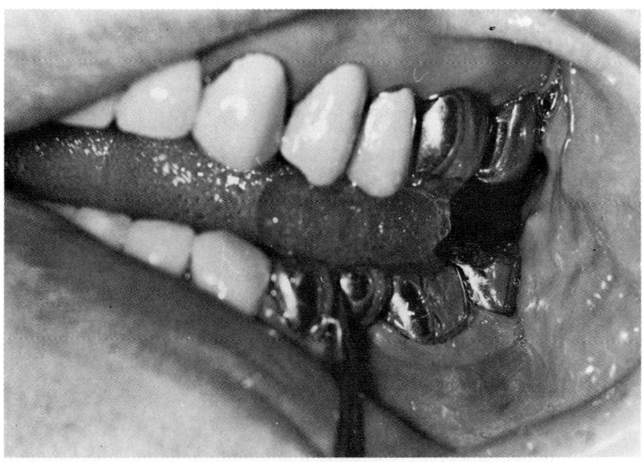

Fig 25–1.—A mandibular three unit bridge with a loose posterior abutment. The patient is biting on an Amurol sugarless fruit drop. A Wiedelstadt chisel is placed under the solder joint and tapped while the patient attempts to open.

*Amurol Products Co., Box 300, Naperville, IL 60566.
**Almore International, Inc., Box 25214, Portland, OR 27225.
***Golden-West Dental, Inc., Box 777. Garden Grove, Ca 92642.

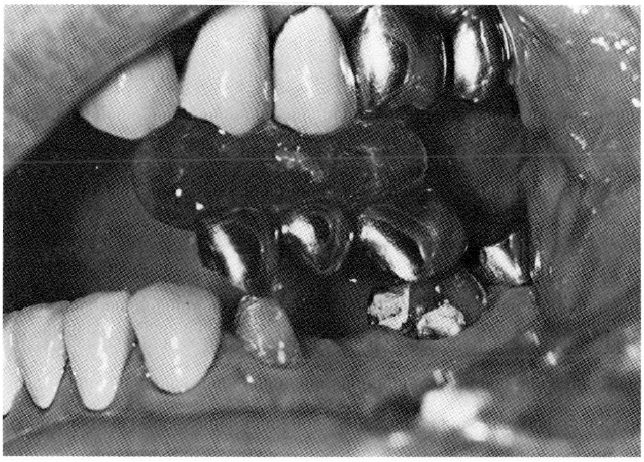

Fig 25–2.—The combination of the negative pressure supplied by the patient and the tapping on the chisel removes the bridge intact.

occlusal of posterior units. A hollow core tap, threaded both inside and outside is tapped into the sized opening and against tooth structure. A pin is inserted into the core of the tap, which engages tooth structure. A small bolt is treaded into the inside of the tap to engage the pin at which point a strong and effective unseating force may be exerted (Fig 25–3). This is much less traumatic than the blow imparted by the crown remover but care must be taken not to drive the pin through foundation or tooth structure into the pulp.

The safest but most destructive method of removing cemented units is by cutting a channel through the restoration to prepared tooth structure on the facial or lingual and occlusal or incisal aspects and gently expanding the casting with a large spoon

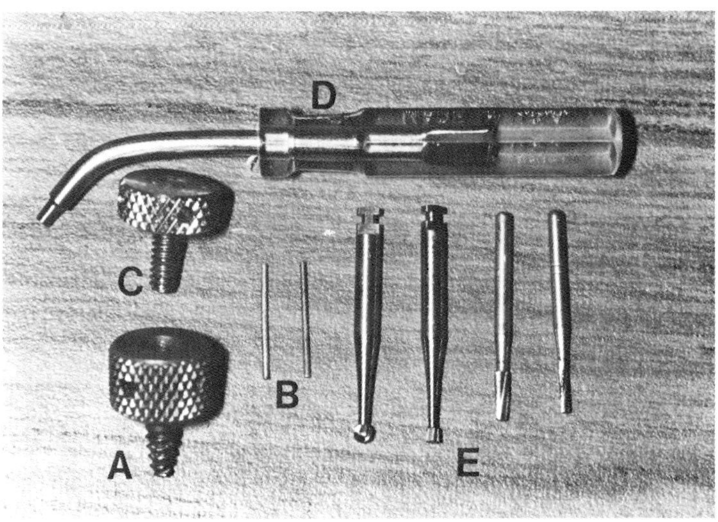

Fig 25–3.—The components of the Golden West crown remover kit include a hollow core tap *(A)*, smooth pins *(B)*, small bolt *(C)*, bolt wrench *(D)*, and drills for occlusal access opening *(E)*.

excavator to break the cement joint.[1] If this technique is used on a porcelain unit, the porcelain is almost certain to fracture and a remake will be required. On an all metal unit it may be possible to repair the slot in the metal with solder and recement the restoration. When this removal technique is used it is advantageous to use a round bur for cutting the metal. The curved cutting leaves of the round bur remain intact and sharper for a much longer time than the angular leaves of a fissure or an inverted cone bur. This results in more efficient cutting and a major saving of time (Fig 25–4).

When the restoration is removed, it is carefully cleaned and examined for suitability for recementation. The abutment teeth are examined for any caries or fracture and the restoration is rechecked. If satisfactory, any damage or altering is repaired and the restoration recemented.

In selected cases, it may be possible to recement one loose abutment without removing the entire fixed partial denture.[2] This is only advisable when the cement failure is recent, if it is quite certain there is no caries in the tooth under the loose abutment, and the patient has excellent oral hygiene. After thorough cleaning with hydrogen peroxide and sodium hypochloride, a permanent cement or a low viscosity composite resin may be successfully injected through an access opening made in the lingual or occlusal of the loose abutment. With care, skill, and a pumping action while injecting, it may be possible to fill the retainer until excess appears on all gingival margins and then allow the cement to set under biting pressure.

Failure of the cement joint between posts and cores and tooth structure may occur. If no caries or tooth fracture has occurred, the restoration may be recemented as is. If remaining tooth structure must be altered, or if it is necessary to lengthen the post, a new cast post and core may be fabricated with a resin[3] or wax[4] pattern of the prepared canal, tooth and internal surface of the existing restoration.

If the fractured post remains in the tooth, a technique has been described[5] where a part of the post is exposed mechanically. Acrylic resin in a copper tube is applied and allowed to polymerize to firmly attach to the exposed post and aid in removal.

Cases where the entire restoration is lost should be carefully examined to deter-

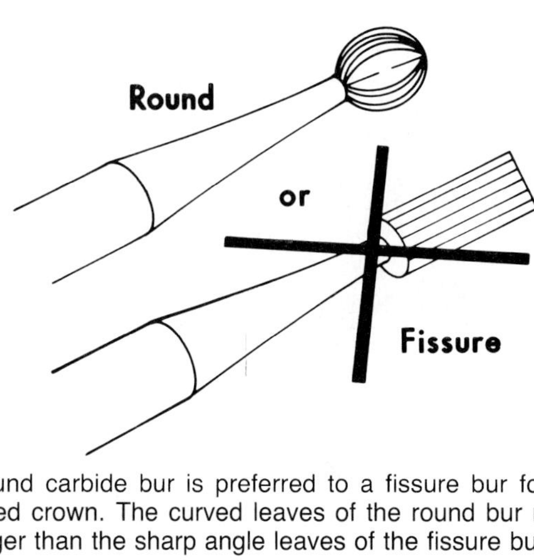

Fig 25–4.—A round carbide bur is preferred to a fissure bur for cutting metal when removing a cemented crown. The curved leaves of the round bur remain sharp and cut efficiently much longer than the sharp angle leaves of the fissure bur.

mine the reason for cement failure. If no obvious reasons exist, the restoration may be recemented. If there is little or no remaining frictional retention of the casting on the tooth, a resin cement or composite material may be the medium for recementation.[6]

Preparation Fractures

Tooth fractures occur on single unit castings as well as fixed partial denture abutments. Fractures of single units where the fracture does not extend apically from the margin of the crown can usually be salvaged by making a wax or Duralay pattern of the prepared canal and internal surface of the crown.[7] The cast post and core can then be cemented, followed by the salvaged crown (Fig 25–5,A–F).

Similar procedures may be used when abutment teeth fracture. A situation where the abutment tooth fractured during try-in is described.[8] A Duralay post and core pattern was made and the cast post and core and the fixed partial denture cemented simultaneously. A Duraly pattern may be made to develop copings between amalgam buildups and exiting restorations[9] where the tooth is still vital but cement failure and recurrent caries necessitate a foundation buildup. Also described is the remake of a coping for a sleeve-coping prosthesis using Duralay to fabricate the pattern for the new coping.[10]

Amalgam is considered the strongest and most stable material for crown foundations. However, it does not lend itself to repair procedures nearly as well as composite. Even though composite has a heavy consistency it still exhibits some flow. In cases where caries or fracture has destroyed a major portion of the crown of a restored tooth, pins or posts can often be placed in the remaining tooth structure, the inner surface of the failed restoration lubricated with vaseline, filled with composite and seated to place over the pins or post. Care is taken to prevent major overfilling or underfilling of the restoration so that the composite will fill all spaces and be compressed around pins, posts, and prepared tooth structure without large amounts of excess. If there is gross excess, it will be difficult to seat the restoration completely because of the flow resistance of composite. The vaseline on the casting will allow the restoration to be removed after setting of the composite. This will allow access for removal of excess composite from preparation margins. It will also allow adjusting or remake of the foundation if it was not possible to seat the casting fully while the composite was setting. When the foundation is satisfactorily completed and adjusted, the restoration is cemented with any preferred final cement.

Acrylic Veneer Wear or Loss

Abrasion can result in loss of severe amounts of acrylic on acrylic veneer crowns and pontics. Even though acrylic is less popular than it once was, wear of these restorations is still a problem. Abrasion can be caused by functional loading or abrasive foods and habits, but probably toothbrush abrasion is the most common cause (Fig 25–6,A). Repairs may be effected by replacing lost contours with autopolymerizing resin (Fig 25–6,B). This can be done without removing remaining resin. It may or may not be necessary to add mechanical retention in the form of undercuts or threaded posts. The composites are now becoming more popular for these repairs. They require mechanical retention but are probably more resis-

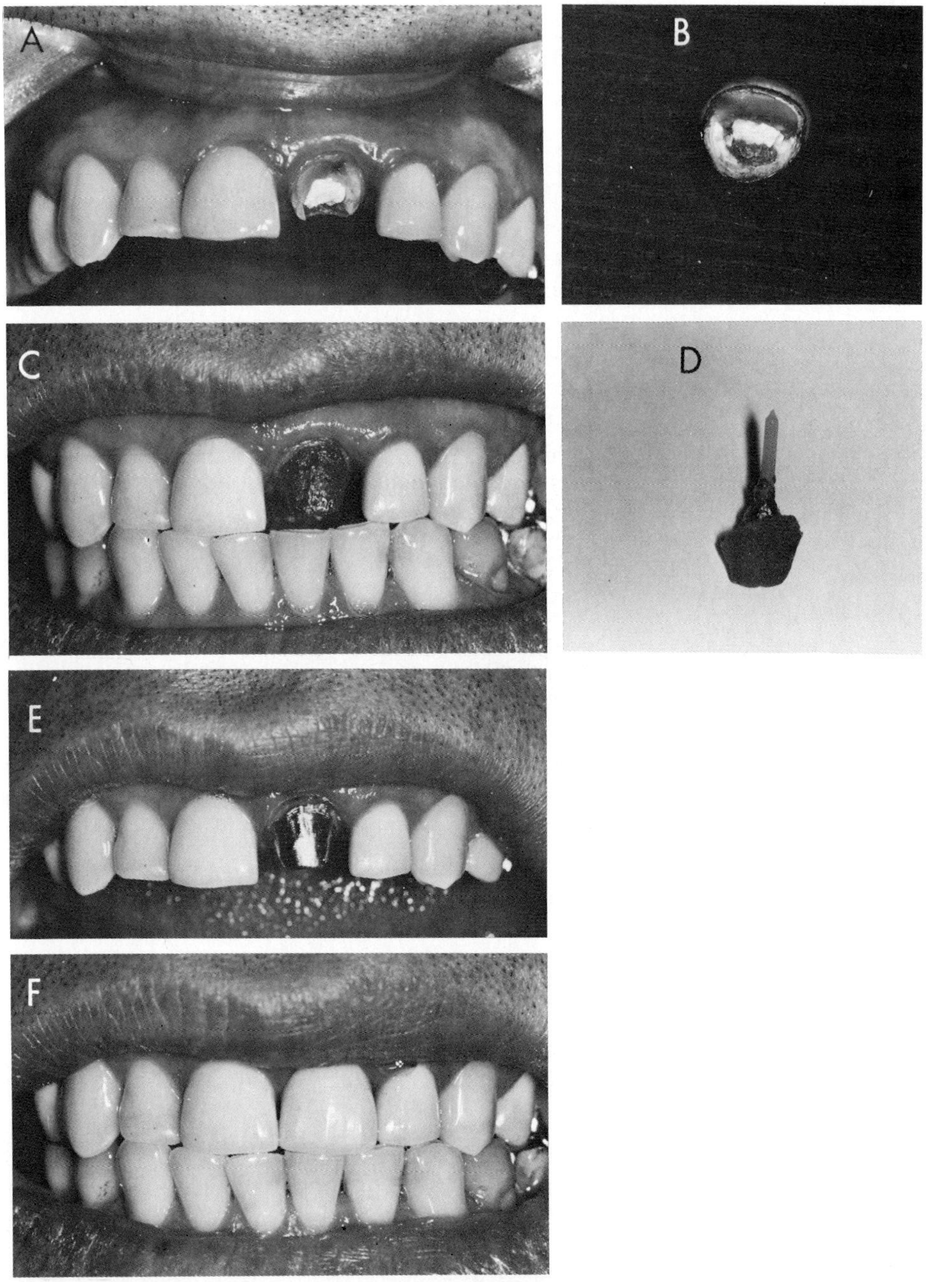

Fig 25–5.—A, the crown and part of the prepared tooth fractured from a nonvital tooth that was restored without a post and core. **B,** the crown with fractured tooth structure inside. The tooth fracture did not involve the margin of the crown preparation at any point. **C,** after removal of the gutta-percha and preparation of the root canal and removal of tooth structure and cement from the crown a Duralay pattern for a post and core is formed by seating the crown over the unset Duralay until all crown to tooth margins are closed. **D,** the complete post and core pattern ready for sprueing and casting. **E,** the cast post and core cemented to place. **F,** the completed repair using the original porcelain-fused-to-metal crown that is now supported and retained with a cast post and core.

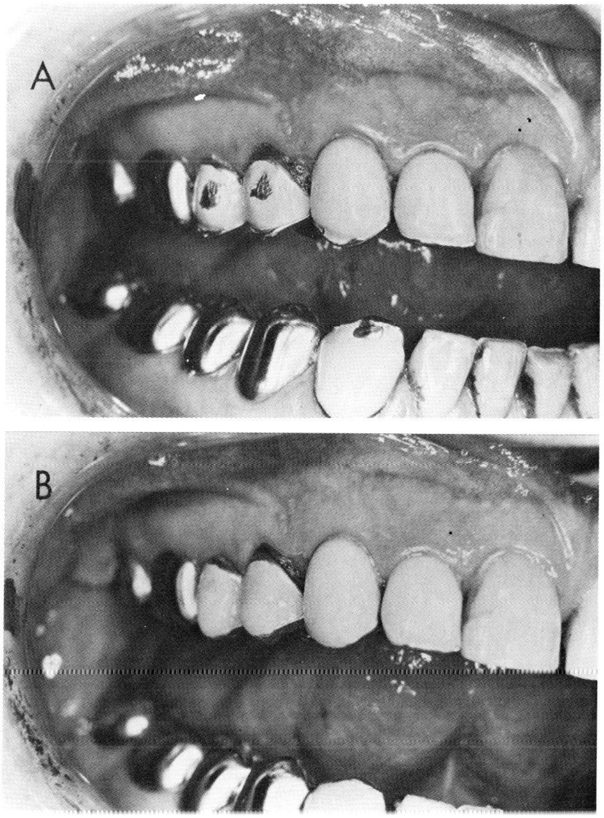

Fig 25–6.—A, acrylic veneer crowns showing toothbrush abrasion on facial of maxillary premolars and mandibular canine. Acrylic wear is also seen at metal-acrylic junction on incisal of maxillary canine and occlusal of maxillary premolars. **B,** worn areas are repaired with addition of tooth-shaded autopolymerizing acrylic resin.

tant to wear and maintain function and appearance longer than acrylic resin repairs.

Porcelain Fracture

Porcelain fractures remain a persistent problem with porcelain-fused-to-metal restorations. As more and more of these units are in service the total number of fractures increases. There are many causes for these fractures. Some are laboratory related, some dentist, and some patient.

A common laboratory cause of failure is metal surface contamination that interferes with the oxidation and bonding of the opaque porcelain. Resultant failures will show clean loss of porcelain from large areas of the casting. When a bright yellow gold surface appears in a fracture area the probable cause is overuse of britecoat, a material designed to enhance shading. This material is no longer in popular use. Other laboratory related failures occur when the porcelain-to-metal junction on occlusal surfaces is improperly designed or placed. Metal-porcelain junctions should be placed well away from any eccentric functioning contacts with opposing teeth. These are the areas where wear, burnishing, and slight deformation of the metal is most likely to occur. If the metal deforms or changes shape, the porcelain will fracture. The cavosurface angle of the coping at the metal-porcelain junction should be obtuse or at most a right angle. If an acute angle is designed, the porcelain will shrink away from the undercut area in the metal and result in a weaker bond. During the firing process porcelain will shrink onto convex and flat surfaces and away from concave or undercut surfaces. Another serious laboratory related failure occurs when there is a major difference in the thickness of the porcelain from one area to another. The best example is when the porcelain thickness is increased on pontics. This commonly occurs when the proper tooth shaped metal framework is not developed (Fig 25-7,A,B). Where porcelain is fused with large variations in thickness, internal strains are set up and fractures can occur under little or no load.

Dentist related failures most often result from improper tooth preparation or inaccurate impressions and fit. There must be occlusal reduction on posterior teeth to allow for a uniform thickness of porcelain when the occlusal surface is designed in porcelain. Uniform and adequate facial reduction is important also. Failure can result from esthetic as well as strength problems. Restorations where metal is exposed during equilibration of the restoration, such as lingual surfaces of maxillary anteriors, do not usually present a major concern. If the porcelain was fused to a relatively uniform thickness originally, no internal strains will be present and the

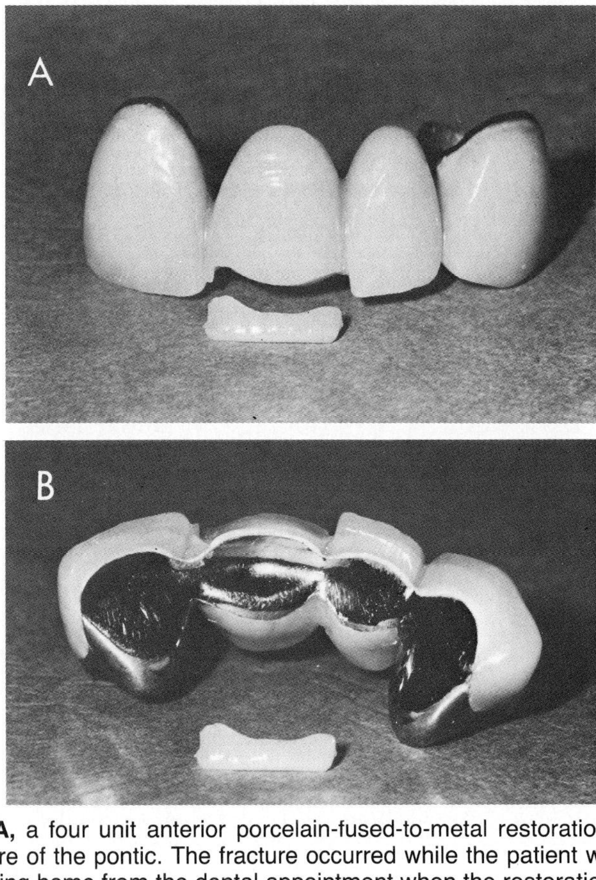

Fig 25–7.—A, a four unit anterior porcelain-fused-to-metal restoration with an incisal porcelain fracture of the pontic. The fracture occurred while the patient was sitting quietly in his car returning home from the dental appointment when the restoration was cemented temporarily. **B,** the fracture probably resulted from improper metal framework design.

bond between the opaque and the oxidized metal surface is as strong or stronger than the porcelain itself.

Some patient failures occur from patient abuse. Unnecessary loads and strains should be routinely avoided. A major uncontrolled cause of fracture is bruxism. When this is a problem from the standpoint of porcelain fracture, or if wear on the restoration or opposing restorations or teeth occurs, a night guard should be considered. A high glaze on the porcelain will minimize wear but, in bruxism, the glaze can be worn away rather rapidly. The only concerns with abrasion occur when the teeth contact in eccentric positions and excursions. If a canine protected occlusion exists on natural teeth, there is little or no concern for fractures of porcelain on posterior teeth. Neither is there concern regarding abrasion resulting from differing surfaces (gold, porcelain, or natural tooth structure), contacting in opposing arches. Little or no wear results from vertical contacts. When contacts are present in horizontal movements abrasion can occur rapidly between dissimilar material surfaces. The final major cause of patient fracture is trauma. This may result from accidental or occupational blows or from foreign particles or objects in food. These are frequently unavoidable and are truly accidental in nature.

Repair of any porcelain fracture can be difficult. If the fractured fragment is complete and intact, it may be recemented with an unfilled composite resin.[11] This is a temporary measure at best. It is only recommended until a more definitive solution can be effected. Before any definitive solution is undertaken an attempt should be made to establish the cause of the fracture so that such factors can be eliminated or minimized in the repair or remake. Several commercial products, such as Fusion,* have been marketed but these products have met with limited success. The most effective one appointment repair has been the use of composite resins combined with mechanical retention gained from undercut metal substructure or threaded or cemented pins. Light and chemically curing composites work equally well. Frequently, composite material may be formed with a festooned and contoured celluloid tooth form.[12] This can greatly reduce the finishing time and enhance the final resultant contour (Fig 25–8,A-C).

Pontics can sometimes be effectively repaired using a slipper type porcelain-fused-to-metal restoration over the remaining metal framework after all porcelain fragments are removed.[13] Pin retained porcelain-fused-to-metal units can be used as repairs with high quality results. Surface and esthetic qualities comparable with the original can be attained. A repair of this nature involves as much or more time and laboratory cost as a single unit so it is only feasible when there is a failure of one or two units of an extensive restoration (Fig 25–9,A-C).

Solder Joint or Major Connector Failure

Solder joints or connectors of multiple unit restorations cast in one piece occasionally fail. This is usually the result of improperly designed and weak frameworks or incomplete flow or crystalization of solder joints. Porosities can result in either soldered or cast connectors that may lead to failures. If the abutment castings can be removed, they can be indexed, resoldered and recemented. If removal is unsuccessful it may be necessary to remake some or all of the units of the restoration. In special situations or where extensive restorations are involved innovative techniques may be used with good success[14] (Fig 25–10,A-C).

---

*George Taub Products and Fusion Co. Inc., 227 New York Ave., Jersey City, NY. 07307.

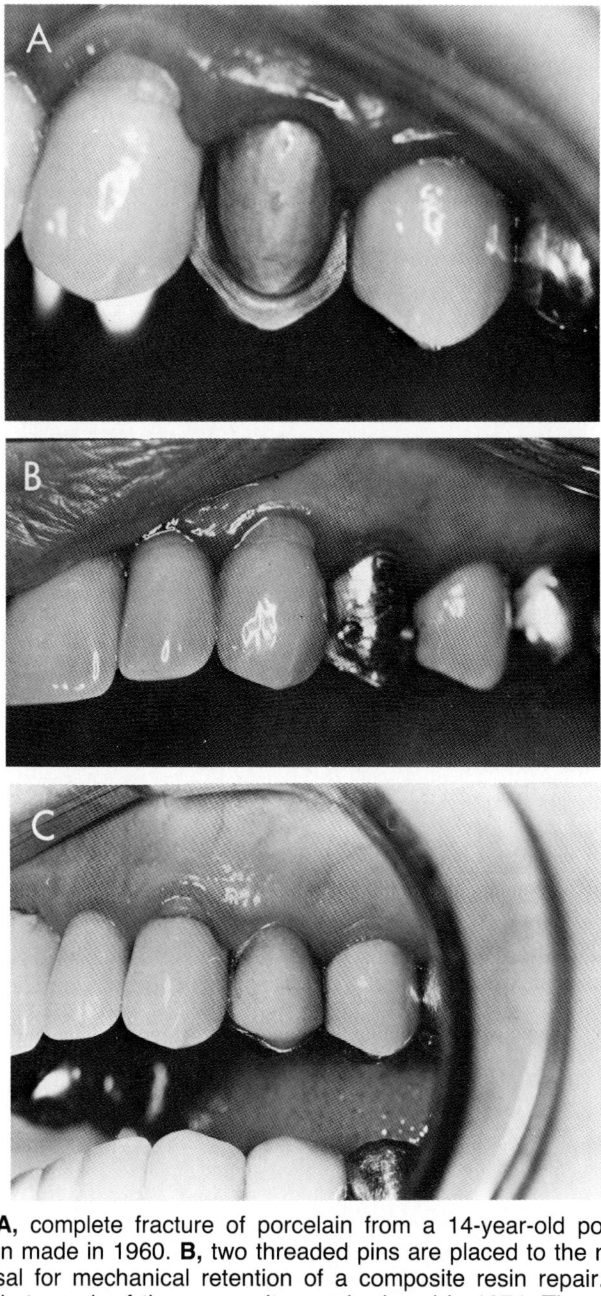

Fig 25–8.—A, complete fracture of porcelain from a 14-year-old porcelain-fused-to-metal restoration made in 1960. **B,** two threaded pins are placed to the mesial and distal near the occlusal for mechanical retention of a composite resin repair. **C,** a nine-year postoperative photograph of the composite repair placed in 1974. There is some discoloration and surface roughness but it still serves esthetic and functional requirements.

Periodontal Involvements

Multiple abutment extensive fixed partial dentures are frequently made for periodontally compromised patients. Because the periodontal prognosis for some teeth is somewhat guarded, it may become necessary in the future to extract the roots of one or more of the abutment teeth. Providing these teeth are not key teeth to the

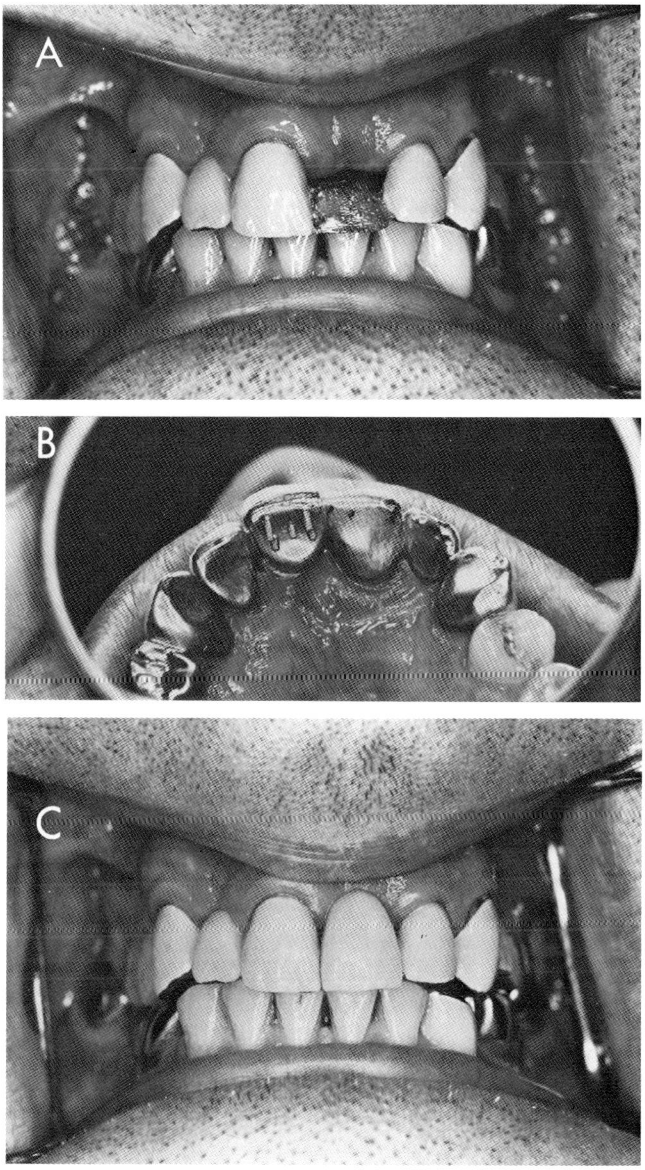

Fig 25–9.—**A,** a five unit anterior bridge from right canine to left lateral with porcelain fractured from left central framework. The framework is poorly designed and contaminated with britecoat. **B,** the repair is a thin metal casting with five parallel pins for retention and porcelain fused to the labial surface of the casting. The pins are cut and polished from the lingual after cementation. **C,** the finished repair from the labial with good gingival adaptation and esthetics and a durable porcelain surface.

support of the fixed partial denture, it is sometimes possible to remove remaining tooth structure from the retainer casting. This can then be filled with amalgam or composite and formed in the shape of a pontic.[15] If preplanning for such eventualities can be done when the restoration is initially fabricated, contours and relationships may be unharmed.

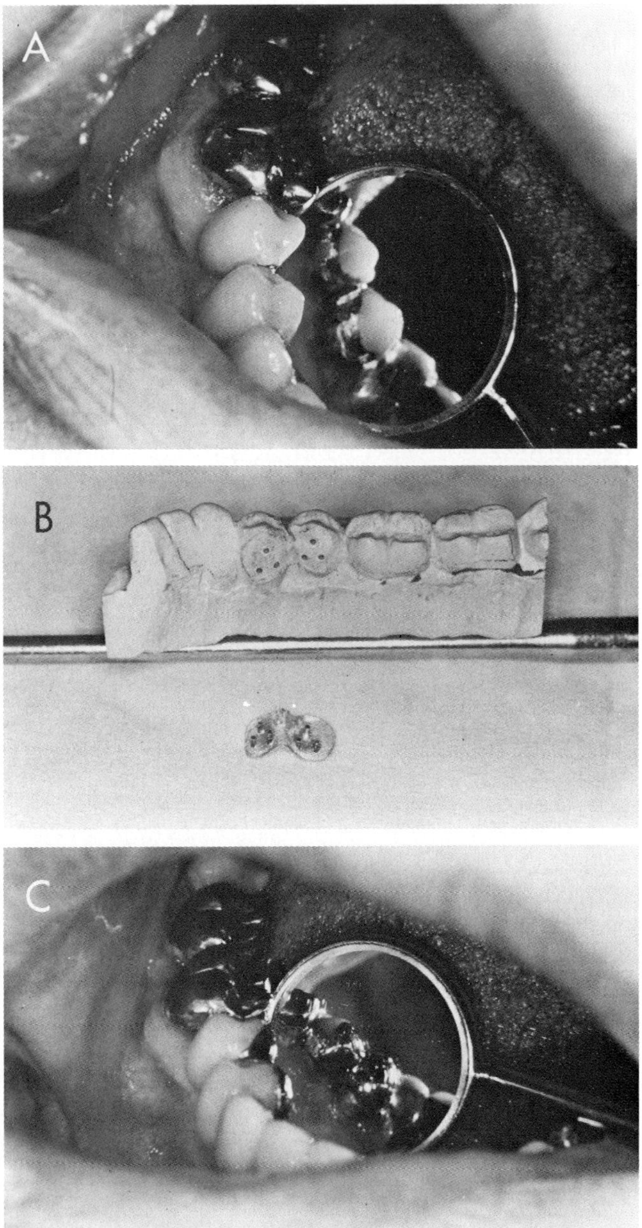

Fig 25–10.—**A,** 13 unit lower fixed partial denture extending from left first molar to right second molar fractured between the right premolar pontics after seven years of service. **B,** the lingual surfaces of the pontics were prepared and a metal casting with three parallel pins in each pontic was fabricated. **C,** the casting with pins parallel to the occlusal surface for optimum resistance to occlusal loads was cemented to place. It served to reunite the two segments of the appliance until the patient's death 11 years later.

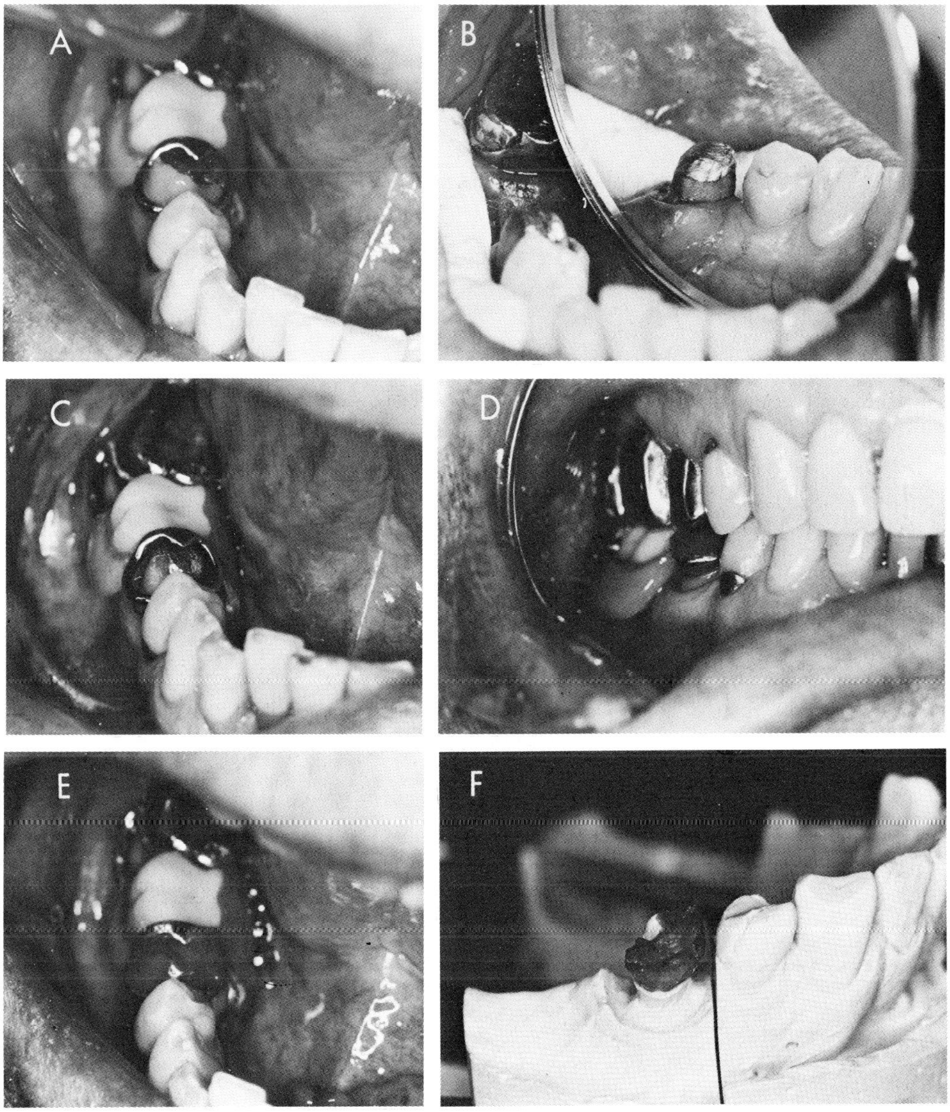

Fig 25–11.—**A,** there is extensive caries beneath a large distoocclusal amalgam on a clasped abutment tooth. The tooth requires a full cast crown for adequate restoration and the partial denture is functioning satisfactorily. **B,** caries has been removed, an amalgam foundation placed, and the tooth prepared for a full cast gold crown. **C,** the partial denture is inserted and the preparation carefully checked for adequate clearance from all clasps, rests, and struts of removable partial denture. **D,** the patient closes lightly in occlusion to stabilize the removable partial denture while Duralay is flowed between the preparation and the buccal clasp and allowed to polymerize. **E,** the patient may then open for access to flow Duralay between the preparation and remaining clasps and rests. **F,** the Duralay pattern is trimmed and placed on the working die so that the margins, occlusion, and remaining axial contours may be finished in wax.

Crowns for Existing Partial Dentures

A repair situation sometimes arises in relation to existing serviceable removable partial dentures. This may be a result of the fracture of the abutment tooth.[16] The need may also arise when the removable partial denture abutment tooth was previously crowned and for one or more reasons requires remake or when extensive caries occurs on abutment teeth requiring full coverage.

An effective technique for this restoration is to establish a foundation for a new crown that is prepared to provide clearance from all struts, rests, and clasps of the existing partial denture. The foundation may be a pin amalgam buildup, a preformed post with amalgam buildup, or a cast post and core depending on the need of the tooth being treated. With the foundation completed and the crown preparation finished the removable partial denture is inserted and positioned by the patient's occlusion. Duralay is then flowed between the preparation and an accessible clasp or rest to establish the relationship of the clasp to the preparation. The patient may then open and the dentist will have access to flow Duralay between all remaining portions of the partial and the preparation. The preparation is recorded in any final impression material and a die is prepared. The Duralay pattern is placed on the die and incorporated into the wax pattern for the crown (Fig 25–11,A-F). The Duralay preserves the partial-to-preparation relationships and the wax finalizes the margins, occlusion, and general contours of the pattern for the crown.

SUMMARY

The first consideration when confronted with any failure or repair situation is to ascertain the cause or suspected cause. Sometimes this is easy and obvious. If there is a cause that is correctable it should be taken care of first. Care should be taken not to become involved in repairs that should have been remakes. Repairs are usually second best to the original in one or more ways. The patient should always be aware that there is a contingency plan and that the contingency plan is usually remake in the event of repair failure. Imagination and innovation are key factors in successful repairs. Most failures are unique and present varying challenges to the dentist. Great satisfaction can be achieved in meeting a situation and solving it in an effective and economical manner.

REFERENCES

1. Hall D.L., Connor R.J.: Removal of partially loosened fixed partial dentures. *J. Prosthet. Dent.* 45:221, 1981.
2. Grunwaldt D.C.: Simplified technique for removal of a fixed bridge. *Dent. Surv.* 49:32, 1973.
3. Tebroch O.C.: Technique for post-core removal from a crown and a new post-core fabrication. *J. Prosthetic. Dent.* 43:463, 1980.
4. Beheshti N.: Fabricating a post and core to fit an existing crown. *J. Prosthet. Dent.* 42:236, 1979.
5. Samani S.I., Harris W.T.: A procedure for repairing fractured post-core restorations. *J. Prosthet. Dent.* 39:627, 1978.
6. Robb R.G.: Recementation technique for loose appliances. *Dent. Surv.* 48:41, 1972.
7. Richardson J.T., Padgett J.G.: Repair technique for a fractured, crowned anterior tooth. *J. Prosthet. Dent.* 31:409, 1974.
8. Priest G., Goerig A.: Post and core fabrication beneath an existing crown. *J. Prosthet. Dent.* 42:645, 1979.

9. Johnson E.T.: Saving a bridge. *Dent. Surv.* 55:44, 1979.
10. Stern N., Redah A.: Repairing a crown and sleeve-coping prosthesis. *J. Prosthet. Dent.* 43:286, 1980.
11. Rehany A., Zalkind M., Revah A.: Repair of fractured porcelain jacket crowns with a composite resin. *J. Prosthet. Dent.* 45:455, 1981.
12. Aspes T., McIlwain J.E. Jr.: Restorative technique to repair pontics. *Dent. Surv.* 49:24, 1973.
13. Bruggers H., Jeansonne E.E., Grush L.: Repair technique for fractured anterior facings. *J. Am. Dent. Assoc.* 98:947, 1979.
14. Miller T.H., Thayer K.E.: Intraoral repair of fixed partial dentures. *J. Prosthet. Dent.* 23:382, 1971.
15. Sarrett D.C.: Fabricating fixed partial dentures using existing restorations. *J. Prosthet. Dent.* 46:142, 1981.
16. Thurgood B.W., Thayer K.E., Lee R.E.: Complete crowns constructed for an existing partial denture. *J. Prosthet. Dent.* 30:507, 1973.

Index

A

Abrasion: pinlay casting for, 77
Abutment
  preparation, 319–321
  teeth, rotating, 292–293
  tilted, 316
Acid etch, 70
Acid-etch resin
  application in occlusal treatment, 250–251
  bonded cast restorations, 246–263
    advantages of, 249
    canine risers in, 251–252
    case reports, 255–262
    contraindications, 254–255
    design, etched metal, 248–249
    design, perforated, 248
    designs for retainer, 253
    disadvantages of, 249
    at first appointment, 247–248
    indications for, 254–255
    laboratory fabrication, 251–252
    laboratory procedures, 252–255
    at second appointment, 248–249
    technique, description of, 247–249
    work authorization for, 251
  splint, 257
Acrylic
  guide planes, 289
  index, 76
  provisional restoration, customized, 120–121
  resins, autopolymerizing, 135–136
    tray resin, 101
  spring space regainer, 291
  template technique, vacuum formed, 125–129
    indirect, 129–130
  veneer
    crown, 333
    loss, 331–333
    wear, 331–333
Adhesive: for impression tray, 103
Adrenaline
  chloride, 85
  gingival retraction and, 83
After-image, 269
Alginate impression technique: for provisional restoration, 130
Alum: and gingival retraction, 85
Aluminum
  chloride, and gingival retraction, 83
  shell, 117
    crown, 117, 118
Alveolar process, 10–11
Amalgam, 28, 331
  build-ups, 284
  caries beneath, 339
  in cast post and core, 282–284
  foundation, 318
Amputation: root, 300
Amurol, 328
Anatomical structures, 5–11
Anterior
  closure, 160
  reference point, 149
Aqua regia, 229, 241
Arcs of closure, 153, 158, 181
Articulation (*see* Cast, articulation)
Articulator, 178–189
  arbitrary, 179
    crown and bridge, 179
    Stephens, 179
  fully adjustable, 178, 186–189
    Denar D5A, 186
    Stuart, 187
    TMJ, 187
  Hanau-Mate, 180
  positional, 179–180
  semi-adjustable
    arcon type, 182, 183
    Hanau, 183
    slot type, 183
  Whip-Mix, 182
Autopolymerizing resin, 188
  acrylic, 101, 135–136
Axis-orbital plane, 148, 149, 152, 153, 157

B

Bar shaped pontics, 221
Bennett
  angle, 168, 181
  movement, 167

Bevel
  with chamfer, in porcelain fused to metal restorations, 55
  gingival margins, 35
  shoulder with, for porcelain fused to metal restorations, 55
BIS-GMA, 240
Bite
  crossbite (*see* Crossbite)
  planes, 287
Blood pressure: and gingival retraction, 83
Blue Cement Spacer, 209
Boley gauge, 199
Bridge
  and crown articulator, 179
  nineteenth century, 2
  pontics in porcelain fused to metal restorations, 57–59
Bristles: nylon, 74
Broken-stress restorations, 19
Bullet shape pontics, 221
Butt joint, 36

C

Canine risers: in acid-etch resin prosthesis, 251
Cantilever fixed partial denture, 19
Caries, 327
  beneath amalgam, 339
Case fabrication, 319–325
Cast
  articulation, 134–145
    materials for, 143
    methods for, 143
    working cast, 210–211
  centric adjustment, 231–232
  contact adjustment, 230–231
  diagnostic, 15
  excursive adjustment, 232–233
  finishing, 233–234
    armamentarium for, 234–235
    laboratory procedures, 228–230
  fit, marginal, 231
  fitting of, 228–233
    armamentarium for, 234–235
  gypsum, 190
  impression for, rinsing of, 192–193
  metal crown, full, reduction for, 37–38
  occlusal adjustment, 231
    gross, 230
  opposing, 210
  patient procedures, 230–233
  polishing, 234
    after cementation, 234
  porcelain-fused-to-metal, 254
  post and core (*see* Post, and core, cast)
  split cast technique, 158
  sprue removal, 228
  working, 190–217, 323
    articulation of, 210–211
    base of, reduction of, 199
    base technique, and die, 197–201
    clinical considerations in, 213–215
    fitting on, 229–230
    laboratory considerations in, 213–215
    lined with rope wax, 202
    mounted, 215
    mounting of, 210–211
    with removable dies, 190–217
    with removable dies, criteria for, 190–191
    sectioning of, 201–203
Casting
  of impression, 193–195
  procedures for porcelain fused to metal restorations, 62
Cavity
  filling of, 28–29
  floors made perpendicular, 24
Celluloid crown, 123
  form, 122
Cement, 325
  Blue Cement Spacer, 209
  failure, 327–331
  film thickness of, 240
  final, 238–239
  glass ionomer, 240
  handling of, 244
  polycarboxylate, 240
  selection of, 241–242
  silico-phosphate, 240
  spatulation of, 242
  zinc phosphate, 237
Cementation, 236–245
  of dowel pins, 197
  permanent, materials for, 237–240
  in pin retained restorations, 80
  polishing after, 234
  procedures, 242–245
  of provisional restoration, 131
  recementation, 330
  techniques, 240–241
  temporary, 236–237
Cemented pin, 26
Cementum, 8–9
Centering guide, 100
Centers of rotation, 153
Centric
  interocclusal centric records, 15
  occlusion, 13
    records, 143–144
Centric relation, 12, 136, 158, 165
  definition, 167

position, 139
records, 140–143
Chamfer
gingival margins, 35
in porcelain fused to metal restorations, 54–55
Chart: tooth, 15
Checkbite records, 185
Chroma, 265, 268–269
Cleaning: of impression, 193
Closure
anterior, 160
arcs of, 153, 158
posterior, 160
Clutches
to cover teeth, 167
for kinematic location of hinge axis, 155
for pantography, 174
Color, 266
Composite, 331
build-ups, 284
in cast post and core, 282–284
Condylar determinants: of occlusion, 165
Condylar guidance, 153
Condyle: translatory movements of, 163
Connectors, 57, 324
major, failure of, 335–336
pontic (*see* Pontic, connectors)
Copings, 60
Copper bands and tubes: for gingival retraction, 84, 86
Cord for gingival retraction, 87–88
instrument for placing, 88
Core (*see* Post, and core)
Crossbite, 287–288
anterior, 288
elastics, 290
posterior, 289–290
Crown
acrylic veneer, 333
aluminum shell, 117, 118
and bridge articulator, 179
cast metal, full, reduction for, 37–38
celluloid, 123
form, 122
design preparation, periodontal considerations in, 299
foundations, 21–30
indications for, 21
half, mesial, 48
Kurer crown anchor system, 283
lengthening, 317
nineteenth century, 2
for partial denture, existing, 340
polycarbonate, 117, 122
form, 122
porcelain-fused-to-metal, 256, 274
reduction for, 41–48
remover, 328
Golden West, 328–329
Golden West, kit for, components of, 329
resin, custom-made, 117
root relations, 294
after root removal, 302
seven-eighths, 48
three quarter, reduction for, 38–41
Cusp: stamp, 165
Cyanoacrylate resin, 197, 200, 209

D

Degassing: in porcelain fused to metal restorations, 63, 67
Degree of taper, 32
Denar
D5A fully adjustable articulator, 186
face-bow transfer, 161
Dental
history, 12, 314–315
pulp (*see* Pulp)
Dentin, 7
rectangular channels in, small, 24
sclerotic, 7–8
secondary, 7
Dentist-laboratory interaction, 325–326
dentist's needs, 325–326
laboratory needs, 326
Dentistry: early, 1–2
Denture
-base type contact, in pontics, 219
partial
cantilever fixed, 19
existing, crowns for, 340
fixed, provisional, 124–131
fixed, three unit, 309
Deplating: electric, 241
Deprogrammer, 141–142
Detrusion, 171
Diagnosis, 12–20
variety of factors involved in, 14
Diagnostic
casts, 15
mounted, 315
wax-up, 17, 213, 318–319
for pontics, 224
for provisional restoration, 130
Diastema, 256, 290
Dichromatism, 266
Die(s), 323
electroformed silver, 191
epoxy resin, 191–192
gypsum, type IV, 192–195, 203

Die(s) *(cont.)*
keyed matrix die technique, 212–213
material, selection of, 191–195
removable, 190–217
with dowel pins, 196–197
fitting on, 228–229
from preformed tray systems, 212–213
systems of, 195–206
working cast and, 190–217
working cast and, criteria for, 190–191
spacers
materials for, 241
use of, 206–209
trimmed, largest diameter of, 208
working
sectioning of, saw blade for, 204
trimming of, 203–206
working cast base technique and, 197–201
Diffraction, 267
Di-Lok tray, 195, 197, 212
Dowel pin, 195
cementation of, 197
hole for, 200
placement systems, commercial, 211–212
with removable dies, 196–197
shapes and sizes of, 196
technique, 196–206
Drill(s)
breakage in pin retained restorations, 79
twist, 76
Duralay resin, 255

E

Ear face-bow, 151, 161
Egg shape pontics, 221
Elastics: crossbite, 290
Electric deplating, 241
Electroformed silver die, 191
Electrolytic relief, 229
Electrosurgery, 256, 318
for gingival retraction, 86
Embrasures: gingival, 58, 79
Enamel, 6–7
Endodontic considerations: in fixed prosthodontics, 298–299
Endodontic fill techniques, 298–299
Endodontic treatment
diagnosis after, 276–278
molar after, 277
preplanning in, 278–279
restoration after, 276–285
final restorations, 284–285
Endodontically treated tooth: protection for, 130–131
Epimine plastic, 121
Epinephrine: in gingival retraction, 83, 85
Epoxy resin die, 191–192
Equilibration: occlusal, 317
Esthetic requirements: determining of, 12
Ethyl methacrylate, 121
Examination
clinical, 12
intraoral, 315–316
radiographic, 315

F

Face-bow, 134, 136, 178
ear, 151, 161
kinematic, 134
measurement type, 162
regular, 134
transfer, 15, 146–163, 213
Facing
lap facing pontics, 220
Steele's, 218
Fatigue: retinal, 270
Feather edge gingival margins, 35
Filling: of cavity, 28–29
Films: hardening, 206–209
Finishing lines, 320
Fisher's angle, 176
Fixed-fixed restorations, 19
Fixed-movable restorations, 19
Fixed prosthodontics
case fabrication, 319–325
cementation (*see* Cementation)
diagnosis in, 313–316
endodontic considerations in, 298–299
failures
causes of, 327–340
periodontal involvements in, 336–339
history of, 1–4
impressions for (*see* Impressions)
mouth procedures for, preliminary, 316–319
orthodontic considerations in, 286–295
occlusal considerations, 295
pulpal considerations, 293–294
patient management for, 316
periodontal considerations in, 296–312
case reports, 300–310
historical background, 296–297
problems in, 313–326
repairs of, 327–341
tooth preparation, 319–325
treatment expectations in, 313–314
treatment planning in, 313–316
treatment restoration, 321–322
in twentieth century, 3
Foundation, 331

Fracture
  of porcelain, 324, 333–335, 337
  of preparation, 331
  tooth, 278, 284, 332
Frankfort plane, 148, 153
Frenum attachment, 317
Full shoulder gingival margins, 35
Functionally generated path, 179, 180

G

Gauge: Boley, 199
Gingiva, 9
  embrasures, 58, 79
  margins, 32–36
    bevel, 35
    beveled shoulder, 35
    chamfer, 35
    design of, 34–36
    feather edge, 35
    full shoulder, 35
    knife edge, 35
    position of, 32–34
  retraction, 83–90
    chemical, 84–86
    copper bands and tubes for, 84, 86
    cord, 87–88
    cord, instrument for placing, 88
    electrosurgery for, 86
    mechanical, 84
    modes, 84–86
    techniques, clinical, 86–89
  tissue management, 83–90
Glass ionomer cements, 240
Glaze: natural, in porcelain fused to metal restorations, 66
Glazing of porcelain fused to metal restorations, 66
  staining after, 66–67
Golden West crown remover, 328–329
  kit for, components of, 329
Gothic arch tracings, 141
Guide planes: acrylic, 289
Guide table
  custom, 213
  incisal guide table technique, custom, 213, 214, 215
Gypsum
  cast, 190
  die, type IV, 192–195, 203

H

Half crown: mesial, 48
Hanau-Mate articulator, 180
Hanau semi-adjustable articulator, 183
Hard tissue
  anatomy, 6–9
  treatment, 317–318
Hardening films, 206–209
Hawley palatal appliance: conventional, 290
Health questionnaire, 13
Heart shape pontics, 221
Hemisection: of mandibular molar, 305–307
Hinge axis, 150, 165
  kinematic location, 150, 151, 154
    clutch for, 155
  location, 146–163
    arbitrary point and, 153
  pantograph oriented toward, 166
Hinge position: terminal, 154, 165
History
  dental, 12, 314–315
  of fixed prosthodontics, 1–4
  medical, 12, 314–315
Hole: occlusal vent, 241
Homogeneity: of impression materials, 105
Horizontal axis, 181
  of rotation of mandible, 147
Hue, 265, 268
Hydrocolloids for impression material, 93–94
  reversible, 93
Hygiene: mouth, 316

I

Impression(s)
  adhesive for tray, 103
  alginate, technique, for provisional restoration, 130
  blocking out of embrasures for, 79
  casting of, 193–195
  cleaned tray, 102
  cleaning of, 193
  cleaning the preparation, 92
  compound, 93, 135
  custom trays for, fabrication of, 99–103
  final, 109
  first pour base, thickness of, 195
  good, prerequisites for, 91–92
  handle of tray, 102
  hydrocolloids for, 93–94
    reversible, 93
  isolation of preparation, 92
  materials for, 91–99
    dispensing, 103–113
    homogeneity of, 105
    manipulation of, 99–103
    mixing, 103–113
  polyethers for, 97–98
  polysulfides for, 94–95
  procedures, final, 322
  putty-wash systems, 110–113
  rinsing of, 192–193

Impression(s) *(cont.)*
silicones for, 95–97
syringe, injection, armamentarium for, 106
techniques, 99–113
putty-wash, 96
tissue management during, 92
trimmed tray, 102
two paste systems, 103–110
vinyl polysiloxanes for, 98–99
wax, technique, for provisional restoration, 130
acrylic, 120–121
Incisal guidance, 181
Incisal guide table technique: custom, 213, 214, 215
Incisors
congenitally missing, 258
in labioversion, pin retained restorations for, 78
Index
acrylic, 76
soldering, 324
Infraorbital notch, 148
pantograph oriented toward, 166
Initiating position: of movement, 155
Insertion: path of, 320
Interocclusal records, 134–145, 157, 213
centric, 15
material selection for, 140
ready for mounting, 136
Intraoral exam, 315–316
Intraoral records, 315
Investment, 241

J

Jackscrew space regainer, 292
Jelenko Verticulator, 180
Joint
butt, 36
slip, 36

K

Keyed matrix die technique, 212–213
Kinematic location of hinge axis, 150, 151, 154
clutch for, 155
Knife edge gingival margins, 35
Kurer crown anchor system, 283

L

Laboratory (*see* Dentist-laboratory interaction)
Lap facing pontics, 220
Laterodetrusion, 170, 173
Lateroprotrusion, 171, 173
Lateroretrusion, 171, 173
Laterosurtrusion, 170, 173
Laterotrusion, 166, 168, 170
Lentulo spiral, 75
Ligament: periodontal, 10
Light
physics of, and optics, 267
waves, 267

M

Malocclusion, 286
Mandible
rotation of
horizontal axis, 147
rotational axes, 147
sagittal axis, 147, 148
vertical axis, 147
side shift of (*see* Side shift)
Mandibular splint, 287
Margins
designs for porcelain fused to metal restorations, 53–54
gingival (*see* Gingiva, margins)
subgingival, 32
supragingival, 33
Materials: for restorations, 27–28
Matrix, 27
vacuformed, 127
Medical history, 12, 314–315
Mediotrusion, 166, 168
Metal
crown, full cast, reduction for, 37–38
deformation of, 333
porcelain-fused-to (*see* Porcelain-fused-to-metal)
Metamerism, 270
Methyl methacrylate, 121
Minigraph, 139, 141
MOD onlay, 48
Molar
cast post and core for, 281
after endodontic treatment, 277
mandibular
hemisection of, 305–307
root resection, 298
root separation of, 307–310
maxillary
partially resected, improper restoration, 304–305
root of, buccal, 300
root, palatal, 303–304
root resection, 297–298
uprighting, alternatives to, 294–295
Mounted diagnostic casts, 315

Mouth
  hygiene, 316
  procedures, preliminary, 316–319
Movement
  initiating position of, 155
  timing of, 186
Munsell Color System, 265, 268
Myomonitor, 139

N

Natural glaze: in porcelain fused to metal restorations, 66
Ney Parallel Pin Technic, 76
Nylon bristles, 74

O

Occlusal
  adjustment of cast, 231–232
    gross, 230
  anatomy, 303, 306
  considerations in prosthodontics, 294–295
  equilibration, 317
  scheme, 213
  splints, 139
  stops, 100
  surfaces of pontics, 223–226
  treatment, acid-etch application in, 250–251
  vent hole, 241
Occlusion
  analysis of, 17
  centric, 13
    records, 143–144
  condylar determinants of, 165
  interocclusal records (*see* Interocclusal records)
  management of, 146
  questionnaire, 12, 16
Opposing cast, 210
Optics: and physics of light, 267
Orbital: axis-orbital plane, 148, 149, 152, 153, 157
Orthodontic considerations in fixed prosthodontics, 286–295
  occlusal considerations, 294–295
  pulpal considerations, 293–294
Orthodontic retainer, 259
Overglaze: in porcelain fused to metal restorations, 66

P

Pantograph, 139, 163, 166
Pantographic tracings, 15
Pantography, 164–177
  technique, 173–177
Paste
  registration, 138–139
  zinc oxide and eugenol, 138
Path of insertion, 320
Patient management: for fixed prosthodontics, 316
Periodontal considerations
  in crown preparation design, 299
  in fixed prosthodontics, 292–312
    case reports, 300–310
    historical background, 296–297
Periodontal disease, 260
Periodontal involvement: in fixed prosthesis failure, 336–339
Periodontal ligament, 10
Periodontal splints, 250, 259
Perio-prosthesis, 257, 260, 261
Physics of light: and optics, 267
Pin(s)
  angulation, 25
  cemented, 24, 26
  channel preparation, 25–26
  diameter, 24–25
  dowel (*see* Dowel pin)
  insertion, 26
    threaded, 25–26
  length, 25
  location, 25
  Ney Parallel Pin Technic, 76
  noncemented, 24
  number, 25
  problem solving with, 80
  retained restoration, 70–82
    blocking out of embrasures for impressions, 79
    cementation, 80
    contraindications, 78–80
    drill breakage in, 79
    for incisors in labioversion, 78
    indications, 78–80
    for overlapped teeth, 78
    pin angulation, 79
    pin location, 78–79
    pinhole, temporary protection, 79
    pulp exposure in, 79
    uses of, 78–80
  selection, 24–25
  size, 24–25
  use of, 72
  veneer, lingual, 72–77
    insertion path, 73
  veneer, preparations, 76
Pindex, 211
Pinholes
  direction of, 72
  locations of, 72
  temporary protection of, 79

Pink porcelain, 224–225, 260
Pinlays, 77–78
  casting for abrasion, 77
Pinledge, 71, 77–78
  preparations, 74, 75
    schematic diagram identifying salient feature of, 75
Plaster of Paris, 135
Plastic: epimine, 121
Polishing of cast, 234
  after cementation, 234
Polycarbonate crown, 117, 122
  form, 122
Polycarboxylate cement, 240
Polyethers: for impressions, 97–98
Polysulfides: for impressions, 94–95
Pontic(s), 218–227
  axial contours of, 223–226
  bar shaped, 221
  bridge, in porcelain fused to metal restorations, 57–59
  bullet shape, 221
  connectors
    broken stress, 223
    design, 222–223
    rigid, 223
  contact, 324
  denture-base type contact, 219
  design of, 219–226
  diagnostic wax-up, 224
  egg shaped, 221
  formed, 218–227
  heart shape, 221
  ideal, 226–227
  lap facing, 220
  materials for, 218–219
  occlusal surfaces of, 223–226
  repair of, 335
  ridge adaptation in, 219–222
  ridge contact, fused type, 224
  ridge contour, 219–222
  ridge-lap, 220
    modified, 220
  saddle, 219
    modified, 220
  sanitary, 221
    modified, 221
  space, regaining, 291–292
  spheroidal, 221
    modified, 221
  types of, 220
Porcelain fracture, 333–335, 337, 324
Porcelain fused to metal cast, 254
  crown, 256, 274
    reduction for, 41–48
  restorations, 53–69
    anterior teeth, 55–57
    axial designs, 53
    bridge pontics, 57–59
    build-up, 64–65
    burnout, 61
    casting procedures, 62
    chamfer, 54
    contouring, 64–65
    degassing, 63, 67
    failures, reasons for, 67–68
    finishing procedures, 62–63
    framework design, 55–59
    glazing, 66
    inadequate incisal reduction, 54
    inadequate labioincisal reduction, 54
    inadequate lingual reduction, 54
    investing, 61
    margin designs, 53–54
    metal framework, 59–64
    metal framework, on dies, 59
    metal-porcelain junction, 57
    porcelain application, 64–67
    posterior teeth, 57
    restoration considerations 53–54
    shoulder, 55
    shoulder with bevel, 55
    soldering, 63–64
    sprueing, 61
    staining, 65–66
    staining after glazing, 66–67
    waxing, 59–60
Porcelain: opaque, 64
Porcelain: pink, 224–225, 260
Post
  cast, 280–281
  and core, 318
  and core, cast, 332
    amalgams in, 282–284
    composites in, 282–284
    construction of, 279–285
    for molar, 281
    pattern, 280
  and core, pattern, 280
  length of, 279
  prefabricated, 281–282
  Whaledent parapost system, 282
Posterior closure, 160
Postural position: and axis location, 155–156
Prefabricated posts, 281–282
Preformed tray systems: removable dies from, 212–213
Premolar: longitudinal cross section of, 5
Preparation(s), 31–52
  fracture of, 331
  of tooth, 22–24
Problem solving, 327
Proprioceptive guidance, 157
Prosthesis: perio-prosthesis, 257, 260, 261

Prosthodontics (*see* Fixed prosthodontics)
Protrusion, 172
Provisional fixed partial denture, 124–131
Provisional restoration, 116–133
  acrylic, customized, 120–121
  cementation of, 131
  requirements for, 116–117
    esthetic, 117
    mechanical, 116–117
    physiologic, 117
  single posterior, 118–120
  types of, 117–124
Pulp, 9
  exposure in pin retained restorations, 79
  protection, 26
Pulpal considerations: in prosthodontics, 293–294
Pulse rate: and gingival retraction, 83
Putty-base material, 110
Putty: silicone putty materials, 137–138
Putty-wash
  impression technique, 96
  systems, 110–113
  technique, 96

Q

Questionnaire
  health, 13
  occlusion, 12, 16

R

Radiography: for examination, 315
Radix anchor system, 283
Range of motion, 164
Recementation, 330
Recording
  devices, 139
  techniques, 139–140
Reduction: tooth, principles of, 36–48
Reference point: anterior, 149
Registration pastes, 138–139
Removable dies (*see* Dies, removable)
Repairs: of fixed prosthodontics, 327–341
Reservoirs: adequate, 61
Resin
  acid-etch (*see* Acid-etch resin)
  acrylic, autopolymerizing, 135–136
    tray, 101
  autopolymerizing, 188
  composite, 29
  crowns, custom made, 117
  cyanoacrylate, 197, 200, 209
  Duralay, 255
  epoxy, die, 191–192
Resistance form
  pins and, 80
  retention form and, 31–32
Restorations
  acid-etch resin (*see* Acid-etch resin, bonded cast restorations)
  broken-stress, 19
  design modifications for, 48–51
  after endodontic treatment, 276–285
    final restoration, 284–285
  fabrication techniques, 241
  final, 321, 323–325
  fixed-fixed, 19
  fixed-movable, 19
  improper, of partially resected maxillary molar, 304–305
  intermediate
    anterior single unit, 121–124
    removal of, 132
  materials for, 27–28
  of partially resected multi-rooted teeth, 300
  permanent, 321
  pin retained (*see* Pin, retained restorations)
  porcelain fused to metal (*see* Porcelain fused to metal restorations)
  provisional (*see* Provisional restoration)
  "temporary," 116
  tooth, 21–22
  treatment, 321–322
Retainer, 324
  designs, 253
  orthodontic, 259
  selection, 319
Retention, 70
  form
    pins and, 80
    resistance form and, 31–32
  grooves, auxiliary, 32
Retinal fatigue, 270
Retrusion, 172
Richwil, 328
Ridge
  adaptation, and pontics, 219–222
  contact, in pontics, fused type, 224
  contour, and pontics, 219–222
  ideal, 227
  -lap pontics, 220
    modified, 220
  modifications, 226–227
Rigid materials, 135–136
Rinsing: of impression, 192–193
Root
  amputation, 300
  buccal, of maxillary molar, 300
  crown relations, 294

Root *(cont.)*
palatal, of maxillary molar, 303–304
removal
crown after, 302
distobuccal, 302–303
mesiobuccal, 300–302
resection, 296, 304, 306
molar, mandibular, 298
molar, maxillary, 297–298
principles for, basic, 297–298
separation of mandibular molar, 307–310
Rope wax: to line working cast, 202
Rotation: centers of, 153
Rotational axes: of rotation of mandible, 147
Rubber base impression: polysulfide, 94

S

Saddle pontics, 219
modified, 220
Sagittal axis: of rotation of mandible, 147, 148
Sanitary pontics, 221
modified, 221
Saw blade: for sectioning the dies, 204
Sclerotic dentin, 7–8
Seven-eighths crown, 48
Shade
guide, 264
tab, 271, 272–273
matching, 271
selection
mechanics of, 264–275
problems, 264–275
variation between tabs of same number, 271
Shoulder
with bevel in porcelain fused to metal restorations, 55
beveled, gingival margins, 35
full, gingival margins, 35
in porcelain fused to metal restorations, 55
Side shift, 171
disturbed, 169
early, 169
immediate, 169
progressive, 169
Silicone
for impressions, 95–97
putty materials, 137–138
Silico-phosphate cement, 240
Silver die: electroformed, 191
Slip joint, 36
Soft tissue
anatomy, 9
treatment, 316–317
Solder joint: failure of, 335–336
Soldering
index, 324
of porcelain fused to metal restorations, 63–64
Space regainer, 291
acrylic spring, 291
jackscrew, 292
Spatulation: of cements, 242
Spheroidal pontics, 221
modified, 221
Splint
acid-etch resin, 257
mandibular, 287
occlusal, 139
periodontal, 250, 259
Split cast technique, 158
Split tooth, 277
Sprue, 61
removal, of cast, 228
Sprueing: in metal fused to porcelain restorations, 61
Staining of porcelain fused to metal restorations, 65–66
after glazing, 66–67
Stamp cusp, 165
Steele's facings, 218
Stephens articulator, 179
Stuart fully adjustable articulator, 187
Subgingival margins, 32, 299
Supporting tissues: anatomy of, 9–11
Supragingival margins, 33
Surtrusion, 171
Syringe: injection, for impressions, armamentarium for, 106

T

Taper: degree of, 32
TDI system, 211
Teeth
abutment, rotating, 292–293
chart for, 15
clutches to cover, 167
endodontically treated, protection for, 130–131
fracture, 278, 284, 332
furcated, 296
movement, minor, 288–293
management of, 293
multi-rooted, partially resected, restoration of, 300
overlapped, pin retained restorations for, 78
preparation, 22–24, 319–325
reduction, principles of, 36–48
restoration of tooth, 21–22
split, 277
surface characteristics, 265

"Temporary" restoration, 116
Terminal hinge position, 165
Three quarter crown: reduction for, 38–41
Tilted abutment, 316
Timing: of the movement, 186
TMJ fully adjustable articulator, 187
Tooth (*see* Teeth)
Tragus-canthus line, 150
Transtrusion, 166, 168
Tray
  Di-Lok, 195, 197, 212
  preformed, systems, removable dies from, 212–213
  Typadon, 195, 197, 212
Treatment
  expectations, 313–314
  planning, 12–20, 313–316
    proposed treatment should be prioritized for sequence and need, 18
    variety of factors involved in, 14
  restoration, 321–322
Twist drill, 76
Two paste systems: for impressions, 103–110
Typadon tray, 195, 197, 212

V

Vacuformed matrix, 127
Vacuum formed acrylic template technique, 125–129
  indirect, 129–130
Value, 265, 268
Veneer (*see* Pin, veneer)
Vent hole: occlusal, 241
Vents, 61
Vertical axis: of rotation of mandible, 147
Vinyl polysiloxanes: for impressions, 98–99

W

Waves: light, 267
Wax, 136–137
  diagnostic wax-up (*see* Diagnostic wax-up)
  impression technique for provisional restoration, 130
    acrylic, 120–121
  rope, to line working cast, 202
Whaledent parapost system, 282
Whip-Mix articulator, 182
Work authorization, 326
  for acid-etch bonded cast restorations, 251
Working
  cast (*see* Cast, working)
  dies (*see* Dies, working)

Z

Zinc
  chloride, and gingival retraction, 85
  oxide
    and eugenol paste, 138
    reinforced, 240
  phosphate cements, 237